Hospital
Library
Management

Hospital
Library
Management

Jana Bradley
Editor

Ruth Holst
Judith Messerle
Associate Editors

Medical Library Association, Inc.
CHICAGO, ILLINOIS   1983

Grateful acknowledgement is made to the Joint Commission
on Accreditation of Hospitals for permission to reprint the
professional services section from the 1983 *Hospital Survey
Profile,* and the standards for professional library services
from the 1983 *Accreditation Manual for Hospitals,* © 1983
Joint Commission on Accreditation of Hospitals, Chicago,
IL.

National Library of Medicine Cataloging in Publication

Hospital library management / Jana Bradley, editor ; Ruth Holst,
    Judith Messerle, associate editors. — Chicago,
    Ill. : Medical Library Association, 1983.
    ISBN 0-912176-15-6

    1. Library, Hospital - organization & administration
I. Bradley, Jana. II. Holst, Ruth. III. Messerle, Judith.
IV. Medical Library Association.

Z 675.H7 H8295

HOSPITAL LIBRARY MANAGEMENT

Preface

A hospital is a stimulating and challenging environment for providing library service, as most hospital librarians will agree. The needs for information in a hospital are theoretically almost limitless, but in practice the translation of this potential into actual library service frequently calls on the highest levels of the librarian's professional, interpersonal and political skills.

Hospital Library Management was designed as a comprehensive guide to providing library service in hospitals. It was planned as a sequel to the extremely influential *Library Practice in Hospitals: A Basic Guide,* edited by Harold Bloomquist, and is intended to be especially useful for the librarian newly entering the profession or transferring from another library specialty. We also hope it will be valuable for experienced hospital librarians as they plan new services or undertake new activities.

Fundamental to the design of *Hospital Library Management* is the assumption that library practice in hospitals has unique characteristics, shaped by the hospital environment. And further, that each hospital is itself unique, with its own intricate web of information needs. We have attempted, therefore, to analyze the issues involved in each chapter and describe some of the diversity of current practice existing in hospital libraries. We have, at the same time, tried to provide practical advice about specific methods that can be used effectively. Our goal was that hospital librarians could use the book in two ways, as a cookbook providing specific ideas on what to do and how to do it, or as an analytical guide stimulating the formulation of tailor-made approaches to problems and issues.

Hospital Library Management is divided into four sections. The introductory chapters provide an overview of the purposes and functions of hospital libraries and a general description of the hospital environment. Chapters three through ten cover the provision of library services in hospitals, including public, technical, and audiovisual services. The next section focuses on management issues, and the final section discusses special types of services which can be provided by hospital libraries.

The twenty-eight authors who have contributed to *Hospital Library Management* bring to their chapters extensive experience in hospitals and hospital libraries. Without their knowledge, hard work, and commitment, this project would have been impossible.

We are also indebted to Judith L. Biss, MLA's energetic Manager of Publications, and the members of the association's Publication Panel for shepherding this manuscript to completion. Finally we would like to thank the many reviewers who read chapters in various stages and offered invaluable advice.

Jana Bradley
Ruth Holst
Judith Messerle

Introduction: Libraries in Hospitals*

Today's hospital library is an active, service-oriented special library. Like other departments within the hospital, the library contributes to the hospital's primary mission of providing patients with the best possible care. The library supports the delivery of patient care by providing physicians, nurses, and other health care professionals with library services to meet their informational, educational, and in many cases, research-related needs.

Although hospital libraries are developing rapidly today, they are by no means a product of the 1970s and 1980s. Many have their roots in medical staff libraries founded half a century ago. Others trace their lineage through nursing libraries that supported hospital-based diploma programs for nurses. During the 1960s and 1970s, many of these separate nursing and medical libraries merged, due in part to difficulties in maintaining adequate space and funding for separate facilities. The need to support expanding continuing education programs and the closing of many hospital schools of nursing resulted in further consolidations. These mergers centralized library activities in the hospital, increased the availability of resources, and encouraged improved services.

Perhaps the biggest push for the development of hospital libraries has come during the last decade from health sciences librarians. In order to provide effective support for the burgeoning educational programs in hospitals, many librarians have felt that hospital libraries need strengthening. The Regional Medical Library Program of the National Library of Medicine (NLM) has placed considerable emphasis on increasing the hospital librarian's ability to respond to the hospital's recurring information needs. This program has systematized the channels for identifying and obtaining resources that cannot be reasonably provided locally. The resource improvement grants of the NLM have also been extremely influential in the development of many hospital libraries.

Much attention has also been paid to strengthening hospital library standards. When the Joint Commission on Accreditation of Hospitals (JCAH) revised its standards for library services, the Medical Library Association (MLA) and individual health sciences librarians provided considerable input. The revised standards were published in the 1978 *Accreditation Manual for Hospitals*. In another effort relating to the establishment of standards, the MLA formed a committee on hospital library standards and practices. It charged the committee with identifying areas of need for hospital library standards, developing standards for hospital library services, and reviewing and revising standards as appropriate.

The literature of the profession also reflects the increased interest in the development of hospital libraries.

PATTERNS OF HOSPITAL LIBRARY SERVICE

Although it is tempting and often expedient to talk about hospital libraries as a homogeneous group, in reality they differ in many ways. This tremendous variety is important for hospital librarians to recognize as they assess the patterns of library service most appropriate for their institutions.

Staffing

The first and most obvious difference among hospital libraries is in staffing. While many hospital libraries are staffed by one person, others have three or more full-time staff members. The educational background of library employees also varies. In the past more frequently than today, hospital personnel with training and responsibilities in other areas, such as medical records, were placed in charge of the library. More than a decade ago, with graduate librarians in short supply, many hospital library positions were filled by individuals without formal library training. Although both of these practices continue, today the trend is to provide qualified medical librarians in hospital libraries, whenever possible. The 1978 JCAH library standards have reinforced this trend.

A number of creative solutions have arisen to the problem of providing a medical librarian's services to hospitals that cannot justify a full-time librarian. Some hospitals have employed a part-time librarian or assigned a full-time librarian to related professional tasks, such as community information. Other hospitals have engaged a library consultant, shared a circuit-riding librarian, or tapped the resources of the extension librarian at a larger health sciences library.

Organizational Position

A second major difference among hospital libraries is the position they hold in the organizational structure of the hospital. Some libraries are independent departments, while others are organizationally part of another department, such as Medical Records, Medical Education, or Education and Training. The range of decisions librarians make vary from program and budgetary planning decisions, through policy and procedural decisions, to responsibility for carrying out established operations. Usually, being part of another department is less desirable than being independent. Occasionally, however, the library can function effectively as an independent section of a larger department, as long as the library retains direction over its programs and its budget.

*The editor gratefully expresses her appreciation for substantial contributions to the preparation of this chapter from Barbara Coe Johnson, Director of Libraries, Harper-Grace Hospitals, Detroit, Michigan.

Library Users

Almost all hospital libraries today provide services primarily to physicians and nurses. Residents, post-doctoral fellows, and medical students form part of the library's clientele in hospitals affiliated with medical schools. Students in other professional programs affiliated with the hospital, or sponsored by it, may also have access to the library. In addition, many hospital libraries provide services to the hospital administration, professionals in other departments, and other hospital employees.

Some hospitals have also opened the doors of their libraries to people not on their staffs, such as patients and their families, attorneys, and physicians in the local area. Due to increased consumer advocacy and interest in promoting healthful living habits, some hospitals have recently begun to provide health information to the community at large.

Services

The range and variety of services that hospital libraries provide reveals the individuality of hospital libraries most dramatically. Although the broad categories of service are similar, the number of creative variations practiced in hospital libraries can be appreciated by attending a "sharing session" among hospital librarians.

Hospital libraries provide standard library services, primarily in the area of the health sciences. These services include the provision of a journal collection, a reference collection, and often a circulating book collection; interlibrary loan services; reference services, including both answers to factual questions and literature searches; and awareness services of various kinds, including routings, table-of-contents scans, newsletters, and notification of recently published materials on specific topics. In addition to providing these services to walk-in users or to clients via the telephone, some librarians function as clinical medical librarians, participate on committees as information experts, assess formal information needs, and support other outreach efforts.

Hospital libraries also provide a variety of information services needed by the hospital in all aspects of its organizational operation. Providing total information services, however, means extending the standard library services beyond the subject matter of the health sciences to include any information needed by hospital personnel in the performance of their jobs. Such an expanded mission requires a collection that covers basic references in selected fields outside the health sciences. While hospital operations touch on almost every conceivable discipline, library funding is usually limited, making extensive interdisciplinary book and journal collections not feasible. Therefore, librarians have taken other approaches to provide total information services in hospitals. Hospital librarians are using local information sources, both formally and informally. Much needed information can be obtained from nearby public and academic libraries, local agencies, institutions, and businesses. When use of other libraries or information agencies is extensive, formal agreements may often evolve. In these formal, cooperative efforts, hospital libraries contribute to and benefit from the agreement. Consortia of hospital libraries constitute the most popular approach to expanding services, and one that fits in well with the overall hospital thrust toward shared services. Finally, initiating total information services is often made more manageable by focusing on one particular need at a time. Limiting the scope of a program to one area, such as government regulation of health care, or to one department, such as social services, can result in a highly visible, successful program within an initially limited context.

Expanding the library's role to include total information services also involves increasing hospital awareness of the library's potential. Many libraries are experimenting with a variety of promotional and marketing techniques, including one-to-one selling, bookmarks, posters, newsletters, open houses, and direct mailing of promotional material. Conducting a highly visible and successful pilot project can serve as one of the most effective public relations techniques.

Many hospital libraries are expanding their services to include various audiovisual services. In some, audiovisual involvement means extending the standard services to nonprint media: providing a software collection, a viewing area, interlibrary loan and rental of software, and basic media reference services. Other libraries have expanded the concept of media services to include equipment distribution, projectionist services, and production of such audiovisual materials as slides, transparencies, graphics of various types, videotapes, and slide-tape programs.

Providing library and information service to hospital and clinic patients, and even to the community at large, is another area in which hospital libraries are expanding. Historically, many hospital libraries have provided recreational reading materials to patients. Staff members or volunteers distributed reading material during ward rounds. Today, however, many libraries are discovering additional ways to provide health science information to patients. Hospital library services may now include identifying and acquiring pamphlets, books, articles, and audiovisual materials on both general health topics and on specific diseases. These services are provided to health care professionals who use the material with patients in a variety of teaching situations. Some hospital libraries provide the resources directly to the patients or public, who have been referred by practitioners or who walk into the library and request help. Libraries may also participate in outreach programs in public libraries, health fairs, and schools.

EXPANDING INFORMATION NEEDS OF HOSPITALS*

Obviously, hospital library roles, staffs, and services can vary from extremely limited to comprehensive. Even though some hospital libraries offer limited services because of a variety of circumstances, most librarians feel that the unique hospital environment creates enormous information needs. These needs challenge librarians to provide better and better library and information services, no matter on what level the library currently finds itself. Many factors contribute to these expanded information needs in hospitals.

Acceptance of Librarians as Medical Information Experts

The continued growth of health science information, combined with increasingly sophisticated access to that information through health science libraries, has produced a growing acceptance of medical librarians as medical information experts. As this attitude is fostered in academic medical institutions and filters into hospitals, it encourages more active library participation in rounds, on committees, and in other educational efforts.

Expansion of Educational Programs

Educational programs in hospitals are continuing to expand to meet the needs of health sciences students, medical students, and residents who are often located in hospitals distant from the libraries of their academic institution. Hospitals are also expanding their continuing and in-service education programs for employees on all levels, both to respond to increasing certification and regulatory requirements and to improve the quality of professional performance. Patient education programs of many types are blossoming. Some hospitals are initiating educational programs directed to the general needs of their employees: physical fitness programs, stop-smoking clinics, parenting classes, and seminars on topics such as rape prevention, stress, and relaxation.

Increasing Professionalism in Health Occupations

Increased professionalism in areas that used to be called health occupations is resulting in broader-based educational preparation, a greater variety of specialized education programs, more stringent credentialing or licensing requirements, and a greater use and production of professional literature. All these developments may increase the need for information by a greater number of health care professionals.

Interdisciplinary Nature of Hospitals

Closely allied to the increased professionalism of hospital personnel is the multidisciplinary nature of the modern hospital. Over 30 autonomous disciplines may

* The editor gratefully expresses her appreciation for ideas and assistance with the preparation of this section to James P. Reber, Senior Assistant Administrator, Wishard Memorial Hospital, Indianapolis, Indiana.

practice in today's modern institution with relative independence. They may have separate professional structures, including tools and channels for information. Yet coexisting with this comparative freedom are the demands of the hospital for centralization of certain services and functions, dictated by the need for uniformity, efficiency, regulation, and cost containment. Library and information services can be perceived as one of many services that are more cost-effective when provided centrally.

Increasing Regulation of Hospitals

Regulatory forces increasingly influence the hospital environment. In addition to the trend of many health care disciplines toward self-regulation, hospitals are continually establishing policies and procedures that conform to external guidelines. Government regulations come from many sources and are directed toward many goals. The issue of cost containment also continues to exert regulatory influence on the programs of the hospital. In view of the complex and rapidly changing nature of regulations and their tremendous impact on hospital operations, effective monitoring becomes essential. Hospitals are coping with the need to manage this large and complex body of new information by hiring administrative assistants, subscribing to newsletters and information services, and sending employees to seminars. However, no effective system of monitoring regulations has become dominant as yet. Thus libraries have the opportunity to demonstrate that they can meet this critical information need effectively.

CONTEXTS FOR HOSPITAL LIBRARY DEVELOPMENT

Given both the wide range of possible services and the expanding library and information needs of hospitals, the library program for an individual institution must be tailored to match the needs of the institution, its current resources, and its potential for expansion and development. In designing this tailor-made blend of information services, hospital libraries face a number of common situations that deserve consideration.

Staff Size

Since many libraries have small staffs, effective management of both the time and the skills of the staff is essential. Much time is needed to carry out all the routine jobs necessary to maintain even a small collection and to provide basic services. Therefore, it is often difficult to reserve time for more formal management activities, such as assessing needs, planning, justifying, and evaluating. The time squeeze can also threaten the librarian's ability to participate in meetings, continuing education, or local cooperative programs. It is an ever-present irony in hospital libraries that the effort to provide thorough, daily service can interfere with activities which would improve that service.

To deal with the problems of limited time, hospital librarians need to consider new technologies and alternate methods for performing necessary procedures. They must also become aware of opportunities to share projects, services, and even such products as forms, proposals, or searches. Adapting another library's needs assessment form may take fifteen minutes; designing an original may take several hours. More importantly, librarians need to take a hard look at the real needs of their users and direct library efforts toward services that are needed and used.

Managerial vs. Service Role

No matter how small the library is, the hospital librarian has to interact with the administrative structure of the hospital on such management issues as goals, policies, and budgets. Librarians who are part of another department may be dealing with these issues through their department head. Directions for any decisions, however, should come from the librarian and eventually filter up to the administration. Librarians who are department heads work directly with an administrative representative. In addition to their involvement with administrative decision making, hospital librarians are also resource managers. They work with financial personnel to monitor expenses, with the purchasing department to obtain materials, and with the personnel department to manage their human resources. Although librarians may view themselves primarily as service providers, they are probably more visible to the administration as managers. Therefore, achieving an effective balance of these two roles is critical.

Administrative Support

Hospital librarians sometimes perceive a lack of administrative support for library programs. Administrative attitudes toward the library vary widely from institution to institution and often reflect the historical role of the library in the hospital, its present place in the organizational structure, and the present activity of the library staff. A few generalizations seem to apply to many institutions, however. Frequently, the administrator who determines the library's budget views the library as a support service primarily for medical education programs, which are not the administration's direct responsibility. Even though these programs are important to the hospital, their value may not seem to justify, in times of cost containment, the degree of budgetary support requested by the librarian.

Administrative reluctance to support a program not viewed as relevant to the entire hospital intensifies if physician advocacy for the library is not broad-based or strong. Hospital librarians have attempted to broaden the administration's perception of the importance of library and information services by encouraging advocacy from physicians in all medical departments and from a broad base of hospital staff. Librarians have tried to create advocates by establishing services that departments perceive as essential to their operation. In addition to creating a wide spectrum of users who require library services, librarians have attempted to identify and provide information services that respond effectively to the needs of hospital administration. Another approach is to increase the visibility of library programs and, therefore, promote the value of the service.

Centralized Library Services

In hospitals where several libraries serve different user groups, the trend today is to move toward centralizing library management and resources into one hospital library. This trend, occurring at varying rates in different institutions, makes sense for a number of reasons.

Cost Effective Use of Library Resources and Staff

Many of the same key resources are required by physicians, nurses, administrators, and personnel in support services. Consolidation of these materials minimizes duplication of these costly resources. It also improves hospital control over purchases by ensuring that materials are stamped as hospital property and kept in a secure environment.

Promotion of the Team Concept

Maintaining separate medical, nursing, and administrative collections supports an older structural model in which the physician was the sole health care decision maker. The consolidation of disparate collections and diverse clientele, however, fosters the health care team concept and recognizes the contributions, interrelationships, and needs of all those involved in providing health care services.

Establishment of an Information Focal Point

Centralized library services for all members of the health care team identifies the library as a focal point for information gathering. This reduces the time spent by team members in tracking elusive information, increases communication effectiveness, and ultimately facilitates all health care decision making.

THE HOSPITAL LIBRARIAN

The hospital librarian is the key to effective library service. He or she is responsible for planning library services, for securing administrative approval for those services, for providing them effectively and efficiently, and for modifying them as institutional needs change. In many hospitals, the librarian works alone at the tasks neccessary for the operation of a successful library. When the library staff expands, however, the librarian assumes an additional supervisory role. These varied responsibilities require a variety of skills and abilities.

Professional Competence

Since many hospital libraries have only one staff member, the librarian may perform all functions of the library from checking in journals to providing manual or computerized literature searches. This breadth of responsibility requires that the librarian be knowledgeable in many aspects of librarianship, including provision of service, management of the library, cooperation with other libraries, and the applications of computer technology in a small library. In addition, a successful hospital librarian must be able to analyze and solve problems, work independently, communicate clearly both in person and in writing to a wide variety of people, and perform as a peer with other health care professionals in management jobs.

Institutional Understanding

Although most hospitals have similar information needs, each institution's response to these needs is somewhat different. Hospitals differ widely in size, in scope of programs, in governing process, in educational affiliation, and in financial support.

To be effective, hospital librarians must understand the operational and organizational structure of hospitals in general and must be able to analyze the specific process, including the political dynamics, in their own institutions. If the hospital is involved in educational programs, the librarian needs to understand the structure of education for medicine, nursing, and other health profes-sions, particularly in a clinical setting. If the librarian is working in a hospital for the first time, several months should be spent learning functions and procedures. Only a librarian who thoroughly understands the goals, functions, procedures, and organizational dynamics of the institution can provide context-oriented library services.

Interpersonal Skills

In order to perform the wide range of activities necessary to plan, operate, and expand a successful hospital library, a librarian must possess additional, less tangible abilities. He or she needs self-confidence, assertiveness, and adaptability combined with good judgment and political awareness. A spirit of cooperation, a commitment to both library and hospital goals, and a strong sense of service are also important. The librarian must also possess interpersonal skills and intellectual and physical stamina if he or she is to be a force in the positive growth of the library.

This introduction has presented an overview of the common patterns of library services in hospitals, the expanding health care information needs that are fostering these services, and some of the contexts within which hospital libraries provide these services. The following chapters will consider in detail the techniques, services, and strategies needed to meet the increasingly complex information needs of the modern hospital.

Jana Bradley, editor

Hospital Library Management
List of Abbreviations

AACR2, *Anglo-American Cataloguing Rules, 2nd edition*
ABI/INFORM, Abstracted Business Information INFORM
AGRICOLA, AGRICultural Online Access
AHA, American Hospital Association
AHEC, Area Health Education Center
ALA, American Library Association
ASIS, American Society for Information Science
AVLINE, Audio Visuals onLINE
BCN, Biomedical Communication Network
BIOSIS, BIOSciences Information Services
BIP, *Books in Print*
BRS, Bibliographic Retrieval Services
CANCERLIT, CANCER LITerature
CANCERPROJ, CANCER PROJects
CAS, Chemical Abstracts Service
CATLINE, CATalog onLINE
CDC, Center for Disease Control
CE, continuing education
CEU, continuing education unit
CHEMLINE, CHEMical Dictionary onLINE
CIP, cataloging in publication
CLENE, Continuing Library Education Network and Exchange, Inc.
CLINPROT, CLINical PROTocols
CML, clinical medical librarian
COD, cash on delivery
COMPENDEX, COMPuterized ENgineering inDEX
CONTU, Commission on New Technological Uses of Copyrighted Works
ERIC, Educational Resources Information Center
FSTA, Food Science and Technology Abstracts
FTE, full-time equivalent
GPO, Government Printing Office
HCFA, Health Care Financing Administration
HESCA, Health Sciences Communication Association
HIM, Health Insurance Manual
HMO, Health Maintenance Organization
HSA, Health Systems Agency
HVAC, heating-ventilation-air-conditioning system
ILL, interlibrary loan
INCOLSA, Indiana Cooperative Library Services Authority
IPA, International Pharmaceutical Abstracts
ISBN, international standard book number
ISI, Institute for Scientific Information
ISSN, international standard serial number
JAMA, Journal of the American Medical Association
JCAH, Joint Commission on Accreditation of Hospitals
LASS, literature attached to staff studies

LATCH, literature attached to charts
LC, Library of Congress
LISA, Library and Information Science Abstracts
LPN, licensed practical nurse
LSCA, Library Services and Construction Act
MAP, Medical Audit Program
MARC, MAchine Readable Cataloging
MEDLARS, MEDical Literature Analysis and Retrieval System
MEDLINE, MEDlars onLINE
MEDOC, MEdical DOCuments
MeSH, *Medical Subject Headings*
MLA, Medical Library Association
NCHS, National Center for the Health Sciences
NICEM, National Information Center for Educational Media
NIH, National Institute of Health
NIMH, National Institute of Mental Health
NLM, National Library of Medicine
OCLC, Online Computer Library Center, Inc.
OHIHP, Office of Health Information and Health Promotion
PAS, Professional Activity Study
PHS, Public Health Service
POPLINE, POPulation information onLINE
PSRO, Professional Standards Review Organization
PSYCHINFO, PSYChological Abstracts INFOrmation service
QA, quality assurance
QRB, *Quality Review Bulletin*
RFP, request for proposal
RLIN, Research Libraries Information Network
RML, Regional Medical Library
RN, registered nurse
RTECS, Registry of Toxic Effects of Chemical Substances
SCISEARCH, Science Citation Index SEARCH
SDC, System Development Corporation
SDI, selective dissemination of information
SDILINE, Selective Dissemination of Information onLINE
SERLINE, SERials onLINE
SLA, Special Libraries Association
TDB, Toxicology Data Bank
TOXLINE, TOXicology onLINE
UPS, United Parcel Service
USBE, Universal Serials and Book Exchange
UTLAS, University of Toronto Library Automation System
WLN, Washington Library Network
YTD, year-to-date

The Hospital: An Introduction

William I. Jenkins
Administrator
Wishard Memorial Hospital
Indianapolis, Indiana
and
Gail Thomalla
Director, Public Relations
Wishard Memorial Hospital
Indianapolis, Indiana

CHAPTER 1

The Hospital:
An Introduction

William I. Jenkins
Administrator
Wishard Memorial Hospital
Indianapolis, Indiana
and
Gail Thomalla
Director, Public Relations
Wishard Memorial Hospital
Indianapolis, Indiana

FUNCTIONS
  Patient Care
  Education
  Research
  Community Outreach Services

CLASSIFICATION OF HOSPITALS

STATISTICAL INDICATORS

HOSPITAL REQUIREMENTS AND
  STANDARDS
  Licensure
  Accreditation
  Other Standards

ORGANIZATIONAL STRUCTURE
  The Governing Board
  The Medical Staff
  The Hospital Staff

FINANCIAL OPERATION OF HOSPITALS
  Income
  Expenses
  Rates and Charges
  Budget

GOVERNMENT ROLE IN HOSPITAL
  OPERATION
  Hill-Burton Legislation
  Medicare Medicaid Legislation
  National Health Planning Legislation
  Professional Standards Review Organizations
  Cost Containment

EDUCATION IN HOSPITALS
  Medical Education
  Nursing Education
  Allied Health Education
  Continuing Education and
      In-Service Education

ORGANIZATIONAL DYNAMICS
  Dual Accountability
  Multiple "Publics"
  Cooperative Arrangements
  Expansion of Health Services
  Stress

The modern hospital is not easily defined. Philosophically, the hospital has been described as the "expression of man's inalienable right to be well and...the formal recognition by the community of its responsibility for providing the means of keeping him well or restoring lost health" (1:29). In more concrete terms, the hospital can be defined as an institution whose primary function is the provision of a variety of diagnostic and therapeutic services to patients, both in the hospital and in outpatient clinics. More pragmatically, the hospital is a partner with the physician in providing health care services needed by the community.

The hospital can be viewed from a number of perspectives. It is the umbrella organization under which many individual health care professionals provide some or all of their services. More than 30 disciplines are represented in most hospitals, each having its own professional structure, body of knowledge, code of ethics, and technical procedures. A hospital is also a social institution, dealing daily with a broad panorama of human hopes, fears, and concerns. Finally, a hospital is a business, responsible for the efficient, cost-effective provision of a wide range of services.

For the hospital librarian whose responsibility it is to provide library service in this complex environment, an understanding of the dynamics of this multifaceted institution is essential. This brief overview of the hospital environment is intended to provide a framework for observation and analysis of the institution in which the librarian works.

FUNCTIONS

The universal function of the hospital is patient care. In addition, many hospitals also have a commitment to the education of health professionals, research, and community outreach services.

Patient Care

A hospital's primary concern is the patient in need of health care services. These may include diagnosis, treatment, rehabilitation, and preventive care. In the past, care was often centered primarily on the hospitalized patient. Today, hospitals provide many services for the outpatient, or ambulatory patient, who receives services without spending the night in the hospital. Patient care, whether delivered to inpatients or outpatients, is usually directed by physicians, most of whom are not employees of the hospital. Physicians are assisted by hospital staff, consisting of a wide variety of health care professionals. Because of this unique arrangement for delivering a service, hospitals and physicians are truly partners in the provision of health care.

Education

The medical and nursing professions have historically depended on hospitals for clinical training and education.

Today, ancillary and paramedical personnel also receive much of their education in hospitals. Written affiliation agreements with teaching institutions commit hospitals to support the education programs and are usually very specific with regard to the resouces and opportunities to be provided. In addition to formal education programs, hospitals also provide continuing education opportunities for their own personnel.

Research

Some hospitals, particularly those with educational affiliations, regard research as an important function of the institution. These hospitals coordinate the work of the scientist and clinician to promote the development of research that may be applied to the practice of medicine.

Community Outreach Services

In the largest sense, hospitals are community servants, responding to the health care needs and desires of the surrounding community. Recently, hospitals have taken a more active role in community service through outreach programs, promotion of good health habits, and emphasis on preventive medicine.

CLASSIFICATION OF HOSPITALS

Hospitals can be classified according to various criteria, including length of stay, types of services offered, control or ownership, levels of care, and the institution's teaching or nonteaching role.

Short term, or acute care, hospitals are those in which the average stay is relatively short. Institutions such as nursing homes and rehabilitation hospitals are defined as long term. Psychiatric hospitals often fall into this category as well.

Types of services offered include general, psychiatric, rehabilitation, pediatric, tuberculosis, maternity, and other specialized care. Some hospitals specialize in only one type of service. Others offer a variety of services.

Type of control or ownership is another criterion for classifying hospitals. Of the 6,000 general hospitals in the United States, 54 percent are voluntary, non-profit institutions, including community hospitals and those affiliated with church groups, religious orders, and fraternal orders. Approximately 12 percent of the country's general hospitals are proprietary, which means they are operated for profit and privately owned, either by a small group or by corporations with stockholders. An additional 29 percent are owned by state or local governments, and the remaining 5 percent are operated by the federal government (2).

"Levels of care" refers to a relatively new concept that involves the type of disease treated, the level of training of the physician treating the disease, and the facilities and services necessary to support the physician. Levels of care include primary (basic), secondary (specialized), and tertiary (highly specialized) care.

Although most hospitals are involved in education to a certain degree, teaching hospitals are those with extensive medical education programs in which residents, also called housestaff, provide a portion of patient care.

STATISTICAL INDICATORS

Hospital size or activity is commonly described by using a variety of statistical indicators. Each hospital calculates its individual statistics. Monthly and annual national averages are published in various statistical sources.

- *Number of beds.* The number of beds is often used as an overall indicator of size, services, and occupancy. A "hospital bed" is defined as one that is available for 24-hour occupancy by inpatients during their period of hospitalization. In 1981 approximately 45 percent of the hospitals in the United States had 6-99 beds; 23 percent listed 100-199; and 12 percent had 200-299. The 300-399, the 400-499, and the 500-plus categories accounted for less than 20 percent of all hospitals (2).
- *Inpatient admissions.* These statistics include number of admissions, average length of stay, and number of patient days. Inpatient statistics are a key indicator of hospital use.
- *Outpatient visits.* The number of outpatient visits has recently assumed increased importance. It points to a national trend toward greater use of clinics for certain conditions and procedures, primarily as a less expensive alternative to inpatient care.
- *Procedures.* The number of procedures, such as tests, x-rays, or treatments, for clinical services is a standard gross indicator of volume in these areas.

HOSPITAL REQUIREMENTS AND STANDARDS

Hospital standards are basic minimum requirements for health care institutions. Some standards are mandatory, such as those established by federal and state agencies. Others are voluntary, such as those developed by associations or voluntary review bodies. Both types of standards are discussed below.

Licensure

In most states, the law requires hospitals to be licensed, usually by the state's health department. The purpose of a state's licensing law is to "further protect the public health through the development and enforcement of standards for the care of individuals in hospitals, and for the construction, maintenance, and operating of hospitals" (3:171). Such a licensing law is usually accompanied by state hospital regulations, which may detail such requirements as sanitary and safety regulations. Hospitals may also be bound by local municipal ordinances that provide another check on the quality of care and facilities.

Accreditation

The Joint Commission on Accreditation of Hospitals (JCAH) is an independent, voluntary, not-for-profit organization formed in 1952 to develop quality standards for hospitals. Any hospital may request evaluation by the JCAH. The evaluation is done for a fee by a survey team that "measures" the hospital's services, organization, and governance against a set of published standards. These standards are periodically reviewed and revised by the JCAH.

Accreditation is awarded for a period of three years to hospitals that comply with the JCAH standards. While JCAH accreditation is voluntary, it is widely recognized and highly desirable.

Other Standards

To be eligible to receive reimbursement for Medicare and Medicaid patients, a hospital must meet minimum standards of care as spelled out in the Medicare regulations. Also, most professional associations have developed standards for hospitals that provide clinical facilities for use in teaching programs. These standards spell out the minimum requirements that must be met for the hospital to affiliate with the teaching program.

ORGANIZATIONAL STRUCTURE

The hospital's organizational structure can be divided into three parts: the governing board, the medical staff, and the hospital itself.

The Governing Board

The legal status of a hospital is derived from a charter granted to it, or to its parent body, by the state. A governing body, known variously as the board of directors, board of trustees, board of commissioners, or board of governors, exercises the powers granted by this legal status (4). The governing body has the ultimate legal and moral responsibility for the policies and operation of the hospital, including standards of patient care. This premise has been upheld by numerous legal decisions. The governing board has diverse responsibilities. It determines policies for the hospital in relation to community needs. It also approves the appointment of medical staff and is accountable for the quality of patient care. The governing board also coordinates medical and other professional interests with administrative, financial, and community needs. It provides adequate financing and control of expenses. Finally, the board selects and evaluates an administrator or chief executive officer (CEO) for the hospital, and delegates to this person the responsibility for selection of competent personnel, control of hospital funds, and supervision of the physical plant.

The Medical Staff

The medical staff of a hospital is an organized group of physicians who are primarily responsible for the care of the sick and injured, in conjunction with a team of nurses and other professionals. Osteopaths, dentists, podiatrists, and psychologists may also be members of the medical staff. The medical staff governs itself by adhering to written bylaws. The staff also provides for its continuing education, evaluates its professional work and efficiency, and makes recommendations to the board of directors. The JCAH *Accreditation Manual for Hospitals* states that "there shall be a single organized medical staff that has the overall responsibility for the quality of all medical care provided to patients and for the ethical conduct and professional practices of its members, as well as for accounting therefor to the governing body" (5:93).

While the hospital governing board has ultimate legal and moral responsibility, it cannot practice medicine and must depend on the medical staff for quality patient care. However, a physician cannot provide care without the permission of the board, and the board approves all medical staff bylaws and all rules and regulations governing the conduct of physicians. Careful balance of these two powers is critical to the well-being of the hospital.

The board's permission for a physician to practice medicine in a hospital is called a privilege. With this privilege, the physician "is authorized to select whatever accommodations in the hospital that he feels are best suited to his patient, subject to the availability of such accommodations, and subject to admitting rules approved by the board" (3:25). The extent of this privilege varies with the type of appointment, which generally fits into one of the following categories:

• *Active staff:* the physician or dentist members who are responsible for the bulk of medical practice and who perform all significant organizational and administrative functions of the medical staff.
• *Associate staff:* practitioners being considered for advancement to active status; often less experienced members or those who have not been actively interested in the hospital.
• *Courtesy staff:* practitioners who have privileges to admit and treat an occasional patient; often active or associate members of another hospital's staff.
• *Consulting staff:* practitioners of recognized professional ability who come to the hospital to consult on other physicians' cases.
• *Honorary staff:* practitioners recognized for their service, reputations, or accomplishments; includes emeritus medical staff members.

Bylaws

The medical staff follows bylaws, which are rules and regulations "that create an atmosphere and framework within which each staff member can act with a reasonable degree of freedom and confidence" (5:103). Bylaws are a code of conduct for the medical staff. They outline how the staff may select members, grant privileges, and discipline members. Bylaws also state what the staff expects of members in terms of ethics, continuing education, and attendance at meetings. The bylaws specify the officers who will govern the medical staff. Typically, these officers include the president, vice-president or president-elect, secretary-treasurer, and immediate past president.

Committees

To govern itself, the medical staff is organized into committees. The chief committee is the executive committee "that is empowered to act for the staff in the intervals between medical staff meetings...and shall serve as a liaison mechanism between medical staff and hospital administration" (5:102).

Additional committees monitor credentials, quality assurance, infection control, utilization, research, medical records, and other areas of concern such as the library. A joint conference committee of board, medical staff, and administration members tackles issues that concern overall hospital operation.

Clinical Departments

Most hospital medical staffs are also organized into clinical departments. These departments can include medicine, surgery, pediatrics, family practice, psychiatry, anesthesia, pathology, obstetrics and gynecology, physical medicine, radiology, dentistry, neurology, urology, ophthalmology, otorhinolaryngology, and emergency services.

Each clinical department is led by a chairperson. Every medical staff member is assigned to at least one department, but may have privileges in other departments.

Quality Assurance

As a self-governing body, the medical staff is responsible for controlling the quality of its members' practice in the hospital, a concept known as peer review. To assure that quality, "mechanisms for the regular review, evaluation, and monitoring of medical staff practice and functions" (5:106) must be in place.

Informal quality assurance may consist of weekly conferences in which current cases are discussed by the medical staff, residents, and medical students. Formal quality assurance is carried out using a medical audit, defined as "the evaluation of the quality of medical care as reflected in medical records" (6:216).

The medical audit may be performed by the staff, by an outside auditor, or by a Professional Activity Study (PAS) and its Medical Audit Program (MAP). The latter are computerized medical information analyses done at a hospital's request by the Commission on Professional and Hospital Activities.

The JCAH requires that an audit include review of surgical cases, drug policies and utilization, medical records, blood utilization, and antibiotic usage. Quality assurance also includes utilization review, a process by which a patient's length of stay is measured against standards for the specific diagnosis. If a certain condition, for example, normally requires a seven-day stay and the patient remains in the hospital beyond that time, the physician must document the need to keep the patient hospitalized.

Continuing Education

The JCAH requires that a hospital's medical staff participate in a continuing education program designed to keep members informed of new developments in the field of medicine. This program must also offer "refresher courses" in certain basic aspects of medical education (5). At its best, continuing medical education is tailored to meet specific needs, especially those identified during the medical audit or utilization review process.

Medical Director

The position of medical director, found in some hospitals, is the result of the evolution of the chief of staff's role into that of a full-time administrator. The medical director works closely with the administrator of the hospital to assure coordination of administrative and medical affairs.

The Hospital Staff

The hospital staff is typically divided into the following categories: hospital administration, clinical departments, nursing services, and administrative departments. Each of these will be discussed below.

The Administration

Over the years, the title of the person who oversees a hospital's operation has changed. A superintendent was replaced by an administrator, who was replaced by an executive director, executive vice-president, president, or chief executive officer. Titles vary considerably among institutions, but in almost all cases there is one individual to whom the governing board delegates the authority to operate the hospital. This person will be referred to in this chapter, and throughout this book, as the administrator.

Hospital administrators are specifically trained for the profession, usually by completing a program that leads to a master's or similar degree in hospital administration. This program often includes a year's residency in a hospital. Since about 1950, administrators with this educational background have steadily replaced physician-administrators and accountant-administrators.

In most hospitals, the administration includes additional staff members who assist in the management of the institution. These staff members have a variety of titles, including associate and assistant administrator, vice-president, and comptroller. Each of these administrative representatives is usually responsible for a group of related hospital departments. The hospital librarian often reports, either directly or indirectly, to the administrative officer responsible for education, audiovisuals, and other activities related to information.

Clinical Departments

A hospital's clinical departments, also called ancillary and allied health departments, are those whose personnel are immediately involved in providing direct patient care and services. These departments employ a wide range of medical professionals and paraprofessionals with varying degrees of education and training.

Clinical departments frequently parallel medical staff services. Clinical responsibility for these departments often rests with a physician under contract to the hospital. This physician may also be chairperson of the department. Administrative responsibilities for a department may be handled by an administrative director or assistant, or a chief technician, therapist, or technologist. The administrative leader is usually recognized as the head of the department, although the physician has greater authority in the department's operations.

Physician-directed departments include laboratory medicine or clinical pathology; radiology; nuclear medicine; radiation therapy; anesthesia; and rehabilitation, which generally encompasses physical and occupational rehabilitation, speech therapy, and audiology. Also in the category of physician-directed departments are psychiatry; emergency medical services, which may include a hospital-operated ambulance service; cardiology; neurology; and in some instances, respiratory therapy.

Additional ancillary clinical departments include pharmacy, chaplaincy services, social services, and dietetics. Each of these departments employs professionals who may be specifically trained to work in a hospital setting. These departments, however, are usually not physician-directed. Department heads, therefore, have full administrative and technical responsibility for them.

Nursing Services

The nursing staff makes up the largest proportion of any hospital's work force. Reasons for this include the need for round-the-clock patient care; demands for highly individualized care (particularly in special care units where the nurse-to-patient ratio may be 1:2); and the obvious fact that nurses are involved in the care of every inpatient and emergency room patient as well as most outpatients.

Nursing is quickly becoming as specialized as the medical profession, creating a growing need for highly educated nurses capable of assuming many responsibilities. Generally, registered nurses (RNs) form the backbone of a hospital's staff. These individuals may have been educated in a hospital-based diploma program that stresses clinical experience; a baccalaureate program that emphasizes academic preparation; or an associate degree program that condenses both types of training into two years. Licensed practical nurses (LPNs) are qualified to care for patients under the direction of a registered nurse after completing an average of one year of training. Nursing assistants or aides are usually trained in the hospital in which they work. Ward secretaries or unit clerks relieve the nursing staff of many administrative duties. They too are usually trained by the hospital, although community colleges are currently developing programs for training unit clerks.

The nursing staff follows a dual leadership, although in a different sense than do allied health professionals. The nurse is functionally responsible to the physician who orders diagnostic or therapeutic services in that the nurse must provide the service or transmit the order for service. However, the nurse is formally responsible to the nursing director, who must see that nursing services are available to the physician and that standards are maintained (3).

This pattern exists whether the nursing service department is centralized or decentralized. In a centralized department, all nurses are part of a single hierarchy under the direction of a nurse who is a member of the administrative team. In a decentralized department, nurses are organized according to clinical service. Depending on the organization, the nursing department may have assistant directors of nursing, evening and night supervisors, or both. In smaller institutions, the evening or night supervisor may serve as the administrative representative who handles problems that arise during that shift.

Categories of nursing service generally parallel those of the medical staff. They typically include the following: intensive care; medical; surgical; maternal and child care; psychiatry; emergency and outpatient care; and operating and recovery room services.

To facilitate the delivery of care, a nursing service department must perform three additional functions: scheduling, to assure adequate staffing at all times in all areas; training and development, to provide orientation and continuing education for personnel; and recruitment and retention, to develop and maintain the work force. In some institutions responsibility for in-service programs and continuing education of nurses rests with a hospital-wide education department.

Administrative Departments

Administrative departments, or support services as they are sometimes called, all have an impact on patient service.

The registration and review of patients and patient services are carried out by the admitting and registration, medical records, and utilization review departments. To maintain a good relationship with patients and the community, a hospital has a public relations department. Some hospitals have a patient representative program as well. Good community relations can also be fostered through volunteer programs or auxiliary groups, which have been an important source of support for decades.

The hospital's environment is monitored by the following departments: infection control, housekeeping, safety, security, and (more recently) risk management. Its facilities are tended by a plant engineering department, which oversees maintenance and renovation. Materials are supplied through the purchasing, receiving, supply, central service, laundry, and linen departments. Specialized equipment may be the responsibility of the medical engineering staff.

Communications are handled by the switchboard, mail room, and printing services. The hospital may also have library, audiovisual production, and medical illustration services.

The hospital's management is served by a data processing system, and, in many cases, planning and marketing departments. The personnel department oversees employment, benefits, and employee policies. An education, training, and development department is responsible for the training needs of the institution. Finally, the financial department or business office handles both patient and general accounts. Additional revenue may be raised by the fund development department.

FINANCIAL OPERATION OF HOSPITALS

Health care financial management has been defined as "the art of manipulating health care resources, i.e., labor, supplies and capital, to ensure financial viability so that the health care institution can meet its immediate and long-range objectives" (7:61). The subject of medical economics is complex. The purchase of medical care is one of the few types of transactions in which the quality of service cannot be adjusted in relation to the purchaser's ability to pay. Hospitals cannot compromise quality of care because of cost.

Income

A hospital relies on three major sources of income: patient services, miscellaneous income, and grants and gifts. In institutions supported by the federal, state, or local government, tax support is included with miscellaneous income.

Income from patient services comes largely from third-party payers, which include Blue Cross, commercial insurance companies, Medicare, Medicaid, workers' compensation, and any other organization contracted to pay all or part of the patient's bill. Additional revenue comes from self-pay patients, those who pay their hospital costs directly.

Miscellaneous income is generated from parking lots, cafeterias, snack bars, building or space rentals, television services, gift shops, and tuition from educational programs. Some hospitals receive tax support for services to indigent patients. In addition, most hospitals receive private or government grants for research or education and gifts in the form of donations, bequests, and legacies.

Expenses

Programs and budget priorities determine a hospital's expenses. Wages, salaries, and benefits make up the largest share of expenses, generally from one-half to three-fourths.

Rates and Charges

Room rates and charges for patient services are set in relation to a hospital's income and expenses. Major third-party payers reimburse only for the cost of patient services, which does not include a variety of nonproduction costs and adjustments for bad debts or free service. Thus, the burden of making up the difference has traditionally fallen on the self-pay patient.

Most hospitals have adopted an all-inclusive room rate, which covers the cost of nursing, housekeeping, dietary services, linen, basic supplies, heat, lighting, and any other costs related to "room and board." Special care rooms, such as those in an intensive care unit, have higher rates.

Budget

A hospital's budget is the bridge between the resources it needs to provide services and what it expects to earn from those services. It is developed with input from department heads and reflects the hospital's plan for the future. For further information on hospital finance and budgeting, see Chapter 13.

GOVERNMENT ROLE IN HOSPITAL OPERATION

The following section describes the government's role in hospital operations at the time of this writing. Changes in the government's activity in the field of health care are being considered, and hospital librarians are advised to follow these developments closely.

Hill-Burton Legislation

Since 1946, when the Hospital Survey and Construction Act was enacted, the federal government has been involved in the support, and later the control, of hospitals. The original law provided support for construction and modernization of hospitals. It has been revised over the years to emphasize outpatient services and underserved areas. One important part of the Hill-Burton legislation is an obligation placed on fund recipients to provide a specific level of free care to indigent patients.

Medicare/Medicaid Legislation

Medicare (Title 18 of the Social Security Act) is a nationwide health insurance program that covers the following groups, all without regard to income: persons over the age of 65; persons who have been eligible for Social Security disability payments for over two years; and certain workers and their dependents who need kidney transplants or dialysis. Medicaid (Title 19 of the Social Security Act) is a federally-aided, state-operated and administered program that provides medical benefits for certain low-income persons, including the aged, the blind, the disabled, and members of families with dependent children in which one parent is absent, incapacitated, or unemployed. The regulations and funding for both programs are constantly changing and require continual monitoring by the hospital's financial and social service departments.

National Health Planning Legislation

The 1974 National Health Planning and Resource Development Act (Public Law 93-641, amended by PL 96-79) places responsibility for hospital program and facility development upon a regional health systems agency (HSA). This agency identifies local and regional health problems, assigns priorities, and develops plans to solve the problems. The act also outlines national health planning priorities, goals, and standards. PL 93-641 followed other, less sophisticated national health planning programs in the United States. Additional changes in these programs are likely to occur in the future.

Professional Standards Review Organizations

The 1972 amendments to the Social Security Act established independent professional standards review organizations (PSROs) composed of physicians. These organizations provide ongoing review of services provided under Medicare, Medicaid, and maternal and child health programs for the purpose of determining reimbursement.

Cost Containment

Much recent legislation has sought to control resources through health planning agencies and to control utilization of care and services through PSROs. The government's major concern, however, is controlling costs. This concern was demonstrated in 1978 when hospitals were threatened with a legally-mandated cap on expenses.

Hospitals responded through the American Hospital Association (AHA) and other organizations, with a voluntary program aimed at maintaining expenses at their current levels or at least reducing the rate of increase. The results of the program have satisfied the legislative interest in cost control for the present and have led to greater overall fiscal efficiency in hospitals.

Costs, however, have continued to rise with inflation, the increasing sophistication of technology, and the growing burden of government regulation. At the time of this writing, "competitive" models for health care systems, encouraged by changes in government regulations, are being actively pursued. Hospitals should be aware of trends in this direction and monitor developments in the area of cost containment.

EDUCATION IN HOSPITALS

Hospitals have always been responsible for a vital portion of the education of physicians, nurses, and allied health personnel. A hospital's purpose determines its involvement in health care education. Many proprietary hospitals concentrate on patient services and provide little or no education, whereas teaching hospitals consider medical education a primary purpose. The latter are usually actively involved in nursing and allied health education as well, all under the auspices of a university or medical school.

Medical Education

Medical school is the first step in a physician's professional education. Students generally spend at least one year of a traditional four-year program in clinical rotation through a hospital's major medical services. At this time, they gain exposure to the variety of medical specialties and to the operations of a hospital.

Upon graduation from medical school, a student usually enters a residency in the specialty of his or her choice. The length of the residency ranges from three to six or more years. It may be sponsored by an individual hospital or by a medical school using the facilities of one or more hospitals. During the residency, the physician-in-training takes an increasingly active role in patient care under the supervision and instruction of the hospital's medical staff or the school's medical faculty.

The benefits to the hospital from a medical education program include intellectual stimulation at all levels and the presence of medical specialists who direct tertiary care units, specialized programs, and research. The hospital also benefits from adequate physician coverage at all times through the use of residents.

Nursing Education

Historically, nurses received all their training in hospitals and, in turn, student nurses provided the bulk of nursing care. Today, the emphasis is on two to four years of academic preparation in conjunction with clinical experience. Most hospitals that continue to operate diploma schools for nurses arrange for a college or university to supply their students' academic training. Conversely, nursing programs offered by colleges or universities establish clinical affiliations with hospitals to round out their students' education. Recently, many hospitals have started "refresher" education programs for nurses who have been out of the work force for a period of time.

Allied Health Education

Hospitals engage in allied health education in a variety of ways. Some hospitals operate their own programs in an allied health specialty with no outside affiliation. Others operate their own schools, arranging for required instructional classes through a technical school, college, or university. A hospital may also serve as the clinical setting for an outside program or accept interns (also called externs or affiliates) from outside programs on an individual basis.

Continuing Education and In-Service Education

The hospital also provides many educational activities other than those leading to professional or technical degrees or certificates. The medical and hospital staff participate in continuing education activities, both formal and informal. In-service training for nurses and other hospital employees is an ongoing concern and often is directed by an in-service or training department. In a decentralized approach, departments with heavy training needs may have a staff member who is responsible for education and instruction.

ORGANIZATIONAL DYNAMICS

The complexity of hospital organization and the wide variation in individual institutions make it impossible to define precisely the issues that shape decision making in hospitals. Some themes, however, seem to be important throughout the health care field.

Dual Accountability

Hospitals are organized around two centers of day-to-day authority—the administrative offices and the medical staff. Both are ultimately accountable to the governing body. Although both have weel-defined spheres of authority, areas of overlap are almost inevitable. Many employees in a hospital, often including the librarian, deliver their services to physicians or are under their direction, but depend on the administration for the resources needed to provide those services. Any professional working in a hospital must be aware of the channels of authority, areas of influence, and political dynamics that operate in the institution and must develop effective ways of working within this environment.

Multiple "Publics"

A hospital has four primary groups, or "publics," which it must consider in any decision: (1) physicians, (2) patients, (3) employees, and (4) the community. A hospital's success depends on how well it balances the needs of each of its "publics." Physicians control the admission of patients, who are the primary source of revenue for the hospital. Patients, however, are gaining a larger voice in selecting a hospital. Employees are the direct providers of daily patient care, and collectively they influence the quality of care patients receive. The community consists of individuals in the service area of the hospital. It determines the acceptance or rejection of the hospital itself. The needs of each "public" require attention, and maintaining an appropriate balance is critical to the provision of quality service and to the stability of the hospital.

Cooperative Arrangements

As costs of health care have continued to rise and as management and technical services have become more sophisticated, hospitals have been forced to reexamine their practices and seek alternative means for providing quality service. Some of these means are discussed below.

Integration of Services into Regional Plans

To prevent costly duplication and gaps in service, hospitals have been working together to institute area-wide planning. Such planning, reinforced by the National Health Planning and Resources Act (PL 92-641), encourages hospitals to meet the needs of the community more efficiently and in some cases to give up duplicated services that are little used. Designing and implementing these plans is sometimes difficult, particularly in areas where there are more beds than are needed or where there is a large overlap in services rendered. Competition between institutions has always been a factor in the cooperative planning process. Emphasis is now being placed on the positive effects of competition in achieving a balance between the demand for a service and its availability and price.

Shared Services and Management

Hospitals have long known the value of cooperative purchasing and are now moving into shared services agreements involving laundry and computer services, equipment maintenance, marketing, and management contract services. Other methods designed to manage the hospital more effectively are also being explored. The most sophisticated shared agreements are found among multihospital groups, whose numbers are increasing steadily.

Expansion of Health Services

Hospitals today are reexamining their role in the community as interest in "wellness" and self-care grows. This reexamination has led to a significant increase in outpatient services. In addition, other markets are being explored to create a continuum of care. Herkimer notes trends toward home care, including nursing care, renal dialysis, rehabilitation therapy, and nutritional care. There is an increased interest in preventive medicine, which may involve outreach clinics, mobile health units, disease screening, health instruction, and physical fitness clinics. Another area of exploration is holistic medicine, which can include crisis intervention, marriage and family counseling, alcoholic counseling, and adolescent rehabilitation (8). These changes are coming about as the community becomes more sophisticated in identifying its own health care needs and as insurance companies begin to reimburse for preventive care services.

Stress

While any organization has problems and conditions that cause tensions among employees, the hospital is unusual in that employees must often deal with life and death situations. This creates an unusually high stress rate among employees, particularly physicians and employees who work in intensive care units, emergency rooms, and other areas in which there is frequent exposure to critically ill patients. This stress may cause a high turnover in personnel. Employees who stay on the job may experience an emotional crisis or even "burnout." Recognition of hospital stress has become more common in recent years and has led to development of stress management programs, which include assignment rotation, flex time, and employee counseling.

REFERENCES

1. MacEachern MT. Hospital organization and management. Rev 3rd ed. Chicago: Physicians Record Company, 1957.

2. Hospital statistics: data from the American Hospital Association 1981 annual survey. 1982 ed. Chicago: American Hospital Association, 1982.

3. Letourneau CU. The hospital administrator. Chicago: Starling Publications, 1969.

4. McGibony JR. Principles of hospital administration. 2d ed. New York: Putnam, 1969.

5. Joint Commission on Accreditation of Hospitals. Accreditation manual for hospitals. 1983 ed. Chicago: Joint Commission on Accreditation of Hospitals, 1982.

6. Eisele CW, ed. The medical staff in the modern hospital. New York: McGraw-Hill, 1967.

7. Berman HJ, Weeks LE. The financial management of hospitals. Ann Arbor, MI: Health Administration Press, 1976.

8. Herkimer AG. Understanding hospital financial management. Rockville, MD: Aspen Systems, 1979.

READINGS

Brown M. Trends in multihospital systems: a multiyear comparison. Health Care Manage Rev 1980 Fall;5:9-22.

Champion JM. General hospital: a model. Baltimore: University Park Press, 1976.

Guthurie MB. Hospital-medical staff collaboration key to survival. Hosp Med Staff 1981 May;10:12-16.

Hamm SJ. The influence of formal and informal communications within a modern hospital. Superv Nurse 1980 Dec;11:38-42.

O'Connor R. American hospitals: the first 200 years. Hospitals 1976 Jan 1;50:62-72.

Rakich JS, Darr K. Hospital organization and management: Text and readings. 2d ed. New York: Halsted, 1978. (Health Systems Management Series, Vol. 11).

Rosenthal CJ, et. al. Nurses, patients and families: care and control in the hospital. New York: Springer, 1980.

Sattilaro AJ. Change challenges traditional hospital/medical staff relationships. Hospitals 1981 Apr 1;55:139,142-144.

Sloan FA. The internal organization of hospitals: a descriptive study. Health Serv Res 1980 Fall;15:203-230.

Snook D. Hospitals: what they are and how they work. Rockville, MD: Aspen Systems, 1981.

Standards for Hospital Libraries

Eloise C. Foster
Director
Library of the American
    Hospital Association
Asa S. Bacon Memorial
American Hospital Association
Chicago, Illinois

CHAPTER 2

Standards for Hospital Libraries

Eloise C. Foster
Director
Library of the American Hospital Association
Asa S. Bacon Memorial—American Hospital Association
Chicago, Illinois

ORIGIN OF STANDARDS

THE JOINT COMMISSION ON
    ACCREDITATION OF HOSPITALS
    The JCAH Standards
    The Accreditation Process
    The Librarian's Role in Accreditation

Appendixes

Figures

Hospitals are understandably concerned about the quality of care provided to their patients. To measure the performance of both the hospital as a whole and its integral parts, standards and guidelines issued by a variety of organizations are utilized. The librarian should be aware of these standards and guidelines and the process through which they are employed.

Although the terms "standards" and "guidelines" are sometimes used interchangeably, guidelines generally define principles basic to the establishment and the operation of service. Compliance with guidelines is generally voluntary. Standards, on the other hand, define the minimum adequacy of facilities and services, and compliance is expected by the issuing body.

Standards are generally established because of a defined need to measure or enhance the quality of all or part of a service. They provide the means by which the size, scope, and efficiency of a service can be judged both by those responsible for providing it and by those assessing it for personal, professional, or managerial purposes (1).

When standards are applied to libraries, a number of issues arise. The issues include the need for standards versus guidelines, agreement on the definition of terms, the difference between qualitative and quantitative measures, the problems inherent in defining minimal levels of excellence, the determination of whether compliance is required or suggested, identifying methods of measurement and enforcement, and the difficulty of applying a single set of standards to a variety of institutions or situations. Resolution of these issues requires a definition of purpose, coupled with analysis and negotiation by all parties involved.

ORIGIN OF STANDARDS

Many library associations, voluntary health associations, and government agencies have been involved in promulgating standards or guidelines for hospital libraries (see Figure 2-1). Each set of standards is slightly different, and analysis and comparison of these documents is recommended for those involved in developing standards or for the serious student of standards. In the 1972 issue of *Library Trends* devoted to standards, Yast presents a historical perspective on the development of hospital library standards (2). In Figure 2-2, selected standards and guidelines are analyzed and compared.

THE JOINT COMMISSION ON ACCREDITATION OF HOSPITALS

The Joint Commission on Accreditation of Hospitals (JCAH) is an independent, nonprofit organization whose standards for voluntary accreditation are widely accepted by administrators of health care facilities. The corporate members of the JCAH are the American College of Surgeons, American College of Physicians, American Dental Association, American Hospital Association, and the American Medical Association.

Accreditation by the JCAH is considered an industry-wide standard of quality. A number of regulatory agencies regard it as a prerequisite for granting certification and licensure. Some insurance agencies make it a condition for honoring reimbursement claims. Many accrediting committees require it. In addition, such accreditation provides a guide to facilities that offer services of a recognized quality. Such guidance is valuable to qualified professionals seeking employment and to the public seeking health care.

The JCAH Standards

Of the hospital library standards that exist, only those published by the JCAH will be discussed here. An overview of the contents of other relevant standards and guidelines may be obtained by studying Figure 2-2; and interested librarians will want to refer to the complete texts.

The standards on which the JCAH bases its accreditation of hospitals are published in its *Accreditation Manual for Hospitals* (3). These standards pertain to hospitals of all sizes and apply to the performance of each function in the overall operation of a facility, including professional library services. They are designed to be valid, optimal, achievable, measurable, and flexible. Accreditation by the JCAH indicates that a facility is in substantial compliance with the existing standards. Specialized health facilities are also surveyed and accredited using pertinent standards. Of these, only the *Consolidated Standards Manual for Child, Adolescent, and Adult Psychiatric, Alcoholism, and Drug Abuse Facilities* mentions library services.

The first set of standards was published by the JCAH in 1953. The standards referred to the medical library as a desirable element but not an absolute prerequisite for hospital accreditation. Several revisions have been made in the standards since 1953. The current standards for professional library services became effective in 1978.

The following is the general principle of the current standards: "The hospital shall provide library services to meet the informational, educational, and, when appropriate, the research-related needs of the medical and hospital staffs." This principle is supported by two standards. According to Standard I, "The professional library services shall be organized to assure appropriate direction or supervision, staffing, and resources." Standard II provides that "The provision of professional library services shall be guided by written policies and procedures." Both standards are accompanied by interpretations (3:147-149). The complete text of the JCAH standards for professional library services can be found in Appendix A.

Like standards for other functions in the hospital, library standards emphasize sound management principles, including organizing, staffing, planning, reporting,

Figure 2-1
**Sources of Standards and Guidelines
for Hospital Libraries Services**

AMERICAN LIBRARY ASSOCIATION
Association of Hospital and Institution Libraries. Hospital Library Standards Committee. Standards for library services in health care institutions. Chicago: American Library Association, 1970.

AMERICAN MEDICAL ASSOCIATION
American Medical Association. Directory of residency training programs. 1981/1982 ed. Chicago: American Medical Association, 1981.

AMERICAN OSTEOPATHIC ASSOCIATION
American Osteopathic Association. 1981-82 Yearbook and directory of osteopathic physicians. American Osteopathic Association, 1981.

AMERICAN PSYCHIATRIC ASSOCIATION
American Psychiatric Association. Standards for psychiatric facilities. Washington, DC: American Psychiatric Association, 1969.

**CANADIAN COUNCIL
ON HOSPITAL ACCREDITATION**
Canadian Council on Hospital Accreditation. Guide to hospital accreditation. Toronto: Canadian Council on Hospital Accreditation, 1977.

CANADIAN MEDICAL ASSOCIATION
Canadian Standards for hospital libraries. Can Med Assoc J 1975 May 17;112:1271-1274.

**CONNECTICUT ASSOCIATION
OF HEALTH SCIENCE LIBRARIES**
Connecticut Association of Health Science Libraries. The Standards Committee. Connecticut Association of Health Sciences Libraries: standards and checklist for health sciences libraries. Bull Med Libr Assoc 1975 Oct;63:417-421.

CONNECTICUT REGIONAL MEDICAL PROGRAM
Connecticut Regional Medical Program. Revised suggested minimum guidelines for Connecticut hospital health science libraries. 2d ed. 1973 June.

**GREAT BRITAIN. DEPARTMENT OF
HEALTH AND SOCIAL SECURITY**
Great Britain. Department of Health and Social Security. Library services in hospitals. London: DHSS, 1970. (H.M. (70)23).

**INTERNATIONAL FEDERATION OF
LIBRARY ASSOCIATIONS**
IFLA/FIAB Libraries in Hospitals Sub-Section. IFLA standards for libraries in hospitals (general service). Unesco Bull Libr 1969 Mar-Apr;23:70-76.

**JOINT COMMISSION ON
ACCREDITATION OF HOSPITALS**
Joint Commission on Accreditation of Hospitals. Accreditation manual for hospitals. 1983 ed. Chicago: Joint Commission on Accreditation of Hospitals, 1982.

Joint Commission on Accreditation of Hospitals. Consolidated standards manual for child, adolescent, and adult psychiatric, alcoholism, and drug abuse facilities. 1981 ed. Chicago: Joint Commission on Accreditation of Hospitals, 1981.

LIBRARY ASSOCIATION
The Library Association. Hospital libraries: recommended standards for libraries in hospitals. London: The Library Association, 1972.

NATIONAL LEAGUE FOR NURSING
National League for Nursing. Criteria for the evaluation of diploma programs in nursing. 5th ed. New York: National League for Nursing, 1978.

National League for Nursing. Guide for the development of nursing libraries. 4th ed. New York: National League for Nursing, 1981.

NEW JERSEY HOSPITAL LIBRARY ASSOCIATION
Standards for New Jersey hospital libraries and interpretation for hospital administrators. New Jersey Hospital Library Association Newsletter 1974 Nov;2-5.

**PACIFIC SOUTHWEST REGIONAL
MEDICAL LIBRARY SERVICE**
Pacific Southwest Regional Medical Library Service. Suggested minimum guidelines for health science libraries. Los Angeles: PSRMLS, June 1978.

SPECIAL LIBRARIES ASSOCIATION
Objectives and standards for special libraries. Spec Libr 1964 Dec;55:671-680.

UNITED HOSPITAL FUND OF NEW YORK
United Hospital Fund of New York. Planning the hospital library, a report. New York: United Hospital Fund, 1957.

United Hospital Fund of New York. Essentials for patients' libraries: a guide. New York: United Hospital Fund, 1966.

**UNITED STATES. DEPARTMENT OF
HEALTH AND HUMAN SERVICES**
Code of federal regulations. Title 42 (Public Health). In: Chapter IV (Health Care Financing Administration, Department of Health and Human Services), subchapter B (Medicare Program). Washington, DC: U.S. Government Printing Office, 1981:262 (Section 405.1030).

UNITED STATES. VETERANS ADMINISTRATION
United States. Veterans Administration. Planning criteria for VA facilities. H-08-9, Chapter 400: Library Service. Washington, DC: Veterans Administration, February 1, 1980.

**WESTERN NEW YORK
LIBRARY RESOURCES COUNCIL**
Hutchinson AP, O'Connell MD, Richards BB, Thompson JC, Wheeler RA. Proposed standards for professional health science library services of New York State. Bull Med Libr Assoc 1981 Jul;69: 287-93.

Figure 2-2
Standards and Guidelines for Hospital Library Services: A Comparison of Selected Documents

ORGANIZATION RESPONSIBLE	YEAR PUB-LISHED	NATURE		AUDIENCE	
		Quali-tative	Quanti-tative	Patients	Profes-sionals
American Library Association	1970	X		X	X
American Medical Association	1981	X			X
American Osteopathic Association	1981		X		X
American Psychiatric Association	1969	X			X
Canadian Council on Hospital Accreditation	1977	X			X
Canadian Medical Association	1975		X		X
Connecticut Association of Health Science Libraries	1975	X			X
Connecticut Regional Medical Program	1973		X		X
Great Britain. Department of Health and Social Security	1970	X		X	X
International Federation of Library Associations	1969		X	X	X
Joint Commission on Accreditation of Hospitals	1982	X			X
Joint Commission on Accreditation of Hospitals (Consolidated)	1981	X			X
Library Association	1972		X	X	X
National League for Nursing. (Diploma Programs)	1978	X			X
National League for Nursing. (Nursing Libraries)	1981	X			X
New Jersey Hospital Library Association	1974	X			X
Pacific Southwest Regional Medical Library Service	1978		X		X
Special Libraries Association	1964	X			
United Hospital Fund of New York. (Hospital Library)	1957		X	X	X
United Hospital Fund of New York. (Patients' Libraries)	1966	X		X	
United States. Department of Health and Human Services	1981	X			X
United States. Veterans Administration	1980		X	X	X
Western New York Library Resources Council	1981	X			X

Note: Complete bibliographic information for current editions appears in Figure 2-1.

DEFINITIONS INCLUDED		AREAS ADDRESSED						
YES	NO	Organization	Personnel	Collection	Services	Space	Equipment	Interlibrary Cooperation
X		X	X	X	X	X	X	
	X			X				
	X		X	X		X		
	X	X	X	X		X	X	X
	X	X	X	X	X	X	X	X
	X	X	X	X	X	X	X	X
	X	X	X	X	X	X		X
	X	X	X	X	X	X	X	
	X	X	X	X	X	X	X	X
	X		X	X		X	X	
X		X	X	X	X	X		X
X		X	X	X				
	X	X	X	X		X	X	X
	X			X				
	X	X	X	X	X	X	X	X
		X	X	X		X	X	
	X		X	X	X	X	X	
	X		X	X	X	X	X	
	X		X	X	X	X	X	
X		X	X	X	X	X	X	
				X		X		
	X					X		
	X	X	X	X	X	X		X

and budgeting (4). Although the standards do not provide specific quantitative measures, they do endorse a number of concepts supported by librarians:

- Service to hospital staff, as well as medical staff
- The employment of qualified personnel on a full-time or part-time basis
- The provision of continuing education opportunities for library staff
- An ongoing assessment of information needs and an evaluation of the effectiveness of services filling those needs
- The acquisition and organization of up-to-date print and nonprint material
- The development of cooperative arrangements with other professional libraries and information systems
- Interdisciplinary participation on the library committee
- The central administration of resources
- Designated space for the library
- Documentation
- The development of policies and procedures

By integrating management and library principles and practices, the standards provide the librarian with a framework for interaction with the administration. The librarian also has a basis from which to participate directly or indirectly in the hospital's accreditation process.

The Accreditation Process

The accreditation process begins when a hospital voluntarily applies to the JCAH for an on-site survey. When contacted, the JCAH forwards the *Hospital Survey Profile* to the facility for self-evaluation. This profile explains the JCAH standards and provides an inventory by which the facility can measure its compliance with the appropriate standards. A copy of the *Hospital Survey Profile* for professional library services appears in Appendix B.

Prior to an on-site visit, the completed self-evaluation profile is reviewed by the hospital administration and the JCAH. When the surveyors arrive at the facility, an initial conference may be held with the administration, major department heads, members of the medical staff, and representatives of the hospital's governing body. The survey visit that follows is conducted with the *Hospital Survey Profile* as a guide. A summation conference at the end of the on-site process reports the JCAH findings. Before completion of the visit, however, JCAH surveyors also invite the public to share information about the facility's compliance with accreditation standards. This occurs in the form of a public information interview.

After the on-site visit, the surveyors submit their report, and an accreditation decision is made based on the evaluation of all available information. Major factors in the decision include evidence of overall compliance with the standards, progressive advancement toward more complete compliance, and the absence of any serious impediments to patient safety or quality care. The JCAH may grant a three-year accreditation, or it may deny accreditation. If accreditation is revoked or refused, a facility may appeal the decision.

The Librarian's Role in Accreditation

Every librarian should be concerned about the hospital's compliance with the standards for professional library services. Familiarity with the current *Accreditation Manual for Hospitals* and the *Hospital Survey Profile* is essential. Keeping abreast of accreditation activities prepares the librarian for effective participation in future hospital surveys.

Keeping Informed

Topper and other members of the Hospital Library Standards and Practices Committee of the Medical Library Association (MLA) have provided a discussion of aspects of the JCAH standards and accreditation process that may be useful for hospital librarians facing their first survey (5). Librarians can also keep informed about accreditation activities by reading the JCAH's official newsletter, *JCAH Perspectives;* its *Quality Review Bulletin (QRB);* and publications issued by library organizations. The hospital librarian should also keep informed of any MLA activities that pertain to standards. Current committees and their charges are listed in the annual *Directory of the Medical Library Association.*

In recent years the MLA has begun a mutually beneficial dialogue with the JCAH. The *JCAH Guide to Professional Library Services for Surveyors* has been developed by the MLA and shared with the JCAH (6). This document lists questions that aid surveyors in evaluating an institution's compliance with standards for professional library services.

In addition, the MLA has issued a statement on the role of hospital library consultants, relating to the use of consultative assistance referred to in the standards (7).

Preparing for the Survey

A librarian can play an active role during the initial planning for the on-site survey. Prior to the survey, a librarian can undertake the following tasks:

- Offer to complete the library section of the self-evaluation profile or request a copy of the completed document from administration
- Plan surveys and reports to document the level of compliance or noncompliance and to keep administrative staff informed
- Collect documents that support compliance or prepare a record of their location
- Note those items listed in the *Hospital Survey Profile* that should be available for the surveyor
- Participate in, or review minutes of, any hospital internal preparations directed to all departments

Participating in the Survey

During the survey period, the library may be visited by a member of the surveying team. Although it is extremely desirable that the surveyors visit the library, various constraints sometimes make this visit not possible. It should be remembered that the library's section of the *Hospital Survey Profile* has been reviewed, even if the library is not inspected. The hospital librarian should work closely with the administration to help ensure that it is knowledgeable about the library and its activities.

In addition to participating in the review of the library, the librarian can serve as a resource person for the hospital staff during the survey process. In this capacity, the librarian may wish to do the following:

• Acquire the *Publications Catalogue* (available from the JCAH, 875 North Michigan Avenue, Chicago, Illinois 60611

• Coordinate acquisition and dissemination of the current edition of the *Accreditation Manual for Hospitals* or appropriate standards released by the JCAH

• Route standards to departments involved, with prior administrative approval

• Circulate publications from the JCAH to administrative staff or to committees involved with quality assurance

• Prepare bibliographies or reference material about the survey process for distribution or for publication in house organs

• Be present at the on-site survey to answer any questions that might arise

REFERENCES

1. Carmel MJ. What standards for standards? Libr Assoc Record 1975 Oct;77:238-240.

2. Yast H. Standards for library service in institutions: B. in the health care setting. Libr Trends 1972 Oct;21:267-285.

3. Joint Commission on Accreditation of Hospitals. Accreditation manual for hospitals. 1983 ed. Chicago: Joint Commission on Accreditation of Hospitals, 1982.

4. Foster EC. Library development and the Joint Commission on Accreditation of Hospitals standards. Bull Med Libr Assoc 1979 Apr;67:226-231.

5. Topper JM, Bradley J, Dudden RF, Epstein BA, Lambremont JA, Putney TR, Jr. JCAH accreditation and the hospital library: a guide for librarians. Bull Med Libr Assoc 1980 Apr;68:212-219.

6. JCAH guide to professional library services for surveyors. MLA News 1980 Sept;6:1-2.

7. Medical Library Association. Hospital library consultants. Chicago: Medical Library Association, 1982.

READINGS

Flower MA. Toward hospital library standards in Canada. Bull Med Libr Assoc 1978 July;66:296-301.

Henderson MM. Standards: developments and impacts. Spec Libr 1981 Apr;72:142-148.

Hoadley IB, Clark AS, eds. Quantitative methods in librarianship: standards, research, management. Westport, CT: Greenwood Press, 1972.

Joint Commission on Accreditation of Hospitals. Hospital survey profile. 1982 ed. Chicago: Joint Commission on Accreditation of Hospitals, 1981.

Lancaster FW. The relevance of standards to the evaluation of library services. In: Lancaster FW. The measurement and evaluation of library services. Washington, DC: Information Resources Press, 1977:288-298.

The Library Association. The Library Association guidelines for library provision in the health service: A consultative document. London: The Library Association, 1978.

Stinson, ER. Standards for health sciences libraries. Library Trends 1982 Summer 31:125-137.

APPENDIX A*
Standards for Professional Library Services

Professional Library Services

The hospital shall provide library services to meet the informa-   **Principle**
tional, educational, and, when appropriate, the research-related
needs of the medical and hospital staffs.

The professional library services shall be organized to assure ap-   **Standard I**
propriate direction or supervision, staffing, and resources.

The extent of services should be related to the needs of the medical and hos-   INTERPRETATION
pital staffs, to the hospital services provided, and to the cooperative arrangements with other professional libraries and information systems. The staffing,
size, contents, and equipment will vary with the extent of services provided.
The interrelationship between the professional library and other hospital   10
units shall be reflected in the overall hospital organizational plan.

Direction/Supervision/Staffing Whenever feasible, all professional library
resources within the hospital shall be under the direction of a qualified
medical librarian. Hospitals requiring extensive library service should employ at least one full-time qualified medical librarian, as well as adequate   15
support staff. A qualified medical librarian is an individual who holds a
graduate degree in library science from a school accredited by the American
Library Association, and who is certified by the Medical Library Association,
or an individual who has documented equivalent training and/or experience.

When employment of a full-time or part-time qualified medical librarian   20
is not possible, the hospital shall secure the regular consultative assistance
of such an individual. Consultative visits should be documented. When the
medical librarian serves only on a part-time or consultative basis, a suitably
trained employee shall be designated and available to provide basic library

*Reproduced from the *Accreditation Manual for Hospitals*, 1983 edition, with the permission of the Joint Commission on Accreditation of Hospitals.

services. This individual should have basic library skills and, whenever possible, should be at least the equivalent of a library technician or library assistant. The individual so designated should have responsibility for ordering, cataloging, organizing, and circulating library resources, and for document reproduction, any required binding, and maintenance of the library collection. In addition, this individual should provide, to the extent possible, document delivery, bibliographic, and reference services.

To enhance the quality of library services offered, the individual charged with responsibility for such services should participate, as appropriate, in relevant in-service and outside educational opportunities. This participation should be documented.

Resources The professional library shall have an up-to-date, authoritative collection of print and nonprint materials, including recent editions of textbooks and current periodicals pertinent to the clinical, educational, and research services offered. The *Index Medicus* or *Abridged Index Medicus* and its cumulations, and, as appropriate, hospital, nursing, and dental indexes should be provided. Document reproduction and delivery service, audiovisual services, and bibliographic sources to facilitate the effective provision of references and information sources should be included in the professional library services available.

It is desirable that all professional library collections within the hospital be under a single library service, at least administratively when not physically possible. The library should be able to provide information concerning library resources located within departments.

Whenever possible, the area designated for the professional library service should be reserved for that purpose only. There should be ready access to all textbooks, other publications, and audiovisual materials and equipment, as well as to facilities for using the audiovisual services. The collection shall be so organized that users can locate materials without assistance. Controlled access to the library may be required when significant loss of library resources occurs during periods when the library is not staffed.

There must be evidence of a continuing effort to study the hospital's needs for professional library services, and to ascertain whether such services are provided. Immediate and long-term goals, as well as the means of providing funding to achieve these goals, should be defined in writing. These needs and goals may be determined through formal written surveys, needs assessments, and structured reviews of the library collection. In order to broaden the availability of community resources and to avoid unnecessary duplication, professional libraries should share their resources through loans or document reproduction/delivery service, consistent with any applicable legal restrictions. Interlibrary cooperation and sharing arrangements shall be documented. Geographically contiguous libraries that share their resources through interlibrary loans should coordinate their selection and retention of library materials.

Standard II   **The provision of professional library services shall be guided by written policies and procedures.**

INTERPRETATION   Written policies and procedures for professional library services shall be current, and shall relate to at least the following:

- The mechanisms for selection and acquisition of library materials;
- Donations to the library;
- Cataloging and classification of library resources;
- The level of reference and bibliographic services to be provided;
- The regulation of access to, and circulation of, library resources mate-   5
  rials, including the mechanisms through which individuals authorized
  to use the library can participate in all library services provided; the
  provision of essential library materials when the library is closed or
  not staffed; and the period that a book, journal, or audiovisual mate-
  rial/equipment may be retained on loan;   10
- The mechanism for informing the medical and hospital staffs of new
  acquisitions and services, and their availability;
- The length of time that library materials shall be retained, and the
  disposition or storage of outdated or unusable books and periodicals;
- The binding of journals, as required;   15
- Any required records or reports; and
- The functions of the professional library committee, when one exists.

When a professional library committee exists, it shall be multidisciplinary
and have representation from at least the medical staff, nursing department/
service, and administration. When a qualified medical librarian serves the   20
hospital on a full-time or part-time basis, this individual shall be a member
of the committee, with a defined role in committee functions. The committee
shall meet as often as required, but not less than twice annually, to review the
library policies and procedures; to evaluate the effectiveness of the library
in meeting the informational and educational needs of its users; and to   25
establish priorities in the selection of new texts, the selection or renewal
of journals, and the acquisition of other library materials. In establishing
priorities, recommendations for library acquisitions made by members of
the medical and hospital staffs and the medical librarian should be considered for their appropriateness and available funding.   30

Refer also to the Medical Staff, Nursing Services, Pharmaceutical Services, and Rehabilitation Programs/Services sections of this *Manual*.

APPENDIX B*
Hospital Survey Profile

Joint Commission on Accreditation of Hospitals
Hospital Survey Profile

22. Professional Library Services

The following items should be available for the surveyor.

1. Written policies and procedures.
2. Written agreements with outside medical library resources.
3. A list of texts purchased since the previous survey.
4. The percentage of texts (supplied for the medical staff) that are less than five years old.
5. Additions/deletions of periodicals since the last survey.

> This section must
> always be completed.

Please respond to each of the following statements by inserting an "X" in the box ☐ beside every statement that describes hospital practice or status at this time.

If additional space is needed, indicate that the answer is to be continued, and complete the answer in the Continuation and Comments space at the end of the section. Carefully identify the answer that is continued by indicating the item number in the left-hand column of the Continuation and Comments section. At the end of each entry in the Continuation and Comments section, draw a heavy line completely across the page.

The individual who has the primary responsibility for the area covered, as designated by the chief executive officer, should complete this section. The name and title of this person, as well as the date of completion, should be provided in the designated space at the end of the section.

1. The following statements describe the status of professional library services in the hospital.
   - ☐ a. A central professional library is available to the medical staff
   - ☐ b. The library is available to the house staff
   - ☐ c. The library is available to nursing department/service personnel and other hospital staff members
   - ☐ d. In addition to a central professional library, the hospital also has small departmental text/journal resources
   - ☐ e. The hospital has no central library; resources are dispersed among the various departments
   - ☐ f. The professional library is open and staffed at all times
   - ☐ g. The professional library is open and staffed only part time
   - ☐ h. The professional library is open only weekdays, but available by key at other times, as required
   - ☐ i. No librarian is on duty at any time
   - ☐ j. The library is conveniently located for those who use it, particularly the medical staff

*Reproduced from the *Hospital Survey Profile,* 1983 edition, with the permission of the Joint Commission on Accreditation of Hospitals.

☐ k. Professional library services are provided entirely by an outside source (please describe) _____

_____

_____

2. Staffing of the professional library is provided by the following.

☐ a. Not assessable because the library is not located in, or operated by, the hospital

☐ b. One or more qualified medical librarians, available on a full-time basis

☐ c. One or more qualified medical librarians, available on a part-time basis

☐ d. A qualified medical librarian, available on a consultative basis and whose visits are documented

☐ e. An individual appointed or authorized through the office of the chief executive officer to provide basic library services during the daytime

☐ f. Personnel of the medical record service or another department/service, as additional responsibility

☐ g. Other (please explain) _____

_____

_____

NOTE: Please refer to Standard I of the Professional Library Services section of the *Accreditation Manual for Hospitals*.

3. The following services are available either in the hospital library or through outside sources.

☐ a. Reference service

☐ b. Document delivery service

☐ c. Reproduction

☐ d. Audiovisual service

☐ e. Bibliographic service

4. Participation of professional library staff personnel in continuing education programs is documented.

☐ a. Not assessable because library services are not located in or operated by the hospital

☐ b. Yes

☐ c. No

5. The library provides *Index Medicus* in either the standard or abridged version.

☐ a. Yes

☐ b. No (please explain) _____

_____

6. The library also provides the following indexes.

☐ a. Hospital

☐ b. Nursing

☐ c. Dental

7. The basic professional library contains at least the following, pertinent to the clinical, educational, and research services offered by the hospital.

  ☐ a. Basic science textbooks

  ☐ b. Reference textbooks

  ☐ c. At least one journal for each professional specialty represented on the medical staff

8. A written plan for further development and growth of the professional library includes

  ☐ a. Immediate goals

  ☐ b. Long-term goals

  ☐ c. No such plan exists (please explain) _____

  _____

9. The professional library committee includes

  ☐ a. Not applicable because the hospital doesn't have a library committee

  ☐ b. One or more physicians

  ☐ c. One or more nurses

  ☐ d. One or more administrative staff members

  ☐ e. One or more house staff members

  ☐ f. Clinical department representatives

  ☐ g. The medical librarian

10. Professional library policies and procedures relate to at least

  ☐ a. Mechanisms for selection and acquisition of library materials

  ☐ b. Donations to the library

  ☐ c. Cataloging and classification of library resources

  ☐ d. The level of reference and bibliographic services to be provided

  ☐ e. Mechanisms through which individuals authorized to use the library can participate in all library services provided

  ☐ f. Provision of essential library materials when the library is closed or not staffed

  ☐ g. The period that the material may be retained on loan

  ☐ h. A mechanism for informing the medical staff and others of new texts and journals and their availability

  ☐ i. The length of time that library materials are maintained, and the disposition or storage of outdated/unusable books and periodicals

  ☐ j. The binding of journals

  ☐ k. Required records/reports

  ☐ l. Functions of the professional library committee, when one exists

11. An annual hospital budget is prepared for the professional library.

  ☐ a. Not for this hospital because the library is not provided in or by the hospital

  ☐ b. Yes, specifically for the professional library

  ☐ c. Yes, but it is subsumed under another hospital budget

  ☐ d. No

  ☐ e. No, the library is underwritten by the medical staff

This section of the *Hospital Survey Profile* was completed by

_____   _____   _____

Name   Title   Date

Item Number	Continuation and Comments

SECTION I:
Selecting, Acquiring, and Organizing Library Materials

Selection of Library Materials

Margaret C. Hardy
Director, Educational Resources Center
Miami Valley Hospital
Dayton, Ohio

CHAPTER 3

Selection of Library Materials

Margaret C. Hardy
Director, Educational Resources Center
Miami Valley Hospital
Dayton, Ohio

Appendixes

Figures

Selecting the resources that belong in a hospital library involves answering three basic questions: Who are the materials for? Who has the responsibility for choosing these materials? Which specific titles will be needed? Unfortunately, the answers are not simple.

Although many hospital libraries originally served only physicians, in recent years the library doors have swung wide to admit students, administrators, nurses, technicians, and in some libraries, patients. The wider clientele, coupled with direction from professional librarians, has changed the focus of the library from purely "medical" to "health sciences." This impact, first felt among the larger hospital libraries, is now being felt by smaller libraries, as they, too, attempt to meet the standards of the Joint Commission on Accreditation of Hospitals (JCAH).

The JCAH standards call for "library services to meet the informational, educational, and when appropriate, the research-related needs of the medical and hospital staffs" (1), yet the standards do not clearly state who is responsible for selecting library materials. Because the involvement of a qualified medical librarian is mandated in the standards generally, the librarian has a role in book selection. The particular blend of responsibility for selection in any individual hospital emerges from the combined action of the librarian, the library committee, and the hospital administrator.

Collection development in a hospital library is a complex activity based on the interaction of many elements: the environment in which selection occurs, the policies which govern selection, and the process which matches user needs to specific resources. This chapter considers each of these in detail.

THE SELECTION ENVIRONMENT

Selection of materials for a hospital library occurs within a broad context which may be termed the selection environment. This environment includes the hospital, the library community, the library itself, and the persons involved with the selection process.

The Hospital

The first step in developing an acquisition program is to study the hospital in which the library exists. What are its services, clinical resources, and patient referral patterns? Answers to these questions provide the focus for the library in meeting specialized needs. The practice of referring all high-risk pregnancies to another hospital, for example, affects the scope of the collection in obstetrics. In addition, what are the teaching programs, research activities, and community service programs in the hospital? What are the hospital's future plans, and what role does the library play in those plans? If three rural hospitals plan to join in a program of shared services, will three libraries be developed, or will one be strengthened to serve all institutions? Understanding the hospital's

present and future programs is essential in identifying potential users of library resources.

The Library Community

Other library collections located in the community are also part of the selection environment. Often the availability of a specific title at a local or regional library can influence the decision to purchase. Since special, public, and academic libraries can provide invaluable back-up services, cooperative arrangements should be considered when developing a plan for hospital library service. Larger hospital libraries can be a vital link in the cooperative effort to support each other, as well as to assist smaller hospitals. Formal cooperative acquisition programs, such as those that require participants to buy books and journals in specified subject areas, can also help to eliminate duplication of little-used materials and stretch meager budgets.

The Hospital Library

The hospital library offers a centralized approach to meeting the organization's need for books, journals, and audiovisuals. Centralizing library services, rather than allowing each department to provide for its own needs, also makes hiring a trained and experienced librarian cost effective. When selection is organized by a librarian, consistent and well-documented principles and procedures can insure a balanced, high-quality collection to meet a wide range of needs. Even when librarians change, the well-established principles and procedures of the library will maintain the focus of the collection and insure its effective development.

The JCAH standards require the services of a professional librarian, either as a staff member or as a regular consultant. They also require written policies and procedures governing selection. When these requirements are met, the smallest library will have a collection developed by a professional, following policies approved by the library committee and supported by the administration.

As a professional educated in book selection and collection development, the librarian consults the medical and hospital staff before selecting books to meet staff needs. These needs are determined in a variety of ways: client recommendations, collection development questionnaires, interviews, collection review by department personnel, and suggestions by the library committee. A librarian who understands the programs and commitments of the hospital can determine the most effective means for identifying user needs. Because the needs of the users often determine the material that is purchased, the medical and hospital professionals are involved in selection. The responsibility for directing, balancing, and guiding that selection, however, rests with the librarian. Once this role is established, it should be defined in the job description of the librarian. Typical phrasing appears below:

Working with the advice of the library committee and other health professionals, the librarian is responsible for the selection and acquisition of all library materials including books, journal subscriptions, and audiovisual materials. The librarian is also responsible for recommending and administering the annual budget for the library.

The Library Committee

Although the JCAH standards do not require a library committee, many librarians find such a committee useful, particularly in providing information and advice for collection development and evaluation. Often the library committee can assist with needs assessments of the groups they represent. They can review materials or find reviewers for the materials; they can evaluate subject areas in the library; and they can offer advice on priorities for acquisitions.

Generally, hospital librarians find that the library committee's most effective role is an advisory one. When the committee reserves selection decisions as its responsibility, however, the librarian should establish the policies concerning the types, balance, and quality of materials. He or she should provide a structure for making regular recommendations to the committee. In this way the librarian can continue to provide the professional direction clearly indicated by the standards of the JCAH.

Further discussion of library committees appears in Chapter 18.

The Hospital Administration

The hospital librarian is responsible, either directly or indirectly, to the hospital administration. The goal of this relationship, in terms of the selection of library resources, is threefold: create an understanding of the value and cost-effectiveness of centralized library service, follow the requirements of the JCAH, and determine the most effective role of the library committee in the selection process. When the hospital administration sees that the selection of materials is based on institutional needs and that organized principles underlie selection and insure quality, administrative support should be forthcoming.

THE SELECTION POLICY

A written selection policy protects the library and the librarian. It helps to assure the orderly development of the collection in a manner that is consistent with the goals of the library and the hospital. It provides valid reasons for the purchase of library materials or justification for decisions not to purchase them and thus helps in the wise allotment of budgeted funds. In addition, a selection policy informs both administration and library users of the scope of the collection, gives evidence of its compliance with the JCAH requirements, and provides continuity in collection development as the library staff changes.

Not only is the selection policy useful, but developing it is often an educational process. It demonstrates to the library committee and to the administration that various considerations are involved in developing a useful collection.

The format, organization, and specific content of the selection policy varies with the institution. Some libraries function effectively with a brief policy statement such as the following: "The library will acquire books and journals to support the programs of the hospital." This is a convenient statement because it allows for continual change in the scope of the collection without requiring a revision of the policy. A more detailed policy, however, is recommended for most libraries to assure the orderly development of the entire collection and to provide a clear guide for the librarian who must interpret the policy.

Elements of a Policy

Major elements included in most selection policies are given below. A sample policy appears in Appendix A.

• A statement on the user population itemizes all groups served by the library.
• A statement on selection responsibility defines the role of the librarian and the library committee.
• A statement on subject coverage itemizes the subject areas in the collection and indicates the extent of the coverage. The levels suggested by Beatty are useful here: exhaustive, research, reference, and skeletal (2). If these terms, or others, are used, definitions should be included.
• A statement on budgetary allotment gives the percentages of the budget assigned to books, journals, and audiovisuals. Beatty's estimate that medical libraries are two-thirds journals and one-third books can be reflected here (2). A percentage specific to the individual library may be preferred.

Although percentages are often assigned to specific areas, the librarian should be able to shift funds when special needs arise. Any alteration in funds, however, should have an administrator's approval.

• A statement on duplicates lists the criteria for determining whether or not to buy duplicate texts and journal subscriptions. The statement can be general or specific. General wording may state that duplicates will be purchased as warranted by use and as funds permit. Specific wording may preclude duplicate purchases except from outside funding sources, or it may actually itemize the conditions under which duplicates will be purchased.
• A statement on gifts requires that the gift meet the selection criteria for purchase. The policy should also give the librarian the right to dispose of the gift later if it no longer meets library needs. The acceptance of gifts is discussed more fully later in this chapter.
• A statement on selection criteria and selection aids lists specific criteria that may be useful for evaluation purposes. Figure 3-1 illustrates detailed criteria for purchase.

Figure 3-1
Considerations for Purchase

Books

1. Determination of need

   a. How thoroughly is subject area covered by selection policy?
   b. What are the weaknesses of the collection in the subject area?
   c. What is the extent of the collection in the subject area?

2. Appropriateness of selection

   a. Timeliness: Is subject covered better in journals?
   b. Usefulness: Is repetitive demand not met by journal articles?
   c. Ratio of cost to use: Should the selection be purchased or borrowed?
   d. Permanent value: Does it support important hospital programs?

3. Guidelines for selection

   a. Previous editions owned
   b. Book reviews
   c. Reputation of author and publisher
   d. Comparative cost with competitive titles
   e. Unique features of book; illustrations, tables appendices
   f. Scope and point of view of the book
   g. Audience level
   h. Usefulness of references and bibliographies

Journals

1. Determination of need

   a. How thoroughly is subject area covered by selection policy?
   b. What are the copyright guidelines?
   c. Are the journals available in area libraries?

2. Appropriateness of selection

   a. Is subject area covered adequately in journals already held?
   b. What is the ratio of cost to use, particularly of journals published outside the United States?

3. Guidelines for selection

   a. What is the reputation of editors and publishers? Is it a "refereed" journal?
   b. Are articles original or reprinted?
   c. Are indexes well done and available on a timely basis?
   d. Do the authors appear to be experts?
   e. Is journal indexed by major indexing and abstracting publications? Does the library have access to these indexes?
   f. Are references accurate and current?
   g. What is the quality of paper, illustrations, text, and binding?

The selection aids used by the librarian should be enumerated in the selection policy. These can include book reviews, core lists, recommendations from users or the library committee, examination of the actual item, and demand in the library.

• A statement on currency of collection explains the purchase of new editions, the retention of old editions and journals, and the weeding of the collection.

The retention policy can also specify different types or levels of retention such as an inactive collection for little-used titles or journal backfiles, or the provision of journal backfiles on microfilm.

The JCAH *Hospital Survey Profile* that is used during the JCAH surveying process requests a statement on the percent of texts for the medical staff that are less than five years old. Therefore, some statement in the policy relating to this requirement is useful (3).

Journal retention policies and policies relating to weeding are discussed in detail in Chapter 6.

• A statement on cooperative collection development refers to both formal and informal agreements. Formal documents should be cited.

• A statement on responsibility for departmental collections includes such topics as selection, prevention of unnecessary duplication, ordering, cataloging, budget, inventory, and accessibility to other users. Collections outside the library are discussed later in this chapter and in Chapter 18.

• A statement on miscellaneous items covers the items not previously dealt with in the selection policy. These may include staff publications, archives, textbook collections, pamphlet collections, and others.

• A statement on revision of the selection policy sets forth the frequency of revision and the approval mechanisms.

Other Library Policies Affecting Selection

The selection and retention of materials are affected by other library policies. A change in the circulation policy, for example, may affect the number of copies ordered, as would the refinement of the reserve system. Obviously, if materials do not leave the library, the need for duplicate copies is minimal. A decision not to circulate journals may reduce the need for duplicates but may also require changes in photocopying policies.

The provision of reference services also directly affects book and journal selection. Is the library going to provide the information resources to meet the research needs of the hospital staff, or will these users be referred to another library? Will the library aim to have available fifty percent of the English language references in a typical MEDLINE search? Policy decisions of other libraries affect the library's users, too. Increased interlibrary loan charges or copyright law requirements, for example, may make it necessary to subscribe to a journal previously considered out of scope for the collection. One final factor directly affecting the selection policy is the increasing number of library users. A rise in the number of library users means additional wear to the collection and may result in increased binding costs or the purchase of replacement copies.

Changes in the use of a collection can occur suddenly or happen gradually over a period of months or years. Major changes, such as the closing of the hospital school of nursing, or the combination of two libraries, will require the revision of policies. The effects of minor change, such as increased use of the library resulting from the initiation of a tuition reimbursement program for all employees, can usually be covered within the terms of a broadly written policy.

THE SELECTION PROCESS

Selection involves determining what is needed, knowing what is already owned, identifying what is available, and choosing what will best meet the identified needs.

Assessing Needs

The importance of purchasing only material that is needed cannot be overstressed. Not only is the budget of the hospital library limited, but many hospital administrators are not entirely convinced that books and journals meet a real hospital need. By clearly identifying needs and appropriate materials to meet those needs, the librarian reinforces the value of library services. When the library is accepted as an indispensable support service for patient care, the librarian can consider purchases that will anticipate programs, rather than just support programs already in place.

There are many ways of determining needs for library materials. Some more common techniques are reviewed here.

Request Forms

A method for requesting books, journals, or audiovisuals is essential. A form or a request slip will insure that the user includes all the necessary information. Libraries that use order slips may want to modify that form. A sample request slip appears in Figure 3-2.

Collection Development Questionnaire

Periodically, the librarian may want to solicit opinions about the library collection. An open-ended questionnaire, such as the one shown in Appendix B, may be useful.

Structured Reviews of the Collection

A review of the library collection by the subject specialists who use the library may be the most effective form of needs assessment. Since all these specialists often do not have time to examine the collection, an alternative method can be used. One member from each department can review subject holdings. The person may be the representative to the library committee, the individual who coordinates educational activities in that department, or just an active library user. Each member that is selected from the appropriate department would make a formal review of the collection, based on a list of the holdings and instructions for the reviewing process that is prepared by the librarian. The instructions may request that outdated titles be deleted and new titles or subject areas be added. If the list is sent to the department head and follow-ups are initiated, response can be quite good.

Needs Assessment Interviews

Many librarians request yearly interviews with department heads, or attend departmental meetings once a year to discuss what materials are used and needed.

Routing Book Announcements, Flyers, and Reviews

When the librarian identifies areas of the collection that need strengthening, he or she may route flyers or reviews of likely titles to subject experts. Evaluating the flyers beforehand and sending only those that are suitable prospects is important. Routing all flyers without screening usually results in indiscriminate selection and nullifies the advantages gained by having the librarian direct selection. Routing flyers to content experts is also useful when deciding whether or not to purchase a revised edition of a title already owned.

Core Lists

Although it is useful to the librarian to know which titles on core lists the library owns, core lists are not generally used to determine areas of need because all institutions may not need materials in all areas. Rather, core lists are an excellent means of identifying standard titles once the need for the subject has been determined.

Librarian's Judgment

Observation and judgment are indispensable factors in determining need. What new programs are being planned for the hospital? What subject areas are in high demand? What requests for books recur frequently? What do interlibrary loan requests show about needs? Whether or not the librarian makes the final decision in selection, the library committee and the administration depend on the librarian's recommendations for directing collection development.

Evaluating the Collection

In order for collection development to proceed systematically, the librarian must know the scope of the existing collection. If he or she is not thoroughly familiar with present holdings, a combined inventory-weeding activity can provide this information. Both these topics are discussed in Chapter 6.

Assessing patron use of library materials is also essential in evaluating the collection. Circulation records provide one of the most helpful tools in collection evaluation and should be used in weighing the merits of a particular title. Whether the title is old or new, if it circulates frequently it is meeting a user need of some kind.

Evaluating the use of materials in the library requires a different procedure. Studying photocopying records will reveal usage patterns. Another helpful practice is keeping records of items as they are reshelved. The person who is shelving the items can record subject, call number, or other useful statistics with hash marks on a daily tally sheet kept on the book truck.

A simple method for studying how the total collection is used involves placing a slip of colored paper in the pocket of every book, or clipping the paper to the flyleaf of every bound journal. The first time the book is re-shelved, the slip is removed. At the end of six months (or any other useful time period), the presence of the slip will indicate that the item has not left the shelf in that length of time. This system is particularly helpful in revealing how materials that do not circulate are being used.

In assessing usage patterns, it is desirable to talk with as many library users as possible. New usage patterns as well as information about lack of use can be discovered in this way. Many of the techniques discussed in determining needs are valuable in evaluating what already exists in the library. The collection should also be assessed in terms of the needs of the library staff who provide reference and bibliographic services.

Using Selection Resources

Bonk and Magrill have described with tongue in cheek the ideal "selection" librarian (4). This paragon possesses

Figure 3-2
Library Purchase Request Form

LIBRARY PURCHASE REQUEST

CALL NO.	AUTHOR (SURNAME FIRST)				
	TITLE				
SEARCHED:					
___ BIP		ISBN:			
___ FBIP					
___ MBIP	PLACE OF PUBLICATION:	PUBLISHER:			DATE:
___ PUBLIC CAT					
___ ORDER FILE	RECOMMENDED/DONATED BY:	EDITION:	VOLS:	COPIES:	PRICE:
REVIEWS:	CORE REF AV CIRC	DATE RECEIVED:			
	SPECIAL INSTRUCTIONS:				

Note: Reproduced with permission of the Hartford Hospital Health Sciences Library.

complete mastery of the subject, has read all books both published and about to be published, and knows the authors and their work intimately.

The average librarian approaches the task of selecting materials without many of these virtues. However, he or she should be able to balance library goals, evaluation tools, and user studies with JCAH standards. The administration and library committee can help the librarian maintain a balance of these elements in selection and acquisition. There are also many selection aids available to make the job easier and help guarantee good results. These aids fall into three categories: evaluation aids such as lists of recommended titles and book reviews, finding aids that supply bibliographic information, and information aids such as publishers' flyers.

Evaluation Aids

Whether one is planning to build up a weak area in the collection or looking for the best title available in a certain subject, the *Selected List of Books and Journals for the Small Medical Library,* compiled by Brandon and Hill, is an excellent place to begin (5). Revised biannually and published in the *Bulletin of the Medical Library Association*, Brandon and Hill's list is reprinted and distributed to libraries by major book dealers. Studying the explanatory notes preceding the listings is important in understanding the intent of the list. These notes also provide vital information regarding library standards, book and journal prices, references to other selection guides, suggestions for effective purchasing practices, and a brief list of book dealers and subscription agents.

Some librarians or library committees think that every library should work toward owning all or most of the titles on the Brandon and Hill list. This is neither the intent of this list nor of the other available selection guides. Lists such as these are intended to suggest titles for consideration and are prepared by subject experts, associations, or librarians based on user preferences. Small libraries will have need for only a few titles from each subject category of the list. User reaction helps in making the correct choice. If the library can afford only one textbook on hematology, for example, the librarian can get both Wintrobe and Williams on approval or loan and ask several physicians for their opinions. If the choice is a difficult one, the second title can be bought the following year or when the next edition is published. Buying one author in one edition and the competitor in the next edition helps to satisfy disagreements about the merits of some expensive standard texts.

If cooperative arrangements exist within a geographic area, it may be possible for a consortium to have access to the entire Brandon and Hill list by assigning specific titles to different libraries. In this way the depth and scope of the list is made available and the expense is shared by several institutions.

Selection aids for nursing literature have been in short supply, but Brandon and Hill's *Selected List of Nursing Books and Journals* appeared in 1979 and was updated in 1982 (6). In addition, Binger and Strauch have both published guides to nursing literature. These, and other sources for book and journal selection, appear in Appendix C. This list is intended as a starting point only. The hospital librarian will need to scan the indexes regularly under the headings "Book selection" and "Bibliography," or do a search of the literature every few months to identify newly published lists.

Book reviews in primary journals are a valuable source of evaluation information. A rave review in the *New England Journal of Medicine* or the *Journal of the American Medical Association,* for example, generally indicates that the book can be ordered without hesitation. Physicians often place great reliance on these reviews, and the library committee will be apt to follow these recommendations when their opinion is requested. The drawback in relying too heavily on reviews for selection, however, is that too much time often will elapse between the publication of a title and the appearance of a review. A general rule in this regard is to look for reviews of titles under consideration, but not to delay the decision by waiting for a review.

In spite of the lists, searches, and reviews, the hospital librarian may still have difficulty locating adequate titles in some subject areas with the tools available. For this reason it is essential to establish a good working relationship with local public and university library staffs in order to use their locating tools and request their professional opinions.

Finding Aids

Books in Print (BIP) is the most complete finding aid for books. It is published annually in six volumes, two volumes each for author, title, and subject listings. Updated with regular supplements, *BIP* may be too expensive for the average hospital library to purchase.

Medical Books and Serials in Print (MBIP) is updated annually and should be in most hospital libraries. At a fraction of the cost of *BIP*, it uses the same databases and includes the major health science disciplines. Listings in *MBIP* will not be as complete as *BIP* because it includes the publications of 1,927 publishers, compared to *BIP*'s 8,400 publishers. Easy access to *BIP* via the telephone or at a local library can satisfy most hospital libraries. If not, *BIP* can be purchased every two or three years.

In addition to the serials section of *MBIP*, *Ulrich's International Periodicals Directory* is valuable as a library tool because it provides information for ordering journals outside the health care field. This added dimension is useful when requests come in for titles in psychology or management, for example.

The *National Library of Medicine Current Catalog* is another useful reference for selection. Materials can be located by subject as well as by author and title. For hospital libraries with access to National Library of Medicine databases, use of CATLINE can be an economical substitute for owning *Current Catalog*. More finding aids are described in the introduction to Brandon and Hill's list.

Information Aids

All materials that inform the reader of current publications are placed in the category of information aids. This category includes book and journal advertisements, acquisition lists from other libraries, listings of "books received" appearing in the book review sections of many journals, book and journal advertisements in journals, publishers' catalogs and flyers, lists of available titles and new editions published regularly by the major book distributors, and lists compiled for special meetings such as those prepared for the American College of Surgeons.

Experience proves helpful in deciding which tools are more useful to a particular library. Perhaps acquisition tools that are not needed every day can be shared among libraries. Also, the online accessibility of acquisition tools is expanding. CATLINE from the National Library of Medicine has proven extremely helpful, and commercial vendors are providing other tools such as *BIP*.

Other Aids to Selections

One of the joys of book selection not often available to hospital librarians is actual hands-on examination of the book itself. Book exhibits at the annual meeting of the Medical Library Association, and at some regional and state meetings, provide this opportunity as do book stores, public libraries, medical school libraries, and book fairs.

Having contact with publishers' representatives may provide another aid in planning library acquisitions. Knowing six months in advance from a representative that a new edition of an expensive set of atlases will be available can help the librarian budget for expenditures. Generally speaking, it is wise to order directly from publishers' representatives only if the advantages outweigh using the library's regular jobber. Further information on ordering is available in Chapter 4.

Selecting Materials for Purchase

Whether the librarian has the responsibility for making the final decision concerning materials for purchase or that responsibility lies with the library committee, the process is much the same. In the latter case, the librarian prepares the list of recommendations and then takes the added step of obtaining approval from the committee before the orders are placed.

Budget limitations will always place constraints on the selection of materials for the library, whether these materials are books, journals, or audiovisuals. The librarian can, however, keep requests for purchases organized and ready for future budget requests. Lists of needed titles, a collection of user requests for purchase, or slips containing complete ordering information can be organized either by title or subject. Such a file provides a quick

source of materials recently published in a subject area or for suggestions for gift purchases.

Books

When a specific book title is under consideration, an evaluation should be made. Some considerations for purchase appear in Figure 3-1. Others may be applicable to an individual library. All considerations should be documented in the selection policy. Careful thought given to each title before ordering can save much time and effort in returning unwanted items.

Knowledge of the reputation of the author and the publisher of a book, as well as an understanding of which subject area the publisher specializes in printing, helps the librarian to choose titles that are best for the collection. A librarian soon learns which publishers to trust, which to buy from "on approval" only, and which to avoid unless they are the only source.

Since the price of medical books and costs of shipping, mailing, and handling the paperwork associated with buying books is continually increasing, the librarian should weigh the advantages of ordering on approval. It is probably no longer cost-effective to order on approval books costing less than $15.00, unless they are part of a larger order that can be returned to a dealer with one return shipment and one invoice. In some cases less expensive titles can be examined on interlibrary loan, if the lending library can supply the material in a timely fashion. Recommendations from trusted users or other librarians may also help reduce the number of items brought in on approval.

When a book arrives, it should be examined carefully. The librarian may use a series of questions during the examination. Is it the book that was ordered? Is it in the format ordered: paper or hard cover, one or two-volume edition? Is it in good condition, or has it been damaged in shipping? Is the cover on properly and securely? Is the paper of good quality, or do the illustrations and printing bleed through? Are pages torn, ink-smeared or missing? Any problems with the book should be noted so that the book can be replaced if it is considered worth adding to the collection. Sometimes problems are not identified until after the book is processed. Reputable dealers will still accept imperfect books for exchange even if they bear the library imprint.

Asking library users to evaluate the quality of a book ordered on approval can provide some useful information. However, the librarian cannot presume that every user's judgment is based on substantive criteria such as subject coverage, quality of illustrations, adequate references, details of indexing, and comparison of this book with others available on the same subject. If users' opinions are sought, it is good policy to ask several people so that a balance can be achieved.

Journals

Selection of journals involves many of the considerations that apply to books. In addition to questions referring to the existing subject coverage in a particular area, the reputation of the publisher, the cost of the journal, and the projected degree of use, the librarian should also consider where the journal is indexed, and whether the library has that indexing tool. Journals that are not indexed may be of questionable value to the collection. Another consideration is the demand the library has for that subject and how many times the journal is currently requested on interlibrary loan. Current issues should be examined on interlibrary loan or by requesting a sample issue from the publisher.

In borderline cases, access to the material can sometimes be obtained without spending budget funds. A cooperative acquisition arrangement can be made with another library, or a gift subscription can be solicited.

Audiovisuals

There are no simple criteria for guidance in the selection of audiovisual materials for purchase. Many types and levels of audiovisual services, from basic to complex, are possible within a hospital. The extent to which the hospital library becomes involved with audiovisual services depends on many factors. These factors are discussed in detail in Chapter 10.

THE ACQUISITION OF GIFTS

Gifts usually are considered the pleasant result of a generous action. Helen Crawford, however, in an article which details the problems encountered by libraries inundated with unwanted and unneeded books and journals, has indicated that this is not always the case (7). Generally, gifts of money and appropriate books and journals should be welcomed and solicited.

Soliciting Gifts

The solicitation of gifts brings several advantages to the library. Budgets can be stretched, and interest and support can be generated among physicians and staff, patients and their families, volunteer groups, and business organizations.

Gift subscriptions should not be relied upon for primary or core journals because continuity is uncertain. The most reliable arrangement is for the donor to pay for a subscription that is sent directly to the library. "Gift" arrangements that allow the user to donate each issue after he or she has read it often result in delayed receipt, missing issues, or involvement of staff time. Gift subscriptions of this type are most useful for filling in missing or damaged issues before binding or for providing second copies of heavily used material. However, as with all gifts, the advantages should be carefully weighed against the staff time involved in processing the gift.

Writing a Gift Policy

The secret of controlling gifts, getting what the library wants and can use, and refusing gracefully what is not wanted lies in a written policy. The section in Appendix A that refers to gifts states that gifts must fit the library's needs, must be judged in accordance with the selection and retention policy, and may be used or discarded at the discretion of the library staff. Internal Revenue Service regulations concerning how gifts are assessed in value stipulate that the assessor should be a disinterested third party (8). Each of these points should be considered when writing a policy. Although the policy states that the librarian will not assess the monetary value of the donation, the librarian can acknowledge the gift with a brief description of what was donated and provide the donor with sources of information concerning prices and appraisers.

The gift policy should be accepted and approved by the library committee and be available to the administration and department directors. This will reduce the likelihood of the hospital staff encouraging donations that the librarian cannot accept.

COLLECTIONS OUTSIDE THE LIBRARY

The need for frequent and convenient access to specific types of library materials sometimes gives rise to collections of materials at several locations in the hospital. These collections can be classified as either unit libraries or departmental libraries.

Unit Libraries

Unit libraries, once called ward libraries, are distinguished from departmental libraries by location and function. They are found in clinical areas and nursing stations rather than in departmental offices. Since everyone from physicians to unit clerks makes use of these convenient collections and they are under no one person's control, the books may often disappear. Yet these collections meet real staff needs. The unit libraries may become core reference collections or include collections of reprints especially prepared for the patient care given in that clinical area.

One guideline for determining the kind of material that should be in the unit library appears in this often repeated comment of unknown origin: If the reader wants to sit down to use the material, it does not belong in the unit library. The implication is that dictionaries, drug reference sources, laboratory and diagnostic test information, and other quick reference sources, should form the basis for most unit collections. When the scope of a collection is limited to this type of material, adequate control is usually possible, and replacement of lost items is not a major budget consideration.

Unit libraries operate most effectively when the following points are considered. Books must be carefully selected with the unique needs of each unit in mind. Discarded publications from the hospital library rarely meet the unit library's needs since currency of reference information is vital. Therefore, the library budget should include funds to purchase current items for the unit library. Many librarians make a special effort to seek financial support for these libraries through donations. The relationship between the main library and the unit library, including policies on selection and funding, should be defined in the hospital library's written policy. Finally, enlisting the interest of the nurses on the library committee is often effective in both controlling and supporting unit libraries.

Departmental Libraries

Departmental libraries are sometimes sources of frustration for the hospital librarian. These libraries can dilute an already inadequate book budget; result in subject collections quite beyond the needs of the institution; duplicate for convenience what is already held in the main collection; and create problems of control and security.

Departmental libraries can be turned into assets rather than liabilities if, as clearly implied in JCAH standards, they are considered a part of the total hospital library service. The acquisition policy should clearly define the categories and scope of materials and how they should be retained by departmental libraries. A commonly used distinction is that books necessary to the performance of daily routines are permanently retained by the department, and those titles that the department refers to only occasionally are kept in the main library. Titles in the second category may reside in the department for an extended loan immediately after purchase and eventually be returned to the main collection. A clear understanding and respect for the unique needs of individual departments and an attitude of compromise and flexibility will work toward a mutually satisfactory arrangement.

Journals, too, can create problems in departmental libraries. Whether paid for out of departmental budgets or library funds, these specialized titles are an extremely valuable information resource. Some library control of these collections is often worthwhile in order to insure availability of all issues. The library may want to order the subscriptions and check in issues as they arrive. Often arrangements can be made for recent issues to be retained in the department for a short period of time and then be sent to the library for binding and storage. By offering to bind and store volumes for permanent access, librarians often acquire personal copies of journals from specialists within hospital departments. Whatever method of journal acquisition the librarian uses, the value of the subscription to the library should be weighed against the time involved in securing it.

Departmental libraries present the librarian with a real challenge when they attempt to bring the demands of influential specialists into balance with overall institutional needs. For more discussion of the issue of departmental libraries, see Chapter 18.

THE FUNDING PROCESS

A steady level of predictable funding is essential for adequate library service. Collection development evolves by planned, steady acquisition over the years and cannot survive the unpredictability of random journal cancellations and inconsistent funding of library activities. Further information on sources of funding and budget preparation appears in Chapter 13.

The librarian who has an adequate budget, written policies, the support of the administration, and both the interest and participation of the clientele in developing the library collection, can enjoy a fascinating job.

The editor gratefully expresses her appreciation of Dr. Gertrude Lamb and the staff at Hartford Hospital for their assistance with the preparation of this chapter.

REFERENCES

1. Joint Commission on Accreditation of Hospitals. Accreditation manual for hospitals. 1983 ed. Chicago: Joint Commission on Accreditation of Hospitals, 1982:147-149.

2. Beatty WK. Technical processing: Part I. Selection, acquisition and weeding. In: Annan GL, Felter JW, eds. Handbook of medical library practice. 3d ed. Chicago: Medical Library Association 1970:71-92.

3. Joint Commission on Accreditation of Hospitals. Hospital survey profile. 1981 ed. Chicago: Joint Commission on Accreditation of Hospitals, 1980:169-171.

4. Bonk WJ, Magrill RM. Building library collections. 5th ed. Metuchen, NJ: Scarecrow Press, 1979.

5. Brandon AN, Hill DR. Selected list of books and journals for the small medical library. Bull Med Libr Assoc 1981 Apr;69:185-215.

6. Brandon AN, Hill DR. Selected list of nursing books and journals. Nurs Outlook 1982 Mar;30:186-199.

7. Crawford H. Treasure or white elephant? Bull Med Libr Assoc 1970 July;58:336-340.

8. Futas E, ed. Library acquisition policies and procedures. Phoenix: Oryx Press, 1977.

READINGS

Boyer CJ, Eaton NL. Book selection policies in American libraries. Austin: Armadillo Press, 1971.

Cramer A. Printed materials: selection and acquisition. Salt Lake City: Network for Continuing Education, Intermountain Regional Medical Program, 1972.

Van Orden P, Phillips EB, eds. Background readings in building library collections. Metuchen, NJ: Scarecrow Press, 1979.

APPENDIX A
Selection Policy: Sample

This sample policy is intended to illustrate the types of decisions that are often documented in a selection policy. The specific details of any policy should be developed to meet the needs of each individual library.

Introduction

This policy has been written in order to formulate guidelines for the selection and acquisition of materials for the library's collection. Approved by the Library Committee on June 12, 1981, it can be changed only by resolution of that committee.

Purpose

This selection policy provides guidelines for building and maintaining a collection of information resources adequate for the current needs of hospital staff. In general the most up-to-date, authoritative materials directly pertinent to patient care and educational and administrative programs and activities will be purchased. Judgment as to whether specific materials meet this criterion is exercised by the library staff in conjunction with physicians, instructors or knowledgeable people in the field, and review articles in journals.

Definitions

The *scope* of the collection refers to its subject content, identifying:

- *Broad,* general subject content
- *Specialized* materials that cover particular areas of interest
- *Topical* materials that give full coverage of narrow subjects

Levels of Coverage

The subject areas of a collection are covered on three levels.
- The *skeletal* level includes a current dictionary and the latest or best edition of one or two texts.
- The *reference* level includes skeletal coverage, plus one encyclopedia, one history, a comprehensive bibliography, an indexing or abstracting journal, one or more journals, and additional texts and reference books.
- The *research* level includes reference coverage, plus monographs, additional journals, pamphlets, research reports and documents necessary to permit independent research on a clinical level.

Scope and Coverage

For each profession and occupational group represented in the hospital, the library will provide, at the minimum, current materials of *specialized* subject scope on the *reference* level.

Topical materials on the *research* level shall be specifically collected in those areas of special interest such as:

Burns	Orthopedics
Cardiology	Psychiatry
Hospital administration and management	Pediatrics
Nursing	

Related or peripheral subject areas that occasionally contribute to the interest and activities of the hospital are generally collected at the *skeletal* level.

Literature in most fields may be considered for acquisition if a reasonable portion of the material is relevant to the needs of the library's user groups. In addition, reference tools necessary for public service or in-house library operations may be acquired.

Criteria for Selection

When selecting books the following criteria should be considered:

- Bibliographic data (year, title, price)
- Authority (author, date, publisher)
- Format (quality, readability, good illustrations)
- Bibliographic aids (index, references, graphs)
- Scope (level of the book, kind of coverage, category of the book)
- Aids in evaluation (book reviews, requests from users, indexed in Index Medicus, requested on interlibrary loan)

When selecting journals the following criteria should be considered:

- Subject (appropriateness to scope of the collection, level of coverage)
- Indexed in major abstracts or indexes
- Language of the journal
- Reputation of publisher and author, journal refereed
- Usage (requested 5 times or more on interlibrary loan)

Special Collections

The library will maintain a collection of archival material that substantially documents the hospital's history and development. These materials may include hospital records, news and press releases, and memorabilia. They will be evaluated by the librarian.

Copies of publications by full-time and part-time staff members will be maintained on file by the librarian.

Departmental Collections

Holdings of books and journals in departmental libraries will be limited to frequently used materials or to specialized reference materials. Items which meet these criteria will be selected and paid for by the individual department but ordered and catalogued by the library staff. Books may be shelved in the department indefinitely, but journals will be bound and shelved in the library. Library users will have access to these collections through the library staff.

Duplicates

The library purchases duplicate monographs and serials when the use of the material demands multiple copies and when funds are available.

Replacements

When current books are lost they should be replaced within six months after the search process has been completed. When current journals are lost they should be replaced one month after the search process has been completed. Books are replaced through the regular book dealer, while journal issues are replaced through the MLA Exchange first and then through back issue suppliers.

Currency of the Collection

New editions of reference books and texts shall be acquired as published. One edition prior to the current edition may be kept for loan as indicated by need.

At least 40 percent of the monograph collection should have been published within the past five years. As a general rule, there must be specific justification for any title held longer than ten years.

Backfiles of medical journals shall be kept twenty years. Journals relating to research materials held by the library (see Scope and Coverage) shall be retained indefinitely as long as space allows.

The collection is systematically weeded when new editions are added to the collection. On a continuing basis, sections will be weeded which show evidence of age, overcrowding, or irrelevance to insure conformity to the policies given in this document. Materials removed from the collection are moved into an inactive collection, sold, exchanged, given to other institutions, or destroyed.

Gifts

Gifts are accepted with the understanding that the library may use the material as needs dictate. This may mean that donated items will be integrated into the collection, used for exchange with other libraries, or discarded by the library staff.

Gifts shall be acknowledged in writing by the librarian. The Director of Development will be notified in writing of each substantial gift so that the hospital may formally acknowledge it.

Upon request the librarian will assist the donor in locating the currently advertised price of items, if one is available. No value shall be estimated on prices not publicly advertised, and no evaluation of gifts for tax purposes will be made by library staff. Donors are encouraged to contact IRS for information regarding deductions applicable to their gifts.

Audiovisual Materials

Selection of audiovisual materials will follow the same scope and coverage criteria as printed materials with the following additions: Only materials available for distribution in the U.S. will be considered. Formats of selected audiovisuals will reflect the equipment available within the hospital and educational facilities.

Microforms

Microform copies may be collected if a hard copy is unavailable or if the microform format would provide a more cost-effective method of acquiring or controlling certain types of publications (e.g., reference tools for in-house library operations). This policy is subject to change with future space limitation.

Extramural Resources

Materials not included in the scope and coverage of the collection are available through interlibrary loans from local, state, regional, and national library collections.

Quality Assurance Program

Quality assurance and evaluation of library policies and services are monitored by regular questionnaires or surveys conducted by the library staff. Those surveyed include medical staff, housestaff, employees, and students. Results are routinely reported to the library committee by the librarian.

APPENDIX B
Collection Development Questionnaire: Sample

Please indicate with a (✔)

1. How often do you use the library?
    Daily _____   Weekly _____   Monthly _____   Rarely _____   Never _____

2. What resources do you use?
    _____ Catalog   _____ Daily newspaper
    _____ Indexes   _____ Leisure reading (magazines, etc.)
    _____ Pamphlets   _____ Dictionaries, directories, etc.
    _____ Reprints   _____ Other (Please Specify)
    _____ New book display   _____
    _____ Media collection   _____

3. What subject area(s) do you frequently need information about?
    _____ Nursing   _____ Patient education
    _____ Nutrition   _____ Other (Please Specify)
    _____ Medicine   _____
    _____ Surgery   _____
    _____ Hospital administration

4. Do you believe this library meets your needs?
    _____ Very well   _____ Well   _____ Adequately   _____ Not well

5. If we could add three new books in your area of interest, what would they be?
    _____
    _____
    _____

6. In your area of interest, how rapidly does information become obsolete?
    1-2 years _____   7-8 years _____
    3-4 years _____   9-10 years _____
    5-6 years _____

7. Would you be willing to assist in the evaluation of the present collection? _____ Yes _____ No
    If yes, in what subject area(s): _____
    _____

8. Would you be willing to evaluate new books and journals as they are considered for purchase?
    _____ Yes   _____ No
    If yes, in what subject area(s): _____
    _____

PLEASE USE REVERSE SIDE FOR COMMENTS.

APPENDIX C
Suggested Sources for
Book and Journal Selection

GENERAL

Allyn R. A library for internists IV: recommended by the American College of Physicians. Ann Intern Med 1982 Mar;96:385-401.

Brandon AN, Hill DR. Selected list of books and journals for the small medical library. Bull Med Libr Assoc 1981 Apr;69:185-215.

Moseley JL. Selected list of family medicine books and journals for the small medical library. Bull Med Libr Assoc 1980 July;68:297-298.

Roper FW, Boorkman JA. Introduction to reference sources in the health sciences. Chicago: Medical Library Association, 1980.

NURSING

Binger JL, Jensen LM. Lippincott's guide to nursing literature: a handbook for students, writers, and researchers. Philadelphia: Lippincott, 1980.

Books of the year. Am J Nurs 1982 Jan;82:70-80.

Brandon AN, Hill DR. Selected list of nursing books and journals. Nurs Outlook 1982 Mar;30:186-199.

Community planning for nursing: a selected bibliography. New York: National League for Nursing, 1975. (NLN Publication, 52-1567).

MacVicar J, Boroch R. Approaches to staff development for departments of nursing: an annotated bibliography. New York: National League for Nursing, 1977. (NLN Publication, 20-1658)

Minority groups in nursing, 1976: a bibliography. Kansas City: American Nurses' Association, 1976. (ANA Publication, M-25).

Nursing administration: a selected annotated bibliography of current periodical literature in nursing administration and management. New York: National League for Nursing, 1978. (League Exchange number 120).

Reference sources for nursing; revised by a committee of the Interagency Council on Library Resources for Nursing. Nurs Outlook 1980 July;28:444-448.

Sleet DA, Stadsklev R. Annotated bibliography of simulations and games in health education. Health Educ Monogr 1977; 5 Suppl 1; 74-90.

Strauch KP, Brundage DJ. Guide to library resources for nursing. New York: Appleton-Century-Crofts, 1980.

Taylor SD. Bibliography on nursing research, 1950-1974. Nurs Res 1975 May/June;24:207-225.

NUTRITION

Casale JT. The diet food finder. New York: Bowker, 1975.

Chicago Nutrition Association. Nutrition references and book reviews. 5th ed. Chicago: Chicago Nutrition Association, 1981.

ADMINISTRATION

Administrator's collection: 1978 ed. Chicago: American Hospital Association, 1978.

American College of Hospital Administrators. Annotated bibliography of management books. (Unpublished, available from the College).

Levey S. Loomba NP. Health care administration: a selected bibliography. Philadelphia: Lippincott, 1973.

SPECIAL SUBJECTS

American Dental Association. Bureau of Library Services. Basic dental reference works. Chicago: American Dental Association, 1980.

Boucher RJ, Dittmar SS. Rehabilitation nursing and related readings. Evanston, IL: Rehabilitation Nursing Institute, 1980.

Cancer Information Clearinghouse. Coping with cancer: an annotated bibliography of public, patient, and professional information and education materials. Bethesda, MD. (NIH Publ. No. 80-2129).

Ennis B. Guide to the literature in psychiatry. Los Angeles: Partridge Press, 1971.

Feller I. International bibliography on burns. Ann Arbor, MI: American Burn Research, 1969. Annual supplements.

Greenberg B. How to find out in psychiatry: a guide to sources of mental health information. New York: Pergamon Press, 1978.

Horton MA, Hammon WE, Curtis T, Horton F. A suggested current literature and reference library for respiratory and chest physical therapists. RC 1979 Feb;24:138-141.

Jonsen AR, Cassel C, Lo B, Perkins HS. The ethics of medicine: an annotated bibliography of recent literature. Ann Intern Med 1980 Jan;92:136-141.

Raskin RB, Hathorn IV. Selected list of books and journals for a small dental library. Bull Med Libr Assoc 1980 July;68:263-270.

Sell IL. Dying and death: an annotated bibliography. New York: Tiresias Press, 1977.

Sewell W. Guide to drug information. Hamilton, IL: Drug Intelligence Publications, 1976.

Sollitto S, Veatch RM. A selected and partially annotated bibliography of society, ethics and the life sciences, 1979-80. Hastings-on-Hudson, NY: Institute of Society, Ethics, and the Life Sciences, 1978.

Sunshine I. Bibliography for a poison center's reference library. Vet Hum Toxicol 1979 Feb;21:54-56.

Wells DP. Child abuse: an annotated bibliography. Metuchen, NJ: Scarecrow Press, 1980.

Acquisition of Library Materials

Kirsten Peterson Quam
Technical Services Librarian
Wishard Memorial Hospital
Indianapolis, Indiana

*Currently:
Coordinator of Library Services
Wishard Memorial Hospital
Indianapolis, Indiana

CHAPTER 4

Acquisition of Library Materials

Kirsten Peterson Quam
Technical Services Librarian
Wishard Memorial Hospital
Indianapolis, Indiana

Appendixes

Figures

Library acquisition is the process of securing the materials that are needed to provide desired library services. In most cases the hospital librarian works with vendors of library materials and with the hospital purchasing department to acquire these materials. Decisions must be made regarding what materials are to be bought, at what price, when and how they will be delivered, and when and how payment will be made.

The librarian's goal is to acquire all selected material within an acceptable period of time and with a minimal investment of time and money. This can best be accomplished by adopting acquisition procedures that work smoothly with both the hospital purchasing system and the marketing systems of library suppliers. These procedures should result in reduced personnel costs and faster turnaround time for orders. Because each library's needs, resources, and set of institutional constraints vary, each librarian must determine individually the procedures that will be most successful.

This chapter will provide the hospital librarian with a framework for developing effective acquisition procedures. The first part of the chapter presents information on acquiring materials in the hospital setting. The second part deals with acquisition of the most common types of library materials.

ACQUIRING MATERIALS IN THE HOSPITAL SETTING

The process of obtaining the goods required to carry on any enterprise, whether it is a hospital, a business, or a factory, is known as "purchasing," "buying," or "procurement" (1:5). It is important for the librarian to thoroughly understand the purchasing procedures followed in the hospital. Therefore, it may be useful to look at some of the general patterns of hospital purchasing.

Patterns of Hospital Purchasing

Hospitals organize purchasing activities in a number of different ways. At one extreme, hospital purchasing is a highly centralized system in which a designated department, or series of departments, coordinates and performs all of the activities for each hospital purchase. Specialists are responsible for each phase of the purchasing process, including selecting products to order; authorizing purchases; placing orders with suppliers; making sure that orders are received; and paying for purchases. At the other extreme, each hospital department or service unit deals directly with suppliers for all its purchases.

The most common patterns of hospital purchasing fall somewhere between these two extremes. In most cases a central staff coordinates hospital purchasing functions and performs some of the necessary activities. Individual departments may then handle some parts of the ordering process for their own materials. The assignment of activities varies among hospitals. Within a hospital, the pattern may vary among departments or for certain types of orders.

Authorization and payment are the two purchasing activities that are most often centralized. Although hospital departments such as the library may deal directly with vendors, authorization and payment for purchases are usually handled by other hospital personnel. Both of these activities are discussed in more detail below.

Authorizing the Order

Each hospital has a system to ensure that responsible people formally authorize expenditures. The mechanisms for authorization may vary depending on the autonomy given to individual departments.

In many hospitals, approval may be required at several levels before an order is placed. A department head or other designated person usually approves a purchase request. Hospital policy may require the signature of at least one administrative representative before a purchase order is typed. In some cases, the fund manager may need to approve the use of specific accounts. The purchasing agent, designated administrator, or financial officer usually must give authorization before the formal purchase order is sent to the vendor.

Special types of orders may receive approval at different stages in the purchasing process. A deposit account, for example, is a sum of money deposited with a vendor so that items may be ordered and charged to the account. Additional approval is not usually required to order individual items on account.

Paying the Vendor

A specific section of the hospital, generally called the accounts payable department, often processes all payments for hospital purchases. Payment is the final step for most orders. At this point, all records of the order are verified. The required records might include the following:

- Proof of the order's authorization (purchase order or other approval form)
- Notice that the materials have been received (packing slip or other form)
- Request for payment (invoice)
- Evidence that the payment is requested in accordance with organizational or legal requirements (claim or voucher)

Any discrepancies in the records are usually reconciled before payment is made. Many hospitals require explanation of differences between items and prices on the original order and those listed on the invoice. A separate authorization or adjustment may be required if all the records do not agree.

Journals and some other materials are paid for in advance. Hospitals usually establish special procedures for these prepaid orders. Prepayment is used if the vendor requires it or if there are advantages to paying in advance. Vendors may require prepayment for small orders, for subscriptions, or to establish credit. Some vendors offer price reductions or free shipping on prepaid orders. Libraries sometimes establish deposit accounts, which are another form of prepaid order, for the convenience of placing multiple small orders with a minimum of paperwork.

Forms

Record-keeping is a very important part of the purchasing process. Whether records are kept on paper or in a computerized system, their purpose is the same. They record and verify all the steps in the purchasing process. They also serve as a means of communication among the various parties involved in the purchasing process. Hospital purchasing procedures specify the forms that are to be used and how they should be routed through the hospital to the vendor. Special forms may be needed for certain types of vendors. The forms used most frequently will be discussed below.

Requisition

A requisition is an authorized request to order an item. It provides the authority to issue a purchase order to a supplier (2). Some hospitals do not use requisition forms. In such cases, the description of the item, the request that it be ordered, and the authorization to do so may be conveyed verbally or in writing to the person who will place the order.

Purchase Order

A purchase order is a written authorization to a supplier to provide certain goods or services at a given price and at a certain time and place. It is usually issued by an authorized employee of an institution. When accepted by the seller, a purchase order becomes a legal contract between buyer and seller. Purchase orders are generally assigned a number. Communications with the vendor and among departments within the hospital often refer to the purchase order number. The department that requested the item, the receiving department, and the purchasing department may all maintain files on the order by vendor name, purchase order number, or both. These files make it possible to monitor the status of a particular order (2).

Invoice

An invoice is the vendor's request for payment. Some hospitals will process payment only for invoices in the exact amount of the purchase order. Others will authorize payment of invoices that cover only part of a shipment or that reflect an adjusted amount. Some hospitals do not require invoices for all payments.

Statement of Accounts

A statement of accounts summarizes transactions between a buyer and a seller over a given period. It generally is not a request for payment but may be accompanied by an invoice. It often lists numbers or dates of all invoices not yet paid. A vendor who offers deposit accounts usually sends periodic statements that show purchases charged to the account and the account balance.

Voucher

A claim or voucher is a signed statement that services have been performed or goods delivered by a vendor. It authorizes payment to be made to the vendor. A voucher may be a separate form or it may appear on a copy of the purchase order. Use of vouchers is required by the governing bodies of some, but not all, hospitals.

Packing Slip

A packing slip is the vendor's statement of what is included in a shipment. The person receiving the shipment, whether in the receiving department or in the department that requested the order, must compare the packing slip to the goods received and to the original purchase order. A signed copy of the packing slip, an annotated copy of the purchase order, or a memo describing the items received may be required to authorize payment to the vendor.

Learning the Hospital's System

The librarian needs to analyze purchasing practices in the hospital based on an understanding of the general patterns described above. The first step is to identify the person or persons who are responsible for each purchasing activity. It is also important that the librarian understand how the purchasing process is coordinated and the types of interaction that should take place between library staff and other hospital personnel. This interaction may be written, verbal, or both.

Written purchasing procedures, formal orientations to the purchasing system, and organization charts can provide some of this information. Informal conversations with those who perform purchasing activities can help the librarian understand the system better. These individuals can clarify written procedures or explain informal practices. This type of information will enable the librarian to acquire library materials more efficiently.

SPECIAL CONSIDERATIONS IN LIBRARY PURCHASING

A hospital's purchasing system may work very well for library acquisition. There are instances, however, when general purchasing procedures must be modified to acquire library materials in the most efficient way. The librarian must demonstrate that modifications in the general system will result in increased efficiency in processing library orders. In order to do this, he or she must thoroughly understand both the requirements of the hospital purchasing system and the marketing system for library materials. A good working relationship with purchasing personnel will also help the librarian in this effort.

Some of the special considerations in library purchasing will be discussed below. This discussion will provide the librarian with a basis for working with the purchasing department to plan the best approach to ordering library materials.

Unique Identification of Materials

Unlike many supplies purchased for hospitals, most items purchased by libraries are unique. There is often no suitable substitute for a selected item. If the third edition of a book is desired, the second edition is usually not acceptable. If a substitution is possible, the choice should be made by the librarian rather than the purchasing staff. Also, the librarian is familiar with the bibliographic elements needed to identify materials and has access to sources of bibliographic information.

Figure 4-1 summarizes the information needed to describe library materials fully. The librarian must determine the kinds of information to include when ordering an item from a particular vendor. Figure 4-2 lists standard sources of acquisition information for each type of library material. Each title is annotated in Appendix A. Two reference works, *Medical Books and Serials in Print* and *Lists of Journals Indexed in Index Medicus*, can probably provide most of the acquisition information needed by hospital librarians.

When a shipment of library materials is received, a close examination is often required to determine that the correct materials have been included. The librarian, rather than the purchasing or receiving department, has the training and the resources to make that determination quickly and accurately.

Pricing

Prices of library materials vary depending on the source, the form of the order, and any special services rendered. The librarian rather than the purchasing department should determine the price for library orders. Prices can be determined from some of the sources listed in Appendix A. Other sources of price information will be included in the discussion of each type of library material. The librarian may wish to use a form letter for requesting price quotations directly from publishers or other suppliers.

Price is often a significant factor in the selection of both vendors and items to be purchased. Based on knowledge of the library's needs and the benefits of a particular payment plan or service, the librarian may sometimes be justified in choosing a higher priced vendor or item.

The hospital purchasing department usually needs to know the exact prices of items to be ordered. When quoted prices change, problems in issuing payment may result. Thus the librarian should monitor the purchasing

Figure 4-1
Standard Information for Identification of Library Materials

BOOKS

Author or editor
Title and subtitle
Publisher's name and address
Date of publication
Distributor
Edition number or name
Library of Congress (LC) number
International Standard Book Number (ISBN)
Choice of binding
Supplier's stock number

JOURNALS

Title and subtitle
Publisher's name and address
Beginning date
Current volume number and date
International Standard Serial Number (ISSN)
Edition
Frequency
Supplier's number
Responsible agency or association

CONTINUATIONS

Author or editor
Title and subtitle of part
Serial title and subtitle
Number or name of part and date
International Standard Serial Number (ISSN)
International Standard Book Number (ISBN)
Library of Congress (LC) number
Supplier's stock number
Beginning date

GOVERNMENT PUBLICATIONS

Author
Title
Issuing agency
Congressional session number
Date of publications and/or date of coverage
Superintendent of Documents number
Government Printing Office stock number
National Technical Information Service report number
Series name
Series number

AUDIOVISUALS

Title
Producer
Distributor
Other responsible agencies or people
Date produced and/or distributed
Format, including medium of accompanying sound
Color or black and white
Sound speed
Length in running time or number of graphics
Accompanying material
Series name and number
Producer's or supplier's stock number
Rights or restrictions of use

Figure 4-2
Sources of Bibliographic and Price Information for Library Materials

BOOKS

American Book Publishing Record
Books in Print
Cumulative Book Index
Forthcoming Books
Library of Congress National Union Catalog
*Medical Books and Serials in Print
Monthly Catalog of United States Government
    Publications
**National Library of Medicine Current Catalog
**National Library of Medicine Current Catalog
    Proof Sheets
Paperbound Books in Print

JOURNALS

*List of Journals Indexed in Index Medicus
**Irregular Serials and Annuals
*Medical Books and Serials in Print
Monthly Catalog of United States Government
    Publications
New Serials Titles
**National Library of Medicine Current Catalog
Index of NLM Serial Titles
Standard Periodical Directory
**Ulrich's International Periodicals Directory
Vital Notes on Medical Periodicals

CONTINUATIONS

*List of Journals Indexed in Index Medicus
**Irregular Serials and Annuals
**National Library of Medicine Current Catalog
**National Library of Medicine Current Catalog
    Proof Sheets
Standard Periodical Directory
**Ulrich's International Periodicals Directory

GOVERNMENT PUBLICATIONS

Documents to the People
ERIC (Research in Education)
Government Publications Review
Health Information Resources in the Department of
    Health and Human Services
**MEDOC
Monthly Catalog of United States Government
    Publications
Monthly Checklist of State Publications
**National Library of Medicine Current Catalog
**National Library of Medicine Current Catalog
    Proof Sheets

*Recommended for all hospital libraries

**Useful for larger hospital libraries

NOTE: See Chapter 10 for sources of information on audiovisual materials.

process closely in order to make any necessary price adjustments.

Selecting a Vendor

The librarian is usually the most appropriate person to select a vendor for a particular item. He or she has the resources and the expertise to identify sources of library materials. In some cases, materials may be available from only one source. When an item is available from more than one vendor, certain criteria should be used in selecting the vendor. These criteria include discounts, shipping charges, payment requirements, type of order required, delivery time, and special services (3). Each of these factors should be considered by the librarian in relation to the hospital's requirements and the library's need for the item. For example, speed of delivery may sometimes be more important than a discount. Services offered by the vendor on orders such as subscriptions may also influence the librarian's choice.

Competitive bidding is not appropriate for most library purchases since so many factors other than price are involved. The librarian should request the right to select a vendor without bidding whenever possible. If the hospital requires bids, the librarian must be sure that the purchasing department includes all the necessary information in the bid specifications. This information might include time of delivery and special services to be rendered. Some hospitals require bids for orders that exceed a certain amount. The librarian may be able to divide large orders to stay under this amount.

Types of Orders

Many library orders can be processed by the standard hospital purchase order system used, but certain library materials and arrangements with vendors require special types of orders. The librarian will need to spend time becoming familiar with the options available in the hospital. They may include the types of orders discussed below.

One-time Order

A one-time order is usually placed by issuing a purchase order in advance. As noted above, a purchase order is a written document legally authorizing a vendor to supply specified materials at a given price. Payment is due upon receipt of the goods and an invoice from the vendor.

Standing Order

A standing order, also known as a blanket order, is a single order placed to meet long-term requirements for specific items. A hospital might place a standing order for a year's worth of stock supplies. The vendor would ship portions of the supplies at stated intervals until the entire amount had been sent. Hospital librarians may place a standing order for all the volumes in a series of books. Larger academic libraries that routinely purchase most material on a given subject may place a standing order with a vendor. The vendor may bill for items as they are shipped or for the full amount of the order at a certain date.

Subscription Order

A subscription is also an agreement to purchase materials to be shipped over a period of time. Payment in full usually must accompany the order. Journals, audiovisual serials, and computer services are usually purchased in this manner. Purchase orders accompanied by payment may be used for subscriptions.

Prepaid Order

A prepaid order is an order that is paid in advance. Certain vendors require prepayment, especially when credit has not been established or the order is small. Deposit accounts, another type of prepaid order, will be discussed below.

Confirmation Order

A written confirmation order follows a verbal order that was placed either in person or by telephone. Written authorization, or confirmation, is necessary to validate a verbal order. The vendor may require that a purchase order number be given with verbal orders. The same number should be used on the confirmation order.

COD Order

A COD, or cash-on-delivery, order must be paid for at the time the goods are received. Vendors with whom credit has not been established may require COD orders. Shipping charges are sometimes handled COD, either as part of the purchase price or as separate charges from the shipper.

Petty Cash Order

Libraries frequently have a petty cash fund used to purchase small items that are needed quickly. The librarian usually authorizes individual purchases and must account for monies spent. In some hospitals there are strict guidelines as to what items may be purchased with petty cash funds. The librarian must be aware of these guidelines and also of the accounting procedures for these funds.

Deposit Account

A deposit account is a form of prepaid order in which a sum of money is deposited with the vendor. Individual items can be ordered at any time and are billed to the account. Deposit accounts are typically used to purchase government documents. They are also used for small repeat orders, especially when speed of delivery is important. Deposit accounts save the hospital the time and money ordinarily spent on processing individual purchase orders.

Receiving and Claiming

The task of receiving orders and claiming missing materials is often more complex in the library than in other hospital departments. A typical library order covers more than one item. A single order often results in multiple shipments, possibly from several different sources. For example, book jobbers may arrange for various publishers to ship individual items directly to the library over a period of several weeks. An order to a subscription agent may involve thousands of items that will be shipped separately over the course of a year. Files of outstanding orders arranged by vendor and order number may be adequate for the hospital purchasing system. The library, however, must usually maintain more detailed records for monitoring receipt of materials. Files arranged by item or date ordered may be useful in providing information on the status of an order.

The problem of claiming missing materials should be handled by direct contact between the library and the vendor. Prompt and systematic claiming is essential for many library materials. Missed issues of journals should be claimed at once since they may not be available after a certain period of time. Audiovisual programs are often needed on a particular date. The librarian should remain in contact with the audiovisual supplier to ensure that materials arrive on time.

Purchased Services

Libraries purchase services from book jobbers, subscription agents, computer search services, cataloging agencies, and equipment vendors. If bids are required, the librarian must determine bid specifications for both products and services. Service fees may be billed separately or along with charges for materials. The librarian must be closely involved in determining prices, verifying delivery, and authorizing payment.

ACQUIRING BOOKS

When ordering books, the librarian must communicate certain information to the supplier. A full description of a book might include all the types of information listed under "Books" in Figure 4-1. Most suppliers, however, will be able to fill orders accurately with much less information.

In selecting vendors, the librarian should consider the amount and types of information required by each vendor to ensure prompt delivery of orders. Many vendors require the following information about a book: author, title, edition, publisher, and copyright date. Other vendors require the ISBN or LC number for a book, as well as their own stock number. Locating such information may be very time-consuming.

Sources of Ordering Information

Bibliographic information and list prices can be determined from the publications that are listed on Figure 4-2 and described more fully in Appendix A. There are many additional sources of ordering information. Some of these sources are discussed below.

Book Jobbers

Book jobbers distribute books from a number of different publishers. Bibliographic information on their book lists may be limited to information the jobber needs to fill orders, including stock or order numbers. Because these lists are generally issued more frequently than standard publications, the information they contain may be more current. Book jobbers occasionally offer listings of editions in progress and their projected publication dates. They frequently issue price lists to reflect vendor's price changes and discounts. Vendors may also be willing to quote prices to jobbers for individual titles.

Publishers' Catalogs and Advertisements

Most publishers issue information on their publications frequently. In fact librarians are often inundated by catalogs and promotional materials. The librarian may wish to arrange these materials by publisher for easy reference when ordering.

Ads and catalogs offer information on prepublication discounts, price advantages for prepayment, shipping charges, and special orders. When using ads and other promotional materials as sources of ordering information, it should be remembered that many of these materials are issued far in advance of publication. Titles, content, publication dates, and prices may change before the products become available.

Reviews

Reviews of library materials frequently include a standard bibliographic citation, although ISBN and LC numbers are rarely included. Reviews gathered during the selection process are useful in completing order information. However, it is often difficult to locate current reviews. Thus the librarian cannot rely on using reviews as the major source of information for most acquisitions.

Online Bibliographic Database

CATLINE, OCLC, RLIN, and other online bibliographic databases can be useful sources of order information. Bowker's *Books in Print* and *Ulrich's International Periodicals Directory* (incorporating *Irregular Serials and Annuals*) are both available as online databases through Bibliographic Retrieval Services, Inc. (BRS) and DIALOG Information Services. These listings have the advantage of many searchable access points that make them particularly valuable in completing sketchy citations.

Correspondence

Correspondence with a publisher or other distributor is sometimes the only way to get information on prices and ordering. Although correspondence is time-consuming, it may help the order move more quickly. Getting information directly from the supplier ensures that orders are submitted in an acceptable form. To save time, the librarian may wish to prepare a form letter requesting price and ordering information. Brief bibliographic information, the supplier's name and address, and any additional questions can be added to each request.

Acquisition Lists

Acquisition lists from other libraries are another source of ordering information. They usually give standard citations sufficient for completing order information. Such lists are, of course, limited to the scope of the library's collection.

Record-Keeping For Book Orders

Libraries usually maintain records for each individual book from the time it is considered for selection until the catalog cards are filed or cataloging data is entered in an online system. Selection, acquisition, and cataloging files can be integrated in most hospital libraries. In this way information gathered during each stage of the process is readily available.

A multiple-copy, three-inch by five-inch book order form can be adapted for both simple and complex library record systems. The standard form shown in Figure 4-3 has five copies, each a different color. They can be separated and used for different purposes after the information has been recorded. Most library supply houses will preprint forms with the library name and address. Space for other information, such as department name or vendor account number, can be added.

The simplest way of placing an order is to send a copy of the order slip to the vendor. Hospital librarians can order books in this way if both the hospital purchasing department and the vendor accept this type of order. Many hospitals require that an order be submitted on a requisition or other form. In these cases the librarian may wish to use order forms for internal records.

Copies of order forms can be arranged in two separate files to monitor the status of book orders. These files would be labeled "on order" and "received." Within each file, forms can be arranged by vendor, date, or title. As each item is received, the order slip should be removed from the "on order" file, marked "received" and dated, and placed in the "received" file. Another copy of the order form can be placed with the book. It can be used as a worksheet for making catalog cards or as an order form for purchased catalog cards. The forms left in the "on order" file allow immediate identification of materials that have not been received. The "received" file becomes a permanent record of orders.

The "on order" file can be used to answer users' questions about the status of a book. Some librarians also file a copy of the order form in the card catalog. When a book is received, the order form is marked. It is removed when the catalog cards are filed. The advantages of having order information in the card catalog should be carefully weighed against the time involved in accomplishing this task.

Multiple-copy order forms can be used in many other ways. For example, copies of order forms can be flagged for routing or special handling of books. Other uses for order forms are discussed below.

• Permanent record of orders. All the order forms for a fiscal year can be placed in a file. The dates on which the order was placed, received, and paid should be recorded. It should also be noted if the order was cancelled or had to be claimed.

• Departmental file. Libraries sometimes order books for other hospital departments. A separate file of order forms can be kept for each department.

• Statistical and financial files. After orders are received, copies of order forms may be used to tabulate expenditures; compile lists of new acquisitions by subject matter;

evaluate vendors; and tally statistics requested by the Joint Commission on Accreditation of Hospitals or other accrediting bodies.

• Vendor file. Arranged by order or by supplier, files can be used to monitor the status of orders for multiple items. This is especially helpful when the library does not keep a file of purchase orders or requisitions.

Since the librarian may be maintaining a number of files on a single order, problems and claims should be noted on one set of records so that the history of the order is clear.

Selecting a Vendor

Book vendors include publishers or issuing agencies, bookstores, publishers' representatives, and book jobbers. Several factors should influence the librarian's choice of a vendor. These factors include price, type of

Figure 4-3
Standard Book Order Form*

Class No.	Author		
Acc. No.	Title		
List Price	Place	Publisher	Year
Dealer	Vols.	Series	Edition
No. of copies	Recommended by	Date Ordered	Cost Other
Order No.	Fund Charged	Date Received	

LIBRARY NAME
LIBRARY ADDRESS

*A new form for hand-written, typed or computer-generated orders, including an alternate 3" x 10" form, was approved by the American National Standards Institute as ANSI Standard Z39.30-1982.

order form required, delivery time, payment requirements, and other services offered. Answers to the following questions may help the librarian select a vendor.

- Price. Is there a discount? How much is it? How is it determined? Is it available on all items? How is discount information provided? Who pays shipping charges? How are they computed? How are they billed?
- Type of order form. Is the vendor's format rigid? Is detailed identification required for each item? How easily can required information be found? Are the vendor's requirements compatible with hospital procedures?
- Delivery time. Is it reasonable for most orders? How are rush orders handled?
- Payment requirements. Is prepayment required? How are items billed? How are credits issued? Are the vendor's requirements compatible with hospital procedures?
- Other services. Does the vendor ship on approval or allow returns? Can a responsive service representative be reached at a local or toll-free number? Are there other services that will save the library time and money on orders?

Publishers or Issuing Agencies

Some books are sold only by the publisher or issuing agency. These often include books published by associations, professional societies, government agencies, and small presses. Even if a hospital librarian prefers to place as many orders as possible through a jobber, some orders will have to be placed directly with the publisher.

Direct orders are usually relatively small because a separate order must be placed with each individual supplier. Small orders have certain disadvantages. The cost of processing them may be high compared to the cost of the materials being ordered. Also, the vendor is more likely to ask that the customer pay shipping and handling charges for small orders. Many publishers do not offer discounts on small orders and often require prepayment. Getting a price quote on shipping charges can delay the order and add to internal handling costs.

The librarian may find it difficult to batch orders effectively if only a small number of items may be ordered from a single publisher in a given year. If the form of the order does not meet the vendor's requirements or is unclear, a delay in shipping the order may result. Many publishers and issuing agencies will not respond to small orders that they can not easily fill. Thus the librarian may not be aware of a problem until the normal claim period has expired. For all of these reasons, many hospital librarians try to keep the number of direct orders as small as possible.

Bookstores

General reference tools and standard medical, nursing, and management texts are usually stocked in bookstores in large cities and cities with colleges or universities. These stores can be an excellent source for rush orders.

Many bookstores will order items that are not stocked. This provides the hospital library with an alternative to direct orders. Although the practices of each bookstore vary, some offer libraries favorable order and payment arrangements to encourage patronage.

Book Jobbers

A book jobber, or agent, is a wholesale agent who can supply libraries with books from many publishers. Book jobbers usually maintain a stock of books. This stock allows them to fill orders rapidly and to offer discounts to customers. The advantages and disadvantages of using jobbers are summarized in Figure 4-4.

Jobbers differ with respect to number and type of publishers represented, order and billing arrangements, and services offered. They may limit themselves to certain subject areas, certain publishers, or a specific geographical service area. There are a number of medical, scien-

Figure 4-4
Advantages and Disadvantages of Using a Book Jobber

Advantages

A single order for books from different publishers reduces the total number of orders.

A jobber usually offers a better discount than a publisher can on direct orders.

Billing arrangements may be more flexible than those of a publisher.

Delivery time is often shorter than for small orders to the publisher.

Additional services may include the following: approvals, return arrangements, free shipping, access to a local sales representative, up-to-date price information and stock lists, toll-free phone numbers for claims and questions.

Disadvantages

Billing requirements may necessitate special arrangements with the hospital purchasing department.

The hospital policy of paying only for complete orders may delay payment on large shipments, complicating credit.

Larger orders may require bidding.

A single jobber may not supply all required titles, subjects, or publishers.

The jobbers' order format may require additional information, such as stock numbers, discounts, or account numbers.

tific, and technical book jobbers who handle major English-language publishers. In general these jobbers are the most appropriate choice for hospital libraries. Several of them are listed in Appendix B. A library that buys foreign-language titles may consider using a second jobber who specializes in distributing books published outside the United States. The services of a general book jobber may also be needed if the library purchases books on subjects not covered by the medical book jobber. These subjects may include psychology, patient education, and consumer health. The geographical location of the jobber may be of concern in terms of shipping costs, claiming, and using special services.

Discounts are an important factor in selecting a jobber, since price savings are a primary advantage of using jobbers. If the jobber does not assume all shipping charges, the librarian should consider the cost of shipping in relation to the discount. Order and billing arrangements must be compatible with hospital procedures. The ability of a book jobber to process an order with minimal identification of each item can save the librarian a great deal of time. If a jobber requires detailed information or has rigid payment requirements, the librarian may need to spend more time processing orders and payments than the discount or other services warrant.

The librarian should consider services offered by jobbers in terms of the library's need for them. The following services may be useful:

- Special orders of nonstock or out-of-stock items
- Current price and stock information
- Rapid filling of orders and ability to process rush orders
- Prompt response to claims
- Acceptance of returned books
- Access to a service representative

Other Distributors

A number of publishers have sales representatives who cover particular geographical areas. Such representatives generally can be contacted directly, eliminating many of the usual problems with small orders to a publisher. Free shipping, discounts, and rush deliveries from stock may be possible. Sales representatives may also be willing to accommodate any special purchasing requirements of the hospital.

Choosing the Most Effective Type of Order

An efficient book order system usually relies on one routine procedure for ordering most books. Following a set procedure reduces the possibility of error. Most books might be ordered on an annual blanket purchase order or several individual purchase orders issued to one or two major suppliers, such as jobbers or bookstores.

Books not available from these suppliers would be ordered from other vendors. These books might be acquired using the customary purchase order or any of the special types of orders discussed above, including COD, prepaid, confirming, deposit account, and subscription. The librarian may decide to use one of these special types of orders because of vendor requirements (COD, prepaid, subscription); ease of processing the order (deposit account); a discount (prepaid or subscription); or speed of delivery (deposit account, confirming order, COD).

Approvals and rush orders are two other types of special orders. They will be discussed below.

Approvals

Certain book jobbers and publishers will ship books "on approval." The librarian has a specified period of time to examine the books and decide whether to purchase them or return them. The librarian should examine the supplier's approval procedures carefully in order to identify any conflict with library procedures or hospital purchasing practices. Answers to the following questions can assist the librarian in evaluating the approval plan.

- Can the librarian select individual titles or subject areas, or will the supplier determine what is sent?
- Is the approval period long enough for reviewing and returning books?
- Who pays the shipping costs?
- Who will approve payment for books selected?
- How will invoices be handled?
- Are the procedures for receiving materials and returning them too time-consuming?

Rush Orders

An occasional rush order may be placed with a vendor if the vendor can provide quick service. If hospital purchasing procedures allow it, orders for immediate delivery can sometimes be placed by telephone. The order may need to be confirmed in writing so that payment can be processed. Some vendors may require that orders be prepaid or delivered COD.

Online Ordering

Computerized bibliographic networks now offer online ordering of books, documents, and reports. The acquisition subsystem, available from OCLC, forwards orders for monographs listed in the system's ONLINE UNION CATALOG to publishers or jobbers according to the library's specifications. Fund accounting and cataloging data are linked to the orders placed at the user's computer terminal (4,5). Online ordering may require the development of special procedures that are compatible with hospital approval and payment procedures.

Document delivery services available through information retrieval systems can be used for library acquisition as well (6,7). Whether the library orders online, by telephone, or by mail, these services can be very useful. They offer hard-to-locate items, including documents and reports. They also handle some out-of-print materials and provide quick service on many items.

ACQUIRING JOURNALS

Journals are periodicals that publish articles of current interest or that contain material directed at a particular group. Continuations, audiovisual serials, and serials issued by government agencies will be discussed separately.

Journals are generally identified by title or issuing body and title. Similar titles can be distinguished by using the standard elements of information listed in Figure 4-1. Bibliographic and price information can be found in the sources listed in Figure 4-2. More current information is usually available from subscription agents and from publishers.

Selecting a Vendor

Journal subscriptions can usually be ordered from a subscription agent or directly from the publisher or issuing agency. Certain titles are not handled by agents or jobbers. These include many association publications and publications from government agencies.

Subscription Agents

Ordering and renewing subscriptions can be extremely time-consuming if all orders are placed directly with the publishers. Hospital librarians can save a great deal of time and paperwork by ordering journals through a subscription agent (8). The advantages and disadvantages of ordering through an agent are summarized in Figure 4-5.

Subscription agents may restrict their services by subject, country of publication, geographical area served, type of publisher, or type of serial. Services offered vary but may include data processing; claiming; bibliographic, indexing, and pricing information; flexible renewal and billing arrangements; and current financial information (9).

When selecting a subscription agent, the librarian should focus on services offered rather than subscription prices. Discounts are rarely available. In fact, agents usually charge a service fee. To justify the selection of a vendor with a higher service fee, the librarian must be able to show that the services performed by the agent will save both time and money. Subscription agents, like book jobbers, offer some services that may not be needed. Thus the librarian should analyze the library's needs in relation to the agent's charges for services.

If the librarian decides to place most subscription orders through an agent, order procedures should be formulated in cooperation with the hospital purchasing department. The procedures should specify the following: the authorization process; how and when renewals will be reviewed; renewal dates for subscriptions; the handling of purchase orders or other order forms; and payment procedures.

Publishers or Issuing Agencies

Ordering subscriptions directly from publishers or

Figure 4-5
Advantages and Disadvantages of Using a Subscription Agent

Advantages

Placing most subscriptions on a single order saves processing costs.

A single expiration date for most titles simplifies library record-keeping and renewal procedures.

All claims can be submitted on standard forms to a single address—the agent's.

Optional data processing services, sometimes available at no extra cost, can provide the library with additional information on the journal collection and expenditures.

The agent usually carries price increases on an account for uninterrupted service.

The agent's arrangements with publishers eliminate need for prepayment of new subscriptions.

An agent can offer current information about serial publications not found elsewhere: price, indexing, new titles, publisher name and address, frequency changes, and so forth.

Some agents handle monographs, serials, annuals, and other multi-volume works in addition to journals.

Disadvantages

A single agent may not handle all titles needed, so some direct orders may be necessary.

Setting up an account with an agent may require changes in the library purchasing procedures.

The agent and the hospital library may have incompatible procedures.

Initial transfer of orders to an agent may cause confusion, including duplications and interruptions in subscriptions for a brief period.

Some subscriptions and claims may take longer to process through an agent than directly to publishers.

Service charges may be difficult to justify to hospital purchasing authorities.

The hospital may require bids for large orders to a single vendor.

renewing existing subscriptions usually requires prepayment for the subscription period. The librarian may be able to place a new subscription on a publisher's reply card and receive an invoice after the subscription begins. The hospital or the vendor may require that a purchase order number be supplied when the order is placed. A written confirmation order should follow.

Introductory subscriptions or those on approval generally must be paid within a short time. The publisher's invoice for continuing the subscription should accompany payment to prevent duplicate subscriptions. Renewals should reach the publisher six to eight weeks before the subscription expires to avoid interruptions. Publishers frequently send an invoice as a renewal notice. Attaching a copy of the invoice to the payment for renewal will help ensure proper credit. Publishers sometimes market subscriptions by using unsolicited invoices, so the librarian must examine invoices carefully before payment is made.

Record-Keeping

Keeping records on journal orders is a complex and time-consuming process. A subscription to a single jour-nal results in the library receiving a number of different items at various intervals during the year.

Check-in File

Most librarians maintain a journal check-in record in a visible file. Preprinted cards similar to the example in Figure 4-6 are commercially available. A well-organized check-in file can be the primary journal record for smaller libraries. It can also serve as an efficient entry point to other records in larger collections.

The check-in file can become the permanent catalog of journal holdings and can include information on inactive titles, title changes, and bound holdings. Larger libraries may wish to keep some of this information in separate files or on lists that are accessible to users. Check-in files can also include information about titles on order, routing of journal issues, and selection or renewal decisions.

Figure 4-6
Journal Check-In Card

TITLE				FREQUENCY						DAY DUE					
PUBLISHER OR AGENT				SUBSCRIPT. DATE								TITLE PAGE			
ADDRESS				NOS. PER VOL								INDEX			
BOUND				VOLS. PER YEAR											
PREPARED				IN BINDERY											
YEAR	SER	VOL	JAN	FEB	MAR	APR	MAY	JUNE	JULY	AUG	SEPT	OCT	NOV	DEC	T.P.	I.
			1													
			2													
			3													
			4													
			5													
			1													
			2													
			3													
			4													
			5													
			1													
			2													
			3													
			4													
			5													
INC.	TITLE															
		JAN FEB MAR APR MAY JUN JUL AUG SEP OCT NOV DEC														

A list of specific information that might be included in a check-in file is given below.

- Journal title
- Source (agent or publisher)
- Frequency of publication
- Dates issues received
- Subscription period
- Renewal date
- Current and previous volume and issue numbers
- Financial and ordering information
- Dates indexes and special issues received
- Binding instructions
- Bound holdings
- Titles on order
- Title changes
- Routing information
- Special handling or shelving instructions
- Titles of free journals received and kept by the library

Claims

The librarian should schedule a monthly or quarterly review of the check-in file to identify and claim any late issues. Missing issues can also be detected during the regular check-in process and claimed immediately. Regular prompt claiming of journals ensures that the library receives all the materials it paid for. It allows the library to request missed issues before the publisher's stock of back issues is depleted. Also, it ensures that complete volumes are available for binding and information services.

Subscription agents often provide a claim form or a means of claiming by teletype or telephone. Libraries can devise a simple form to use for claiming issues of journals ordered directly from the publisher.

Replacements

Gaps in serial holdings result from undelivered, lost, or damaged issues. A library may wish to replace missing issues or acquire back issues of a recently purchased journal. If back issues are not available from the publisher at a reasonable price, exchange systems may be used. These include the Medical Library Association Exchange, the Universal Serials and Book Exchange, and local formal or informal exchange systems.

The Medical Library Association (MLA) operates the Exchange to allow institutional members to obtain back issues of journals at a nominal cost. Member libraries offer items no longer needed on a list published at intervals during the year by the Exchange. Materials may be requested directly from the libraries that own them. The supplying library may request reimbursement for postage. Otherwise, there is no charge for the materials. The MLA is currently studying the feasibility of converting the Exchange to an online computerized system. A copy of the current *MLA Exchange Guidelines* is available to libraries from the MLA, 919 N. Michigan Avenue, Chicago, Illinois 60611.

The Universal Serials and Book Exchange (USBE) collects and distributes books, journals, and documents. Members pay a fee and agree to send unused publications to the USBE. When a request is received from a member, the USBE searches its stock for the item. Information on membership, procedures, and handling fees is available from Universal Serials and Book Exchange, Inc., 3335 V Street, Washington, D.C. 20018.

Hospital employees may be willing to donate back issues of journals. The librarian may wish to compile a list of missing issues and distribute copies of the list throughout the hospital.

ACQUIRING CONTINUATIONS

Continuations are publications issued to update or expand monographs, serials, or other series. Continuations familiar to hospital librarians include numbered and unnumbered monographic series such as *Cardiovascular Clinics* and *Nursing Skillbooks*, annuals such as *Current Therapy*, and multi-volume works published over a number of years such as the American Physiological Society's *Handbook of Physiology*. Because continuations share characteristics of both books and journals, a vendor may choose to treat them as one or the other. This presents special problems to the librarian with regard to identifying, pricing, ordering, and checking in continuations.

Identifying and Pricing

The librarian should provide the vendor with as much information as possible when ordering continuations. The order should include all the elements of information listed under "Continuations" in Figure 4-1. If the information given is incomplete, the vendor may not understand what item is desired.

Cataloging information on continuations can be obtained from the following sources: the *National Library of Medicine Current Catalog*, the *National Library of Medicine Current Catalog Proof Sheets*, and *Irregular Serials and Annuals*. Two databases, CATLINE and OCLC, are also good sources for this type of information.

Pricing information is available in standard sources such as *Medical Books and Serials in Print*, *Irregular Serials and Annuals*, and *Ulrich's International Periodicals Directory*. Book jobbers and subscription agents can also provide pricing information. It is important to clarify whether the stated price is for a single item or for a subscription that may include a number of items to be sent over a period of time. A price quote letter may be required to clarify pricing for new orders.

Selecting Type of Order

Vendors of continuations usually are also suppliers of books and journals, so the same criteria can be applied to selecting the source. To select the most appropriate way to order an item, the librarian needs to consider whether or not subsequent parts will be purchased. The vendor's ordering policies must also be considered.

The librarian may decide to purchase all or most of the parts of a particular item. In this case it would be most convenient for the librarian to purchase it as a standing order or a subscription.

Ordering continuations through a subscription agent with an annual review for renewals or cancellations can be an efficient way to handle orders. Some suppliers, however, do not offer these options, preferring instead to market individual parts as books.

Other suppliers may accept standing orders that can be cancelled at any time. Some will accept returns of individual parts of a work on standing order. This type of arrangement saves the library both time and money, since items do not have to be ordered individually and those that the library doesn't need can be returned. This type of standing order also ensures that the library receives updates as soon as they become available.

Record-Keeping

It is important that accurate records be kept of titles that have continuations. The librarian should consider both the method of ordering these titles and the type of cataloging and processing to be done. All continuations can be logged in a check-in file and routed for cataloging following instructions already noted in the file. To ensure accurate preorder searching, a card might also be placed in the book order files even for continuation items ordered as serials.

ACQUIRING GOVERNMENT PUBLICATIONS

Government publications are issued or authorized by government bodies. They are funded by state, local, federal, or international issuing bodies. Government publications are intended to serve legislative, administrative, reporting, service, research, or information needs (10).

Identifying and Pricing

Government documents can be identified by the elements of information listed in Figure 4-1. Most hospital libraries will not need to purchase any of the specialized sources of bibliographic information for government publications listed in Figure 4-2. This type of information is usually available from other institutions or agencies such as depository libraries (10). Other sources of acquisition information are large libraries with document collections, the Federal Information Service, and state and federal legislators.

One of the most important acquisition tools for the hospital librarian is the annual publication list issued by the National Library of Medicine (NLM) as a supplement to the *NLM News* (11). This list provides full order information for all NLM publications, specifying which should be ordered from the Superintendent of Documents (SuDocs) and which from the National Technical Information Service (NTIS). The monthly issues of *NLM News* announce new publications and price changes throughout the year. This information is essential to ordering new editions of NLM indexes and searching tools.

The *Monthly Catalog of United States Government Publications* provides order and price information on a large range of federal publications. See Appendix A for more information on this publication. A letter to the supplier requesting a price quote is advised before ordering older documents. The Federal Information Center or a Government Printing Office Bookstore may also be able to give a price quote over the telephone.

Selecting Vendor and Type of Order

Some government monographs and serials are carried by general jobbers and subscription agents. A library that has a good relationship with a jobber or an agent should try to order as many publications as possible through that person. Many documents not available from agents are distributed by the SuDocs, the NTIS, or by Government Printing Office bookstores. A deposit account with either SuDocs or NTIS will save time and will prevent problems with price changes for orders. DIALOG Information Services, Inc. offers online ordering of Government Printing Office publications for libraries with access to DIALOG's computerized databases.

Free copies of federal documents are often available on written request to the issuing agency. Local offices of members of Congress will often send copies of documents on request to libraries in their districts. Because most federal documents are not protected by copyright laws, photocopying a borrowed copy of a document is often a good method of acquisition. Documents issued by state and local agencies are often free in limited numbers. The method of ordering them may vary with each agency.

ACQUIRING AUDIOVISUAL SOFTWARE

The term "audiovisual software" refers to all types of audiovisual programs, including films, filmstrips, slides, and videotapes. The process of selecting and acquiring audiovisual software is described in more detail in Chapter 10.

Identifying and Pricing

The identification of audiovisual programs for purchase or rental is closely tied to the selection process and depends on the same sources. The librarian should describe the program in as much detail as possible on the order form using the elements of information listed for audiovisuals in Figure 4-1.

The few commercially available lists of audiovisuals do not contain complete or current price information. Rental catalogs from large audiovisual collections and distributors' catalogs provide the most reliable printed price information. A price quote is advisable on orders even from these sources, particularly if the hospital purchasing department requires firm price quotes.

Price quotes are advisable in any case since pricing schedules for audiovisuals are complex. Charges for preview or rental can sometimes be credited toward purchases made within a stated period. Shipping costs and the method of billing them vary widely. Rush orders may involve additional handling costs. Acquisition of reproduction or rebroadcast rights may require additional royalty payments.

Selecting Vendor and Type of Order

Usually there is only one source for a particular audiovisual program, although occasionally a distributor will rent or sell an item that is also available from the producer or from an audiovisual collection. If there is a choice, the vendor should be selected based on price, turnaround time, order and billing arrangements, choice of formats, and rights of use.

The ordering procedures for audiovisuals are frequently dictated by the vendor and may vary significantly from company to company. In addition, libraries may have special requirements for each order, such as scheduled show dates, the need for previews, or the need to obtain special rights for use. Because of these requirements, the librarian frequently must negotiate directly with the vendor or distributor on each order. A good working relationship with the hospital purchasing department and a knowledge of the requirements of the purchasing system are essential in dealing with the variety of situations that can arise when ordering audiovisuals. For more information, particularly on record-keeping for audiovisual orders, refer to Chapter 10.

ACQUIRING SUPPLIES AND EQUIPMENT

The librarian is often responsible for obtaining general supplies for the library. These may include office supplies, library forms, office equipment, and furniture needed to support library services.

Stock Items

Many standard office supplies, as well as new or used equipment and furniture, may be available from a central hospital inventory. The librarian should be familiar with what is available from stock and with the procedures for obtaining these items. The library can save both time and money if satisfactory products can be acquired from hospital inventory or through internal services.

The hospital may offer printing or duplication services that can be used to produce certain library forms. By working closely with staff from these departments, the librarian may be able to obtain book cards, date due slips, and other forms more economically than through a library supply house.

Using Outside Vendors

If the required products are not available within the hospital, the librarian must order them from outside vendors. He or she may select the item or items from a vendor's catalog and prepare a requisition according to the hospital's requirements. Hospitals frequently have contracts with general office supply houses or are granted discounts by them based on the volume of purchases. Because the librarian may be able to take advantage of the hospital's discount, it is usually best to select a vendor with the help of the purchasing department.

Pricing often depends on the packaging and the volume of the order. Bulky items or those with a short shelf life should be purchased in limited amounts. A discount for a large order, even for frequently used items, is not a bargain if the total price is out of proportion to the library's supply budget.

The library usually orders some supplies from library supply houses such as those listed in Appendix C. Examples include interlibrary loan forms printed with the library's address, journal check-in forms, catalog card stock, and preprinted multiple-copy book order forms.

Equipment

Equipment purchases are frequently subject to the hospital's policy on bids or price quotes because they often involve large amounts of money. The librarian should be aware of hospital policy before signing an agreement with a supplier. Usually the purchase order, bid, or price quote will specify not only the product and price but also any warranty or service agreement, the delivery date, and shipping arrangements. The purchasing staff can help the librarian include essential information in a form acceptable to both the hospital and the vendor. With equipment purchases, the librarian's choice of a vendor may be influenced by agreements the hospital may have with vendors concerning discounts, service agreements, trade-ins, or leases.

Once the equipment is received, the librarian can file and update information on warranties, service agreements, operating instructions, parts, and addresses of service representatives. The librarian should cooperate with any hospital-wide inventory system or insurance plan for equipment.

REFERENCES

1. Aljian G. Purchasing handbook; standard reference book on policies, practices, and procedures utilized in departments responsible for purchasing management or materials management. 3d ed. New York; McGraw Hill, 1973.

2. Ammer C, Ammer DS. Dictionary of business and economics. New York: Free Press, 1977.

3. Woelfl NN. Acquisition of biomedical materials. Chicago: Medical Library Association, 1977. (MLA courses for continuing education, CE 38).

4. Acquisitions subsystem. Columbus: OCLC, 1980.

5. Acquisitions subsystem: fund accounting component. Columbus: OCLC, 1980.

6. Popovich M, Miller B. Online ordering with Dialorder. Online 1981 Apr;5:63-65.

7. Finnigan G, Rugge S. Document delivery and the experiences of Information Unlimited. Online 1978 Jan;2:62-69.

8. Brandon AN, Hill DR. Selected list of books and journals for the small medical library. Bull Med Libr Assoc 1981 Apr;69:185-215.

9. Brown CD, Smith LS. Serials: past, present, and future. 2d ed. rev. Birmingham, AL: EBSCO, 1980.

10. Nakata Y. From press to people: collecting and using U.S. government publications. Chicago: American Library Association, 1979.

11. National Library of Medicine Publications. NLM News 1983 Jan(Suppl);1-28.

READINGS

Ammer DS. Purchasing and materials management for health care institutions. Lexington, MA: Lexington Books, 1975.

Anglo-American cataloging rules. 2d ed. Chicago: American Library Association, 1978.

Bell JA. Methodology for the comparison of book jobber performance. Bull Med Libr Assoc 1982 Apr;70:229-231.

Bloomberg M, Evans GE. Introduction to technical service for library technicians. 4th ed. Littleton, CO: Libraries Unlimited, 1981.

Houseley CE. Hospital materiel management. Germantown, MD: Aspen Systems, 1978.

Morehead J. Introduction to United States public documents. 2d ed. Littleton, CO: Libraries Unlimited, 1978.

Osborn AD. Serial publications, their place and treatment in libraries. 3d ed. Chicago: American Library Association, 1980.

Rueby C. Serials selection and management. Chicago: Medical Library Association, 1980. (MLA courses for continuing education, CE 562).

Wiese F. Health statistics: a guide to information sources. Detroit: Gale Research, 1980. (Health Affairs Information Guide Series, vol. 4).

APPENDIX A
Sources of Information for Acquisitions

American book publishing record. New York: Bowker, 1961-.

The series provides monthly cumulation of lists from Publisher's Weekly. *It cumulates annually into* BPR Annual Cumulative, 1965-. *The record includes books on all subjects by American trade publishers except government publications, subscription books, and periodicals.*

Books in print. New York: Bowker, 1948-.

Annual listing by author and title gives the publisher and price. Title volumes include a comprehensive directory of publishers. Subject Guide to Books in Print is a companion. Both serve as indexes to the more complete Publishers' Trade List Annual.

Cumulative book index: a world list of books in the English language. New York: Wilson, 1928-.

The index is published monthly except August, cumulating at intervals throughout the year and annually. It includes a comprehensive list of books and pamphlets issued in English in the United States and Canada as well as selected titles from other English-speaking countries. The index lists by author, title, and subject with full bibliographic information and prices.

Documents to the people. Chicago: American Library Association, 1972-.

This is a bimonthly publication covering developments on government documents. It is published by the ALA Government Documents Round Table.

ERIC (Educational Resources Information Center). Resources in education. Washington, DC: Department of Education, 1966-.

ERIC is an information network for collecting and distributing educational research. Abstracts are published monthly in Resources in Education. *Documents are distributed in fiche and hard copy from ERIC Documents Reproduction Center. Database is also available online on BRS, DIALOG, and SDC.*

Forthcoming books. New York: Bowker, 1967-.

Bimonthly update of Books in Print *includes books recently published and scheduled to be published. Author and title sections indicate publisher, price, month and year of publication. Companion volume,* Subject Guide to Forthcoming Books, *is published separately.*

Government publications review: an international journal. New York: Pergamon, 1974-.

This review journal covers handling and production of documents from all levels of government, local through international, issued in all countries.

Health information resources in the Department of Health and Human Services, 1980. Washington, DC: US Dept. of Health and Human Services. Public Health Service. Office of Disease Prevention and Health Promotion. Office of Health Information, Health Promotion and Physical Fitness and Sports Medicine, 1980. DHHS (PHS) Publication Number 80-50146.

The publication compiles a list of 76 agencies that provide health information resources. Agency services, contact persons, addresses, and publications are all listed by subject. Also included is an additional detailed subject index.

Index of NLM serial titles. 4th ed. Bethesda, MD: US Dept. of Health Education and Welfare. Public Health Service. National Institutes of Health. National Library of Medicine. 1981.

This keyword index is produced from SERLINE. It indexes over 31,000 serials and numbered congresses owned or on order by the National Library of Medicine.

Irregular serials and annuals: an international directory. 8th ed. New York; Bowker, 1983.

Irregular Serials and Annuals *is a biennial companion to* Ulrich's International Periodicals Directory. *It lists active serials issued annually or less frequently, including yearbooks, transactions, proceedings, and monographic series. It is also a title index to the classified listing of full bibliographic and publisher information, including prices.*

* List of journals indexed in Index Medicus. Washington, DC: Government Printing Office, 1960-.

This is a separate annual publication. It also appears in January issue of Index Medicus *with updates throughout the year and in first volume of* Cumulated Index Medicus *each year. Lists by abbreviation and full title include ISSN and notes about title changes. Subject and country lists are included.*

Medical books and serials in print. New York: Bowker, 1972-.

Medical Books and Serials in Print *provides an annual list of books in medicine, nursing, dentistry, and veterinary medicine available in the United States. The material is arranged in subject, author, and title listings. Entries include author, title, publisher, date, and price.*

** MEDOC; a computerized index to U.S. government documents in the medical and health sciences. Salt Lake City, UT: Spencer S. Eccles Health Sciences Library, University of Utah, 1968-.

MEDOC *is an index of documents received at Eccles Health Sciences Library. Quarterly cumulative issues are indexed by Superintendent of Documents number, title, and subject, and series number. MEDOC is available online through BRS.*

Monthly catalog of United States government publications. Washington, DC: Government Printing Office, 1895-.

This is the official index of GPO publications. Full bibliographic data for items includes Superintendent of Documents number, GPO stock numbers, prices, and order information. Separate listing of serials began in 1977.

Monthly checklist of state publications. Washington, DC: Library of Congress, 1910-.

The monthly publication lists by state all documents of state government agencies received by the Library of Congress. It provides full cataloging data for each entry. Annual index to titles and contents are noted. It also includes a semiannual list of serials.

** National Library of Medicine current catalog. Washington, DC: Government Printing Office, 1966-.

NLM Current Catalog *is computer-produced. It is issued quarterly with annual and five-year cumulations. It provides full cataloging data for books and serials cataloged by NLM and cooperating libraries. Data is available online via CATLINE and the OCLC network.*

*Recommended for all hospital libraries.
**Useful for larger hospital libraries.

National Library of Medicine current catalog proof sheets. Chicago: Medical Library Association, 1970-

Weekly proof sheets of NLM cataloging update the Current Catalog. *The proof sheets include cataloging in publications supplied by NLM and corrections to previous entries. They are cumulated quarterly and annually by* Current Catalog.

National union catalog: a cumulative author list. Washington, DC: Library of Congress, 1953-.

National Union Catalog is printed monthly with quarterly and annual cumulations. It provides a catalog of books in all languages in the Library of Congress collection, government department libraries, and over 700 cooperating libraries throughout the country. Cataloging records are also available in machine readable form from the Library of Congress and via online cataloging networks.

New serials titles: a union list of serials commencing publication after December 31, 1949. Washington, DC: Library of Congress, 1953-.

New Serials Titles is self-cumulating in twelve issues a year. It lists complete bibliographic information and ISSN for new titles and title changes. It also includes changes in the name of corporate authors, interruptions to publication, and holding library information for reporting libraries in the United States and Canada. Cumulations for 1950-1970 and 1971-1975 update Union Lists of Serials, *3d ed., 1965.*

Paperbound books in print. New York: Bowker, 1955-.

This publication is a semiannual listing of currently available paperbacks by author, title, and subject. Entries include publisher and prices.

Publishers' trade list annual. New York: Bowker, 1873-.

The trade list annual is a collection of publishers' catalogs bound together with an alphabetical list of publishers' names. Information for each title varies from minimal to full depending on publisher. Books in Print *and* Subject Guide to Books in Print *serve as indexes to this publication.*

Standard periodical directory: 1981-82. 7th ed. New York: Oxbridge, 1980.

Standard Periodical Directory is an irregularly published guide to United States and Canadian publications. It includes newsletters and house organs not found in other listings. The directory is indexed by title and arranged by subject classification. It gives the name and address of the publisher, beginning year, frequency, circulation figures, and subscription and advertising rates.

Ulrich's international periodicals directory: a classified guide to current periodicals, foreign and domestic. 21st ed. New York: Bowker, 1982.

Ulrich's directory provides a classified list of periodicals from many countries. It is published biennially, alternating with Irregular Serials and Annuals. *Entries include title, subtitle, issuing agency, beginning date, frequency, price, editors, publishers' names and addresses, ISSN, and Dewey Decimal number. It also describes features such as bibliographies, and indicates where titles are indexed.*

United States government manual. Washington, DC: Government Printing Office, 1935-.

This manual is published annually as an official organizational handbook. It provides information on agencies, personnel and activities. It also includes name, subject, and agency indexes.

Vital notes on medical periodicals. Chicago: Medical Library Association, 1952-1982.

This publication was discontinued at the end of 1982.

APPENDIX B
Medical Book Jobbers

Ballen Booksellers International, Inc.
66 Austin Boulevard
Commack, Long Island, New York 11725

Brown and Connolly, Inc.
2 Keith Way
Hingham, Massachusetts 02043

Burns and MacEachern Limited
26 Railside Road
Don Mills, Ontario, Canada

Chicago Medical Book Company
7400 N. Melvina
Chicago, Illinois 60648

Login Brothers Book Company, Inc.
1450 West Randolph Street
Chicago, Illinois 60607

　　　7230 Northfield Road
　　　Walton Hills, Ohio 44146

　　　135 New Dutch Lane
　　　P.O. Box 2700
　　　Fairfield, New Jersey

Majors Scientific Books, Inc.
2221 Walnut Hill Lane
Irving, Texas 75061

　　　3770 Zip Industrial Boulevard
　　　Atlanta, Georgia 30354

　　　3909 Bienville
　　　New Orleans, Louisiana 70119

　　　6632 South Main Street
　　　Houston, Texas 77025

Matthews Book Company
3140 Park Avenue
St. Louis, Missouri 63104

Rittenhouse Book Distributors, Inc.
511 Feheley Drive
King of Prussia, Pennsylvania 19406

APPENDIX C
Library Supply Houses

Brodart, Inc.
Eastern Division
1609 Memorial Avenue
Williamsport, Pennsylvania 17705

　　　Western Division
　　　1236 South Hatcher Street
　　　City of Industry, California 91748

Demco
Box 7488
Madison, Wisconsin 53707

　　　Western Regional Office
　　　Box 7767
　　　Fresno, California 93747

Gaylord Brothers, Inc.
Box 4901
Syracuse, New York 13221

　　　Box 8489
　　　Stockton, California 95208

　　　Furniture Manufacturing Division
　　　Sanford, North Carolina 27330

The Highsmith Co., Inc.
P.O. Box 100, Highway 106 East
Fort Atkinson, Wisconsin 53583

Josten's Library Services
1301 Cliff Road
Burnsville, Minnesota 55337

University Products, Inc.
P.O. Box 101
South Canal Street
Holyoke, Massachusetts 01041

APPENDIX D
Subscription Agents

Ebsco Subscription Services
P.O. Box 1943
Birmingham, Alabama 35201

F. W. Faxon Company, Inc.
15 Southwest Park
Westwood, Massachusetts 02090

Majors Scientific Books
2221 Walnut Hill Lane
Irving, Texas 75061

McGregor Magazine Agency
Mount Morris, Illinois 61054

Read-More Publications, Inc.
140 Cedar Street
New York, New York 10006

Turner Subscription Agency
235 Park Avenue South
New York, New York 10003

Cataloging Library Materials

Olyn K. Ruxin
Head Catalog Librarian
Cleveland Health Sciences Library
Cleveland, Ohio
and
Marlene J. Saul
*Circuit Librarian
Cleveland Health Sciences Library
Cleveland, Ohio

*Currently:
Director, Core Library
University Hospitals of Cleveland
Cleveland, Ohio

CHAPTER 5

Cataloging Library Materials

Olyn K. Ruxin
Head Catalog Librarian
Cleveland Health Sciences Library
Cleveland, Ohio
and
Marlene J. Saul
Circuit Librarian
Cleveland Health Sciences Library
Cleveland, Ohio

Cataloging and organizing are essential for providing full access to library materials. Since efficient use of the library depends greatly on access to the collection, the highest standards for cataloging and organizing materials should be adopted and maintained. Deviations from these standards made because of collection or staff size should be carefully examined to be certain that they do not jeopardize the basic purpose of cataloging: to provide access to materials.

Despite the increased use of automation in the library field, the traditional card catalog will probably remain the chief tool for access to materials in hospital libraries for some time. Moreover, automated cataloging systems will most likely be based on the traditional catalog card format. Thus a proficiency in cataloging will be needed even with automated systems. A well-developed card catalog is vital for library operation today and could be the basis for an automated catalog in the future.

This chapter will discuss the basic decisions involved in hospital library cataloging. It will provide an overview of cataloging procedures for books and other types of materials. It will also present some basic guidelines for developing efficient cataloging and organizing practices.

CHOOSING A CLASSIFICATION SYSTEM

A 1979 survey of health science libraries in the United States revealed that about 65 percent use the National Library of Medicine (NLM) classification system. A total of 2,775 institutions responded to the survey, including 1,800 hospital libraries (1). Most of the other libraries use the Library of Congress (LC) system or the Dewey classification system. A few older health science libraries use systems such as Barnard (British), Bellevue (nursing), Boston (medical), Black (dentistry), or Cunningham (medical). These systems have not been kept up-to-date and do not provide enough detailed information for classification of current materials. If a library has materials already classified according to any of these systems, it is often most economical to leave these materials as they are and to begin classifying current materials using either the NLM or the LC system. In this way, older materials that are least used will be shelved separately from the newer and more frequently used materials.

National Library of Medicine Classification System

The *National Library of Medicine Classification* fourth edition (revised in 1981) is highly recommended for hospital libraries. See Figure 5-1 for a synopsis of the NLM classification. According to this system, preclinical sciences are placed in schedules QS through QZ. Medicine and related subjects are placed in schedules W through WZ. Any materials that do not fit into QS through QZ or W through WZ are classified according to the LC system. According to the *NLM Classification,*

The various schedules of the *Library of Congress Classification* supplement it (the *NLM Classification*) for subjects bordering on medicine and for general reference material. The LC schedules for human anatomy (QM), microbiology (QR), and medicine (R) are not used at all...since they overlap the *NLM Classification*. On the other hand, LC's psychology schedule (BF), sociology (H), science (Q-QP), and bibliography (Z) are used extensively. Other schedules are used as needed (2:vii).

In a hospital library, the LC schedules for sociology (H) and education (L) are frequently used. The fourth edition of the *NLM Classification* has an excellent index that includes LC numbers used by the NLM. The index consists mainly of NLM subject headings with cross-references. Thus the library need not own a copy of the LC schedules. In addition, the introductory material in the *NLM Classification* provides a very thorough guide to the use of the NLM system.

Understanding some of the principles of organization of the NLM schedules makes them easier to use. Diseases are classified according to the organ or organs involved. Diseases that involve more than one body system are in schedules WC and WD. Body systems are covered individually in schedules WE through WL. Schedules WM through WW cover each major medical specialty. Schedule WY covers nursing. Numbers within each schedule are widely separated to allow the addition of new numbers as knowledge develops. Certain numbers are repeated in each schedule, such as 17 for atlases, 32 for laws, 100 for general works, and 141 for diagnosis. Also, each schedule contains many notes that clarify usage and help the cataloger make decisions. A sample page from the *NLM Classification* is shown in Figure 5-2.

Information about new numbers used by the NLM is found in the following sources: *Notes for Medical Catalogers,* the weekly *NLM Current Catalog Proof Sheets,* and the quarterly cumulations of the *NLM Current Catalog.* * Information is also available in the CATLINE (cataloging online) database.

Using the NLM schedules in a specialized collection, such as a nursing school library, may present problems because of the somewhat restricted range of numbers for nursing. The same problems may arise in collections that specialize in psychiatry or dentistry. Several independently published expansions of these schedules are available and may be useful in such cases (see Appendix A). If additional numbers are inserted, such decisions should be documented and applied consistently. Expanding the schedule locally, however, may cause problems later if NLM assigns a different topic to one of the local numbers.

Some hospital librarians have found that nurses prefer that materials on nursing be shelved with the relevant

---

*For more information on sources cited throughout the chapter, see Appendix A.

medical specialty. For example, materials on pediatric nursing can be shelved with other pediatric materials in WS-rather than in WY 159. Books on pediatric nursing can be classified WSY so that they follow the other materials on pediatrics. Once decisions of this type are made, they must be followed consistently by library staff.

Library of Congress Classification System

In the past a number of health science libraries chose the LC system because they depended on the easy availability of LC printed cards. The fourth edition of the LC's *R Classification Schedule* is inexpensive and easy to obtain. However, it can be kept up-to-date only by subscribing to the quarterly *LC Classification: Additions and Changes.* This publication often arrives late and is somewhat cumbersome to use.

There are other disadvantages to using the LC system. Topics that seem unrelated are grouped together in the same schedule. For example, schedule RA includes Public Aspects of Medicine, Public Health and Hygiene, Medical Centers and Hospitals and Clinics, Forensic Medicine, and Toxicology. Most diseases are classified in schedule RC, which also includes Internal Medicine, Practice of Medicine, Psychiatry, Neoplasms, and Tuberculosis. Nursing materials are in schedule RT and are also scattered throughout the other subdivisions of the R schedule. The index of the R schedule can be helpful in locating specific numbers, although the terms used in the index are not necessarily LC subject headings. Finally, the numbers in the LC system tend to be longer and more complex, as shown in a comparison of the LC system with the NLM system (Figure 5-3).

Figure 5-1
Synopsis of NLM Classification

SYNOPSIS OF CLASSES

PRECLINICAL SCIENCES

QS	Human Anatomy	QW	Microbiology and Immunology
QT	Physiology	QX	Parasitology
QU	Biochemistry	QY	Clinical Pathology
QV	Pharmacology	QZ	Pathology

MEDICINE AND RELATED SUBJECTS

W	Medical Profession	WK	Endocrine System
WA	Public Health	WL	Nervous System
WB	Practice of Medicine	WM	Psychiatry
WC	Infectious Diseases	WN	Radiology
WD 100	Deficiency Diseases	WO	Surgery
WD 200	Metabolic Diseases	WP	Gynecology
WD 300	Diseases of Allergy	WQ	Obstetrics
WD 400	Animal Poisoning	WR	Dermatology
WD 500	Plant Poisoning	WS	Pediatrics
WD 600	Diseases by Physical Agents	WT	Geriatrics. Chronic Disease
WD 700	Aviation and Space Medicine	WU	Dentistry. Oral Surgery
WE	Musculoskeletal System	WV	Otorhinolaryngology
WF	Respiratory System	WW	Ophthalmology
WG	Cardiovascular System	WX	Hospitals
WH	Hemic and Lymphatic Systems	WY	Nursing
WI	Gastrointestinal System	WZ	History of Medicine
WJ	Urogenital System		

Figure 5-2
NLM Schedule—Sample Page

WI

GASTROINTESTINAL SYSTEM

Classify general works on the gastrointestinal system and its diseases in WS 310-312 when related to children; in WY 156.5 when related to nursing. Classify works on nursing of patients with specific diseases in WY number also. Classify works on liver and biliary tract treated together in WI 700-740 and in WI 770 if applicable.

Classify works on gallbladder and other specific parts in WI 750-765 as indicated.

WI 1-250	General
WI 300-387	Stomach
WI 400-575	Intestines
WI 600-650	Anus and Rectum
WI 700-770	Liver and Biliary Tract
WI 800-820	Pancreas
WI 900-970	Abdomen and Abdominal Surgery

* 1   Societies (Cutter from name of society)
Includes ephemeral membership lists issued serially or separately. Classify substantial lists with directories. Classify annual reports, journals, etc., in W1.

       Collections (General)
5   By several authors
7   By individual authors

9   Addresses. Essays. Lectures (General)

11   History (Table G)
11.1   General coverage (Not Table G)

13   Dictionaries. Encyclopedias

15   Classification. Nomenclature

16   Tables. Statistics

17   Atlases. Pictorial works
Classify atlases limited to a particular part of the system here also.

* 18   Education Outlines. Questions and answers. Teachers' instructions. Catalogs and discussions of audiovisual materials.   Computer assisted instruction
Classify here works about education and audiovisual materials. Classify textbooks and actual audiovisual materials by subject.

Figure 5-3
Comparison of LC and NLM Classifications

NLM	SUBJECT	LC
WG 298	Angina Pectoris	RC 685.A6
WG 330	Arrhythmia	RC 685.A65
WG 300	Coronary Occlusion	RC 685.C6
WG 285	Endocarditis	RC 685.E
WX 168	Dietary Services	RA 975.5.D5
WX 215	Emergency Services	RA 975.5.E5
WX 165	Housekeeping	RA 975.5.H6

CHOOSING A SUBJECT HEADINGS LIST

Subject analysis is a vital tool in locating information contained in library materials. The number of subject headings that may be applied to library materials depends on several factors. These factors include the skill of the cataloger and the amount of time allotted to the task; the amount of available catalog card space; and the amount of time available for filing.

Subject headings should reflect the content of an item as broadly or as narrowly as the item itself requires. The cataloger must also consider the needs of the library's users. Subheadings are important in a larger collection since they may lead a user directly to the needed information. In a small collection, however, subheadings may be unnecessary.

A controlled, formal list of subject headings is essential for subject analysis. The librarian may choose among several systems of subject headings.

National Library of Medicine Medical Subject Headings List

The NLM's *Medical Subject Headings* (MeSH) is by far the best choice for hospital libraries. The vocabulary of MeSH is used in *Index Medicus, International Nursing Index, Index to Dental Literature, Hospital Literature Index,* and MEDLARS searching. MeSH is therefore familiar to many hospital personnel and to most hospital librarians. It is prepared by experts who deal with current literature. These experts observe the emergence of new terms and the elimination or revision of older terms. MeSH is inexpensive and is updated annually. It accompanies the January issue of *Index Medicus,* and includes many cross-references to older terms and to terms no longer used.

The *Annotated MeSH* is published annually and is used by NLM indexers, catalogers, and MEDLARS searchers. It contains many notes for catalogers, including "see also" and "see related" references and proscriptions for certain subheadings. Its preliminary pages include excellent explanations of its structure and use as

well as tables for quick reference on the coordination of subheadings with main headings.

Additional references such as *Medical Subject Headings Tree Structures* and *Permuted Medical Subject Headings* are available for librarians wishing to do more precise subject cataloging. *Tree Structures* contains a hierarchical arrangement of MeSH terms that shows relationships between broader and narrower subjects. "*Permuted MeSH* takes each significant word that appears in each MeSH term and, indented under that word, lists all the MeSH terms and cross references in which that word appears" (3).

Library of Congress Subject Headings List

LC subject headings are not always appropriate for health science materials. Figure 5-4 shows that although some headings in the LC and MeSH systems are identical, MeSH contains more specific headings. The ninth edition of *LC Subject Headings,* published in 1980, includes only the headings used through December 1978.

Other Subject Headings

The American Hospital Association's list of subject headings for *Hospital Literature Index* was used by some hospital libraries. In 1978 MeSH was expanded to include many more terms needed to describe hospital literature. All terms currently used in *Hospital Literature Index* are MeSH terms. For more information, see "Subject Headings" in the Readings section at the end of this chapter.

Figure 5-4
Comparison of *LC Subject Headings* (7th edition, 1966) and *MeSH* (1982)

MeSH	LC
Menstruation	Menstruation
Menstruation Disorders	
Menstruation Inducing Agents	
Pregnancy Complications	Pregnancy, Complications of
Pregnancy Complications, Cardiovascular	
Pregnancy Complications, Hematologic	
Pregnancy Complications, Infectious	

Terms used in the *Sears List of Subject Headings* are too general for hospital libraries. They do not reflect current medical usage since they are updated only once every six or seven years.

Local lists are likely to be incomplete, inconsistent, or both. The larger they grow, the more difficult they are to manage efficiently.

DETERMINING CATALOGING INFORMATION

Cataloging information can be generated by library staff members using the work itself. This is known as original cataloging. Authoritative sources such as the LC and the NLM prepare cataloging copy and make it available to health science libraries. The hospital librarian may decide to purchase and use cataloging copy "as is." Librarians sometimes make modifications in this source copy.

The costs involved in making such modifications must be weighed against their possible benefits. For example, the librarian may wish to modify source copy to include fewer or briefer access points, entries, or subject headings. Before making such modifications, however, the librarian should consider whether these additional access points may be needed as the collection grows. Another example is the practice of tracing the sponsoring bodies of meetings. Some hospital librarians feel that this type of catalog card is an unnecessary expense. Others find these additional access points useful for locating published proceedings. In general, accepting the fuller and more specific cataloging of authorities such as the LC and the NLM is probably more economical in the long run. The most common sources of cataloging copy are described below.

Cataloging in Publication

Cataloging in Publication (CIP) information is printed on the verso of the title page of a book. This information is provided to publishers from the LC based on prepublication information submitted to the LC. CIP data includes the LC main entry, call number, subjects and some added entries. For some biomedical titles there are also NLM-assigned call numbers and subject headings but no NLM main entry or notes. Because CIP information is brief and sometimes inaccurate due to the limited data available before publication, it is wise to consult the *NLM Current Catalog Proof Sheets* or CATLINE for revised cataloging information from the NLM.

National Library of Medicine Current Catalog

The *NLM Current Catalog* and the *NLM Current Catalog Proof Sheets* are the publications that provide complete cataloging information for materials in the NLM. They include NLM call numbers and MeSH subject headings. The *NLM Current Catalog* contains many "see-references" that lead to the official entry. The *Proof*

Sheets contain no references, so the librarian must look at both personal and corporate names, as well as title entries, to find the official entry. A title index to the *Proof Sheets* accompanies every fourth issue and is very useful in locating official entries.

National Union Catalog

The *National Union Catalog* is an expensive, multivolume publication that provides complete cataloging information for materials cataloged by the LC. Most hospital libraries do not need to purchase this publication.

Other Sources of Cataloging Information

Computerized databases such as those in OCLC, RLIN, and CATLINE may contain cataloging information from the LC, the NLM, or both. These databases may also have cataloging information from other participating libraries.

Card catalogs or acquisition lists from other libraries can also be consulted to determine how these libraries catalog materials. The librarian may be able to save time by adopting some of the cataloging procedures followed in other libraries.

CATALOGING PROCEDURES

It is important that the librarian adopt and maintain standard procedures for cataloging materials. These procedures include choosing a main entry, assigning added entries, determining descriptive information, assigning a call number, and assigning subject headings. Each of these procedures will be discussed below.

Choosing the Main Entry

The main entry is the access point or heading under which the bibliographic description is entered in the card catalog. The main entry may be the title of the work or the name of a person or corporate body.

The definitions of terms and the explanations of the rules for these cataloging practices were first published in 1949 and were reissued in 1967 as part of the *Anglo-American Cataloging Rules* (AACR1). They were extensively revised and published in 1978 as the second edition of the *Anglo-American Cataloguing Rules* (AACR2), effective January 2, 1981. The effective date was set by mutual agreement among the LC, the NLM, and the National Agricultural Library. This date was also adopted by many academic, public, and special libraries. Both the LC and the NLM announce applications and interpretations of these rules in their publications. These two authorities are usually in agreement on choice of main entry, forms of headings, and bibliographic descriptions. They also collaborate extensively in name authority work.

It is usually best to accept the choice of main entry that is indicated in either the NLM's publications and its CAT-

LINE database records or the LC's publications and its MARC (Machine Readable Cataloging) database records. The experts who select the main entries follow the standards of the AACR2.

Assigning Added Entries

Added entries are access points other than the main entry. They provide additional access to materials for which the exact title or author is not known. Coauthors, previous titles, authors of earlier editions, series and corporate names, and subtitles may be useful as added entries.

In larger libraries it is helpful to have a name authority file that lists the forms of the names used in the card catalog. Cross references to other forms of the names should also be included.

Determining Descriptive Information

The International Standard Bibliographical Description for Monographic Publications (ISBD[M]) was published in 1974 by the International Federation of Library Associations. Since ISBD(M) is an integral part of *AACR2*, its adoption is recommended. However, all information on the catalog card can be tailored to fit the needs of the individual hospital library. The cataloger must decide whether to include the publication statement, names of series, printings, or prior titles and authors. The decisions made should be documented to ensure consistency.

Assigning a Call Number

The three parts of a call number are the classification number, the book number, and the date of publication. Both the LC and the NLM schedules have useful notes and directions for assigning classification numbers. If outside sources of cataloging copy are used, the librarian should examine the classification numbers closely before accepting or modifying them.

Proper classification is essential for optimal use of the collection. It is especially important in hospital libraries that are accessible to employees when the library is not staffed. Having books on the same or similar topics grouped together on the shelf will benefit both the users and the library staff.

The book number represents the main entry. It dictates an alphabetical arrangement of authors or titles within the subject area of the classification number. The Cutter-Sanborn tables are used by the NLM and many other health science libraries. They provide three-digit numbers that represent the first major word of the main entry. The LC has its own system of book numbering that may be adapted for use in the hospital library.

In a very small library, a simple system that uses the first three or four letters of the author's surname may suffice. Any book number can be made more specific by adding a work-mark or a letter from the first major word

of the title. The edition number might also be added after the work-mark to aid in chronological shelving. The NLM does not utilize work-marks for title main entries, nor does it add edition numbers.

The third part of a call number is the date of publication. It may not be necessary to include this information in smaller collections. If the material represents proceedings of a workshop, conference, or congress, the date of the meeting rather than the date of publication is most often used.

In general, the complexity of a call number is determined by the size of the library's collection. Figure 5-5 shows that seven different call numbers may be assigned to a single work, depending on how specific the cataloger wishes to be. The fictitious work used in the figure is *Textbook of Pediatrics* by J. Harmon.

Before assigning a call number, the cataloger should consult the shelf list to make sure that the number is not

Figure 5-5
Call Number Construction

WS **HAR**	Simplest call number: WS represents general area of Pediatrics HAR represents author's surname
WS 100 **HAR** or **WS 100** **HARM**	Adds 100 to represent book that treats Pediatrics in general Adding fourth letter to author's name for separation from Harrison, etc.
WS 100 **H2** or **WS 100** **H28** or **WS 100** **H288**	Three cutter numbers indicate degree of specificity of author's surname
WS 100 **H288t**	Adds work mark "t" representing first word of title
WS 100 **H288t3**	Adds edition number so successive editions will shelve in consecutive order
WS 100 **H288t3** **1980**	Adds publication date for greater specificity
WS 100 **H288t3** **v.1** **1980**	Includes volume number so volumes will shelve in consecutive order

Figure 5-6
Sample Page from *Tree Structures* , 1981

CARDIOVASCULAR DISEASES	C14		
HEART DISEASES	C14.280		
ARRHYTHMIA	C14.280.67		
ARRHYTHMIA, SINUS	C14.280.67.93		
ASYSTOLE *	C14.280.67.146		
AURICULAR FIBRILLATION	C14.280.67.198		
AURICULAR FLUTTER	C14.280.67.248		
BRADYCARDIA	C14.280.67.319		
EXTRASYSTOLE	C14.280.67.470		
HEART BLOCK	C14.280.67.558		
ADAMS-STOKES SYNDROME	C14.280.67.558.137		
BUNDLE-BRANCH BLOCK	C14.280.67.558.323		
SINOATRIAL BLOCK *	C14.280.67.558.750		
WOLFF-PARKINSON-WHITE SYNDROME	C14.280.67.558.865		
SICK SINUS SYNDROME	C14.280.67.829		
TACHYCARDIA	C14.280.67.845		
TACHYCARDIA, PAROXYSMAL	C14.280.67.845.695		
VENTRICULAR FIBRILLATION	C14.280.67.932		
CARCINOID HEART DISEASE *	C14.280.129	C4.557.112	
CARDIAC OUTPUT, LOW	C14.280.148		
CARDIAC TAMPONADE	C14.280.155		
CORONARY DISEASE	C14.280.211		
ANGINA PECTORIS	C14.280.211.198		
ANGINA PECTORIS, VARIANT *	C14.280.211.198.955		
MYOCARDIAL INFARCTION	C14.280.211.637		
SHOCK, CARDIOGENIC	C14.280.211.637.667	C23.888.789.	
ENDOCARDITIS	C14.280.282		
ENDOCARDITIS, BACTERIAL	C14.280.282.407	C1.539.328	
ENDOCARDITIS, SUBACUTE BACTERIAL	C14.280.282.407.407	C1.252.890.	
HEART ANEURYSM	C14.280.358	C14.907.55.	
HEART ARREST	C14.280.383		
HEART ENLARGEMENT	C14.280.409		
HEART FAILURE, CONGESTIVE	C14.280.434		
DYSPNEA, PAROXYSMAL	C14.280.434.313	C8.618.326.	C23.888.852.
EDEMA, CARDIAC *	C14.280.434.482		
HEART NEOPLASMS	C14.280.459	C4.588.894.	
HEART RUPTURE	C14.280.470		
HEART VALVE DISEASES	C14.280.484		
AORTIC VALVE INSUFFICIENCY	C14.280.484.95		
AORTIC VALVE STENOSIS	C14.280.484.150		
MITRAL VALVE INSUFFICIENCY	C14.280.484.461		
MITRAL VALVE PROLAPSE	C14.280.484.505		
MITRAL VALVE STENOSIS	C14.280.484.517		
PULMONARY VALVE INSUFFICIENCY	C14.280.484.660		
PULMONARY VALVE STENOSIS	C14.280.484.716		
TRICUSPID VALVE INSUFFICIENCY	C14.280.484.856		
TRICUSPID VALVE STENOSIS	C14.280.484.911		
MYOCARDIAL DISEASES	C14.280.600		
CARDIOMYOPATHY, ALCOHOLIC	C14.280.600.57	C21.613.53.	
CHAGAS CARDIOMYOPATHY	C14.280.600.190	C3.752.935.	
ENDOCARDIAL FIBROELASTOSIS	C14.280.600.281		
ENDOMYOCARDIAL FIBROSIS	C14.280.600.406		
IDIOPATHIC HYPERTROPHIC			
SUBVALVULAR STENOSIS	C14.280.600.608		
AORTIC SUBVALVULAR STENOSIS *	C14.280.600.608.205		
PULMONARY SUBVALVULAR STENOSIS *	C14.280.600.608.714		
MYOCARDITIS	C14.280.600.625		
PERICARDIAL EFFUSION	C14.280.695	A12.383.594	
HEMOPERICARDIUM *	C14.280.695.463	C23.542.433	
PERICARDITIS	C14.280.720		
PERICARDITIS, CONSTRICTIVE	C14.280.720.595		
PNEUMOPERICARDIUM	C14.280.763		
POSTPERICARDIOTOMY SYNDROME *	C14.280.793	C23.814.668	

*INDICATES MINOR DESCRIPTOR

currently in use. If it is, the proposed number should be modified. The easiest way to do this is to add a second letter to the work-mark. The first letter of the second significant word of the title is generally used.

Assigning Subject Headings

The most important aspect of assigning subject headings is deciding how specific the main headings should be and whether subheadings are needed. When selecting main subject headings, *Tree Structures* may be useful in finding broader or narrower terms. The hierarchical arrangement of MeSH headings in *Tree Structures* can aid in making such choices. This arrangement shows the positions a MeSH term may have in relation to broader and narrower terms. Thus a term may appear in several places, depending on its meaning in each context or category. See Figure 5-6 for a sample page from *Tree Structures.*

If the hospital library uses MeSH, it is likely that the subheadings for language and geography will not be needed. However, form subheadings, such as "legislation" and "directories," and topical subheadings, such as "etiology" and "drug effects," may be very useful. Once a policy on the use of headings and subheadings is adopted, it should be documented and practiced consistently.

A local subject authority file is recommended to keep track of subject headings in local use. This information may be recorded on index cards or on a checklist. The use of a printed subject heading list is not recommended because check marks and annotations would have to be transferred to every new edition of the list.

Cross references in the subject catalog can assist both the users and the library staff. Terms that may seem obvious may not be MeSH forms or may be inverted. For example, materials on management are found under "Hospital Administration" or "Organization and Administration." The MeSH heading for shared services is "Hospital Shared Services" (see Figure 5-7). Cross references are also important when MeSH terms have been changed. Many librarians place a copy of the current MeSH near the card catalog so the cross references printed in it can be used.

It is important to check the annual edition of MeSH for information on headings that have been added, changed, or deleted. Ideally, all such information should be incorporated into the card catalog. If this is not feasible, or if the old terms are preferred, cross references should be inserted. For example, in 1980 the heading "Immunology" was changed to "Allergy and Immunology." A cross-reference card should be filed noting this change (see Figure 5-8).

If changes are made as designated in MeSH, a cross-reference card should be inserted to direct the user to the new heading (see Figure 5-9). This type of cross reference should be kept in the card catalog for about one year.

Figure 5-7
Cross References from Unused Subject Headings

MANAGEMENT

see   Organization and Administration

Hospital Administration

SHARED SERVICES

see   Hospital Shared Services

Figure 5-8
Cross References to New and Retained Subject Headings

ALLERGY AND IMMUNOLOGY

see also Immunology

IMMUNOLOGY

see also Allergy and Immunology

Figure 5-9
**Cross Reference to New Subject Heading
from Discontinued Heading**

IMMUNOLOGY

see Allergy and Immunology

Figure 5-10a
"Dropped" Subject Heading Identified by Check Mark

WW
100
T686e
1967

Toronto Hospital for Sick Children. Department
of Ophthalmology.

The eye in childhood. Chicago, Year Book
Publishers [c1967]

537 p. illus.

✔ 1. Eye Diseases—in infancy & childhood
I. Title

PRODUCING CATALOG CARDS

Typing individual catalog cards is extremely time-consuming and prone to error. There are several methods of making multiple copies from a master card. These methods include making copies using a hand-operated duplicating machine, adaptations to photocopy machines to allow duplication of cards, and having the cards printed in the hospital print shop.

Many hospital librarians purchase printed cards from outside sources. LC printed cards are relatively inexpensive but may need considerable modification. Bibliographic utilities such as OCLC and other commercial sources offer card production services. These sources will be discussed in more detail below in the section on automation. Several factors should be considered in deciding whether to use printed cards. These factors include the type of cataloging used in the library, the number of modifications that the source can make on the card, and the number of modifications required once the cards are received.

FILING CATALOG CARDS

The two most common types of card catalogs are the dictionary catalog and the divided catalog. A dictionary catalog contains a single alphabet with authors, titles, and subjects interfiled. This type of catalog may suffice in a small library, but it requires a method of distinguishing subjects from other access points. This is usually done by overtyping the subject headings in red ink or capital letters.

A divided catalog contains two separate sections. The first has authors and titles interfiled in alphabetical order. The second section has subjects only. Subject headings can be overtyped in the subject catalog, or "dropped" headings and guide cards can be used. This method involves using a separate unit card for each subject. The

Figure 5-10b
Guide Card Tabs for Main Heading and Subheading

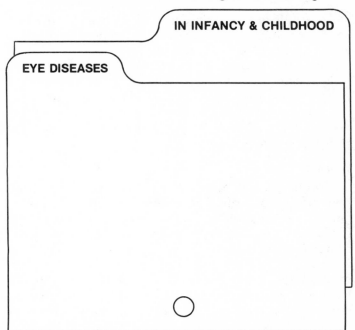

IN INFANCY & CHILDHOOD

EYE DISEASES

subject heading is checked, circled or capitalized in the tracings area of each catalog card so that it stands out from other added entries. All such cards for the same subject may be filed behind a tabbed guide card with the heading typed on the tab. These subject guides also save time when a subject heading is altered or replaced, as often happens with MeSH vocabulary. Only the guide card needs to be replaced in this case. The cards behind it need not be altered (see Figure 5-10).

The separate shelf list, containing catalog cards filed in call number order, is usually the catalog librarian's most important resource. It is consulted regularly to verify that a new call number is not in current use. The shelf list can also be used to record information such as the number of copies owned, replacement cost of items, and accession numbers. The shelf list may also serve as a control for inventory purposes. It functions as a cataloging reference as well. It can be used to compare subject headings chosen for new materials with headings already used for materials having the same or similar classification numbers.

Card filing practices are fairly standardized and are described in such sources as the *American Library Association Filing Rules*. However, there may be local practices that should be documented. These may include interfiling British and American spellings (such as haematology and hematology) and filing the card for the latest edition of a work first. These practices should be noted on cross-reference cards in the catalog or on signs posted near the catalog.

ORGANIZING OTHER LIBRARY MATERIALS

The cataloging procedures described thus far provide a solid basis for cataloging books in the hospital library. Although many of these principles and procedures can be applied to organizing other library materials, these materials sometimes require special handling. Suggestions are given below for organizing the following: journals, government publications, audiovisual materials, microforms, patient education materials, vertical files, and staff publications.

Journals

Most hospital libraries shelve journals separately from books in an alphabetical arrangement by title. The librarian can decide whether journal information should be filed in the card catalog. In many cases, a separate journal reference in the form of a check-in file or a printed list is sufficient. In other cases, it is useful to have complete catalog information filed in the card catalog. This should include a title card, subject cards, and information concerning the volume and year that the library's subscription began (see Figure 5-11).

Certain periodical publications, such as *Medical Clinics of North America* and *DM: Disease-A-Month*, deal with a specific topic in each issue. If the library subscribes to the entire series, the title can be shelved with other journals. However, if the library receives only certain volumes from a series, it may be wiser to classify volumes according to the specific topic and to shelve them with other materials on the same topic (see Figure 5-12).

Government Publications

Many federal, state, and local government publications provide useful information at little or no cost. These

Figure 5-11
Journal Catalog Card

JOUR	Gastroenterology. Baltimore, American Gastroenterological Association.
	v.1- 1943-

LIBRARY KEEPS LAST 10 YEARS

1. Gastroenterology 2. Periodicals—Gastroenterology

publications may be in the form of monographs, serials, or ephemera in print or microform. In most cases, it is best to fully catalog these materials and to integrate them into the collection. Ephemera may be kept in binders or folders.

Many librarians find cataloging such publications difficult, since it is often hard to determine the correct name of the issuing agency. The United States Government Printing Office is the authoritative source for agency names and for descriptive cataloging of federal publications. Cataloging information appears in the *Monthly Catalog of United States Government Publications*.

Audiovisual Materials

Audiovisual materials may be organized in different ways, depending on several factors. These factors include how the collection is to be used, how much shelf space is

Figure 5-12
Single Issue of Periodical Classified

WL **100** **S989s** **1979**	Symposium in clinical neurology: new approaches to old problems. William K. Hass, guest editor. Philadelphia, Saunders, 1979. viii, 260 p. (Medical clinics of North America, vol. 63, no. 4, July 1979)

1. Nervous System Diseases I. Hass, William K., ed. II. Series

available, and the types of special packaging available. Audiovisual materials can be shelved and listed separately, using a catalog or a printed list. They can be cataloged with the cards integrated into the general card catalog, but shelved separately. Audiovisual materials can even be shelved in the main collection, although this is not usually recommended.

The title is usually the main entry for audiovisual materials. The following information should also be noted: type of format, length, color or black-and-white, size, and date issued. Added entries can also be useful for names of producers, sponsoring agencies, or associations. In the subject catalog, it may be useful to establish a file of all audiovisual titles under the main heading "Audiovisual Aids," subdivided by subject (see Figure 5-13).

Authoritative cataloging of audiovisual materials is available from the NLM in its AVLINE database and in the *NLM Audiovisuals Catalog*, which consists of selected citations from AVLINE (Audiovisuals online). This catalog is issued quarterly, and every fourth issue is an annual cumulation. Each issue contains full cataloging information in the name and title sections for both monograph and serial titles. Cataloging information for audiovisual serials also appears in the serials sections of the quarterly, annual, and quinquennial *NLM Current Catalog*. Beginning in 1982, the NLM's weekly *Current Catalog Proof Sheets* include cataloging information for monographic audiovisuals in the English language. These are listed in a separate audiovisuals section. For more information on cataloging and organizing audiovisual materials, see Chapter 10.

Figure 5-13
Cataloging Audiovisual Formats (AACR2)

---

video cassette
WJ
378
C762
1982
Continual ambulatory peritoneal dialysis [video-recording] / presented by Department of Nursing, Grady Memorial Hospital. — Atlanta, Ga. : Emory Medical Television Network, 1982.
1 videocassette (27 min.) : sd., col. : 3/4 in.
Credits: Dee Clowers.
Approved for continuing medical education credit by the AMA.

   1. Ambulatory Care—videocassettes 2. Peritoneal Dialysis 3. Audio-Visual Aids—Ambulatory Care 4. Audio-Visual Aids—Peritoneal Dialysis I. Clowers, Dee II. Emory Medical Television Network III. Grady Memorial Hospital. Department of Nursing

---

motion picture
QV
350
K48
1981
Killing of bacteria by antibiotics [motion picture] — Indianapolis : Eli Lilly, c 1981.
1 film reel (21 min.) : sd., col. : 16 mm.
Credits: Consultant, Gerald L. Mandell.

   1. Antibiotics—pharmacodynamics—motion pictures 2. Bacteria—drug effects—motion pictures 3. Audio-Visual Aids—Antibiotics 4. Audio-Visual Aids—Bacteria I. Mandell, Gerald Lee, 1936-   II. Eli Lilly and Company

---

sound cassette
WF
980
T487
1980
Thoracic surgery [sound recording] / American College of Surgeons. — Chicago : The College, 1980.
12 sound cassettes (720 min.) : 1 7/8 ips + 1 guide — (Postgraduate course ; 1980, 8) (ACS/clinitapes)
Credits: Chairman: Benson B. Roe.
Includes guide (xiii, 115 p.).
Recorded at the 66th annual clinical congress of the American College of Surgeons, Oct. 19-24, 1980 in Atlanta.
   1. Thoracic Surgery—audiocassettes 2. Audio-Visual Aids—Thoracic Surgery I. Roe, Benson B. II. American College of Surgeons III. Series IV. Series

---

slide
WP
870
C929c
1982
Crile, George, 1907-
   Changing concepts in the treatment of breast cancer [slide] / George Crile, Jr. — New York : Medcom, 1982.
45 slides : col. + 1 sound cassette (29 min. : 1 7/8 ips) + 1 guide. — (Medcom famous teachings in modern medicine)
Includes guide (32 p.) and post-test.

   1. Breast Neoplasms—therapy—slides 2. Audio-Visual Aids—Breast Neoplasms I. Title II. Series

Microforms

Because microforms are on cards or reels, they are not usually shelved with books. However, they should be fully cataloged (see Figure 5-14). Information on cataloging and describing microforms is found in the AACR2. There is some disagreement regarding using the AACR2 to catalog microforms that are reproductions of previously published works. Some authorities believe that the original publication should be emphasized as was done in the AACR1. Others believe that the microform itself should be emphasized, as is recommended in AACR2. Pending resolution of the problem, the national libraries have issued a joint statement indicating that they will continue to follow the AACR1 for describing microform reproductions of books and serials. The AACR2 will be applied for choice and form of access points.

Patient Education Materials

It is usually best to shelve patient education materials separately from the main collection. The medical staff sometimes objects to the practice of intershelving patient materials with professional materials, since this brings patients into direct contact with clinical materials. A decision on this matter should be made in consultation with members of the medical staff and the hospital administration.

If patient education materials are shelved separately, subject cards should be interfiled in the main catalog so that these materials are accessible to the professional staff. A separate subject heading such as "Patient Education Materials" could also be added to the card catalog.

Some librarians set up a separate card catalog for patient education materials. Subject cards in this catalog should use terms or headings that are familiar to most lay persons. Unless a standard list of terms is used, it will be necessary to document terms to ensure that they are used consistently. See Chapter 21 for further information on patient education materials.

Vertical Files

Vertical files are an excellent means of organizing special types of materials, such as articles, pamphlets, and copies of laws and regulations. Cataloging of these materials is not usually required. They can be grouped together in folders by topic, issuing body, or title. An index to the file can be arranged by subject, agency, or title. A simple guide to the file allows users to find materials without a librarian's help. In certain cases, materials in the file can be cataloged, depending on the length of time they will be kept and the amount of staff time available for cataloging.

In smaller libraries, vertical files might be sufficient for organizing government publications. All materials from a single source can be kept in one folder. All vertical files should be weeded regularly to discard unneeded materials.

Staff Publications

Hospital librarians have a responsibility to learn of and acquire staff publications. This can sometimes be difficult. In some hospitals, staff members are more than willing to inform the library of their publications and often will donate a copy of their articles or books. In smaller hospitals, the librarian can generally make informal requests for information about staff members' publications. In larger hospitals, more formal methods of finding out about publications may be necessary.

The librarian may wish to scan the tables of contents of journals received in the library to discover staff publications. A listing of staff publications received in the library may be included in the acquisitions bulletin. This may inspire other staff members to inform the librarian of their work. Also, the librarian may wish to remind staff members of the library's interest in their publications. This can be done by issuing a memo or by talking to staff members personally. The librarian may also wish to prepare a special display of staff publications.

Reprints of articles by staff may be kept on a special shelf in folders or in three-ring notebooks. They can be arranged by subject or by author.

PROCESSING MATERIALS

When a new item is received, certain information is usually marked on it. Such information may include accession number, date received or processed, call number, and the name of the library or the department to which the book is permanently assigned. The call number is placed on the upper or lower part of the book's spine. If the spine is too narrow to accommodate the whole call number, it may be placed on the front cover. Whenever possible, the spine should be used so that the call number can be read without removing the book from the shelf.

Figure 5-14
Cataloging a Microform (AACR2)

Micro-	Bush, George Pollock
Fiche	Technology and copyright: annotated bib-
Z	liography and source materials. George P.
642	Bush, editor. Foreword by Lowell H. Hattery.
B978t	Mt. Airy, Md., Lomond Systems, 1972.
1972	viii, 454 p. 24 cm.

Microfiche (negative). 5 sheets (10.5 x 15 cm.)

1. Copyright I. Title

If the library permits circulation of materials, book pockets and cards can be used for control. Book pockets are usually fastened to the inside front or back cover. Care should be taken to avoid covering tables or charts that may be printed on the end papers. The book pocket is a good location for special labels or notices, such as "Reference Only," "Overnight Use Only," or "3-day Loan."

In addition to processing new material, the librarian may also have to mend damaged materials. In most cases, only the most basic repairs should be attempted. It may also be necessary to bind or collect materials to preserve or organize them. Methods for doing so include using file folders, looseleaf binders, in-house machine binding, and commercial binding. See Chapter 6 and Chapter 23 for more information on binding and mending library materials.

PUBLICIZING NEW LIBRARY MATERIALS

The size of the parent institution has direct bearing on bulletins, news items, and publicity about new acquisitions that the library may want to disseminate. Large libraries, especially in teaching institutions, may find monthly acquisitions bulletins, generated from the library, to be extremely helpful to users. In other situations, a selected list of new titles in an in-house publication may be sufficient. In small, community hospitals, a quarterly memorandum is often adequate. In addition, a personal note to interested staff about specific purchases is usually appreciated. For example, when a book is received in a specialty area or when a specific book requested by a staff member arrives, an informal note or phone call announcing its arrival is good policy.

AUTOMATION AND AUTOMATED CATALOGING SERVICES

Automated bibliographic utilities are expanding rapidly and improving their services steadily. All are based on growing databases stored in their computers. Databases for cataloging may be compiled from the LC's MARC tapes, the NLM's CATLINE tapes, and user contributions. Major utilities include Online Computer Library Center, Inc. (OCLC), Washington Library Network (WLN), Research Libraries Information Network (RLIN), and the University of Toronto Library Automation System (UTLAS). The librarian may wish to engage the services of bibliographic utilities directly or through

Figure 5-15
**Cost Comparison Between Manual
and Automated Cataloging**

MANUAL TIME	PROCEDURE		AUTOMATED TIME
(variable)	1. Search for catalog copy		(variable)
5-30 min.	*Manual:*	hand search printed tools	
	Automated:	machine search database	1-3 min.
	2. Copy cataloging if found		
5-10 min.	*Manual:*	hand copy or photocopy	
	Automated:	printout from terminal screen	30-60 sec.
	3. Consult shelf list and catalog to verify call number, names,		
5-20 min.	subjects for new item		5-20 min.
	4. Prepare new catalog unit card		
20 min.	*Manual:*	type master card for reproduction, proofread	
	Automated:	edit on terminal screen and order "produce"	3-5 min.
	5. Receive sets of new catalog cards		
30 min. - ? hrs.	*Manual:*	overtype added entries and subject, sort and alphabetize before filing	
	Automated:	overtyping, sorting, and alphabetizing already done; ready for filing	none
	6. *Costs:*	salaries divided by time used plus charges	app. $1.40/title
$.05-.10/card		for card stock and services	app. $.042/card

vendors who provide indirect access to these utilities.

Automatic catalog card production and authoritative cataloging information are available through bibliographic utilities. The hospital librarian who catalogs as few as two hundred items a year may find that automation saves both time and money. Smaller hospital libraries may wish to join or form a consortium to access a utility. Among OCLC's networks, there are a number of consortia that have been developed by medical center and medical school libraries to assist local hospital libraries (see Appendix B).

Many hospital librarians are already familiar with the advantages of the NLM's MEDLARS services, particularly MEDLINE. They can also query the NLM's CATLINE, AVLINE, or SERLINE databases for information on cataloging books, audiovisuals and serials. Cataloging information available through CATLINE reflects the NLM's standards and can be easily adapted. CATLINE records provide information that can be used for local catalog card production.

There are also cooperative library organizations that provide catalog cards, spine labels, and book card and book pocket labels. Some commercial vendors offer similar services. In general, these services are fast, reliable, and relatively inexpensive. A list of bibliographic utilities, commercial vendors, and cooperative library organizations appears in Appendix B.

The librarian should consider several factors when deciding which of these services are needed. These factors include the size and expertise of the library staff, the size of the collection and its potential for growth, the need for reclassification of materials from an older collection, and the library's budget. The recent expansion of computer technology has lowered the cost of hardware. Thus automation of many library functions is proving to be cost-effective (see Figure 5-15).

The hospital may already own computer equipment or purchase computer services. The librarian may wish to consult with the hospital administration to learn how the library might participate in the hospital's system.

There is no doubt that automation speeds up cataloging and processing. It also relieves both professional and clerical personnel of many repetitive tasks. Even the smallest hospital library can participate in local, regional, national, and eventually international networks of libraries by becoming involved in automated systems. The library may retain some of its individual practices while using these systems. However, it may benefit by abandoning some of its unique practices in favor of the more standard practices utilized in automated networks.

DEVELOPING EFFICIENT CATALOGING PRACTICES

The manner in which cataloging activities are carried out depends on several factors. These factors include the type of collection and its potential for growth, the number of library employees and the type of training they have, the library's budget, and the equipment and space available. Each librarian must develop procedures that are appropriate to his or her situation.

It is important to set aside a regular block of time for cataloging. Postponing cataloging until the librarian has "free" time usually results in information being withheld from the library's users. Batching new materials to be cataloged at one time is efficient. New materials should be cataloged promptly, however, so cataloging once a week probably represents optimal timing, regardless of the size of the batch.

The librarian should develop a cataloging manual containing guidelines for cataloging and cataloging policies and procedures. This manual will ensure consistent practice in making cataloging decisions such as form of names used, kinds of added entries that will be made, type of subject headings, form of call numbers, and treatment of series. The manual should be kept up-to-date and should include examples.

It is suggested that cataloging and processing procedures be evaluated periodically. The librarian needs to determine if cataloging is being done promptly, accurately, neatly, and consistently. Also, he or she must determine if the card catalog functions as a useful tool for both users and library staff.

REFERENCES

1. Rees AM, Crawford SY. Directory of health sciences libraries in the United States, 1979. Cleveland: Cleveland Health Sciences Library, 1980. (Health science information series, Vol. 3, no. 1).

2. National Library of Medicine classification, 4th ed, rev. Bethesda, MD: National Library of Medicine, 1981.

3. National Library of Medicine. Permuted medical subject headings. Springfield, VA: National Technical Information Service, 1982. Annual.

READINGS

AACR2 AND CARD CATALOGS

Chan LM. Cataloging and classification: an introduction. New York: McGraw-Hill, 1981.

Gorman M. The Anglo-American cataloguing rules, 2d ed. Lib Res Tech Serv 1978 Summer;22:209-226.

Gorman M. The concise AACR2: being and rewritten and simplified version of Anglo-American cataloguing rules, second edition. Chicago: American Library Association; Ottawa: Canadian Library Association; London: The Library Association, 1981.

Hagler R. Where's that rule? A cross-index of the two editions of the Anglo-American cataloguing rules. Ottawa: Canadian Library Association, 1979. Distributed in the United States by the American Library Association.

Hunter EJ. AACR2: an introduction to the second edition of the Anglo-American cataloging rule rev. ed. Hamden, CT: Linnet Books, 1979.

Malinconico SM, Fasano P. The future of the catalog. White Plains, NY: Knowledge Industry, 1979.

Maxwell MF. Handbook for AACR2: explaining and illustrating Anglo-American cataloguing rules, 2d ed. Chicago: American Library Association, 1980.

Norie E. False economy: or, sabotage at the catalog! Lib Res Tech Serv 1980 Winter;24:69-70.

Potter WG. When names collide: conflict in the catalog and AACR2. Lib Res Tech Serv 1980 Winter;24:3-16.

AUDIOVISUALS CLASSIFICATION AND PROCESSING

Brantz MH, Forsman R. Classification and audiovisuals. Bull Med Libr Assoc 1977 April;65:261-264.

Fleischer EB, Goodman H. Cataloguing audiovisual materials: a manual based on the Anglo-American cataloguing rules II. New York: Neal-Schuman, 1980

Kaufman J. A system for cataloging and classifying visual resources. Lib Res Tech Serv 1979 Spring;23:168-174.

Mann TJ. A system for processing and shelving works of mixed media format. Lib Res Tech Serv 1979 Spring;23:163-167.

Olson NB. Cataloging of audio-visual materials: a manual based on AACR2. Mankato, MN: Minnesota Scholarly Press, 1981.

AUTOMATION AND NETWORKS

Allison AM, Allan A, eds. OCLC, a national library network. Short Hills, NJ: Enslow Pub., 1979.

Braden S, Hall JD, Britton HH. Utilization of personnel and bibliographic resources for cataloging by OCLC participating libraries. Lib Res Tech Serv 1980 Spring;24:135-154.

De Gennaro R. Research libraries enter the information age; The 1979 Richard Rogers Bowker memorial lecture. Lib J 1979 Nov 15;104: 2405-2410.

Jacob ME, Woods R, Yarborough J, comps, Martin SK, ed. Online resource sharing II: a comparison of OCLC, Incorporated, Research Libraries Information Network, and Washington Library Network. San Jose, CA: California Library Authority for Systems and Services, 1979.

Martin SK. Library networks 1981-82. White Plains, NY: Knowledge Industry, 1981.

Matthews JR. The four bibliographic utilities: a comparison. Lib Tech Rep 1979 Nov/Dec;15:665-838.

COSTS IN TECHNICAL SERVICES

Allen CW, Branson JR. OCLC for the hospital library: the justification plan for hospital administration. Bull Med Libr Assoc 1982 Jul;70: 293-297.

Angold L. Cost and time analysis of monograph cataloging in hospital libraries: a preliminary study. 1969. Detroit, MI: Wayne State University, School of Medicine, Library and Biomedical Information Center, 1969. (Wayne State University, School of Medicine, Library and Biomedical Information Service Center, Rep. no. 51).

Dolby JL, Forsyth VJ. An analysis of cost factors in maintaining and updating card catalogs. J Libr Automation 1969 Dec;2:218-241.

Tesovnik ME, DeHart FE. Unpublished studies of technical service time and costs: a selected bibliography. Lib Res Tech Serv 1970 Winter;14:56-67.

West MW, Baxter BA. Unpublished studies of technical service time and costs: a supplement. Lib Res Tech Serv 1976 Fall;20:326-333.

GOVERNMENT DOCUMENTS

Heck LA. Organizing and maintaining a document collection in a health systems agency: suggested resources. Washington: National Health Planning Information Center, 1978. (DHEW publication no. [HRA]79-14011) (Health planning methods and technology ser. 9).

PATIENT EDUCATION MATERIALS

Sorrentino S, Goodchild EY, Fierberg J. Cataloging procedures and catalog organization for patient education materials. Bull Med Libr Assoc 1979 Apr;67:257-260.

PROCESSING CENTERS

American Library Association Resources and Technical Services Division, Commercial Processing Services Committee. Checklist for commercial processing services. Lib Res Tech Serv 1979 Spring;23:177-182.

Cooperative regional centralized processing centers directory. Salisbury, MD: Maryland Materials Center, 1978.

RECLASSIFICATION

Compton A. Reclassification of a small hospital library collection. Bull Med Libr Assoc 1977 July;65:379-381.

Tong JG, Brennen PW, Byrd GD. Reclassification in a small decentralized medical library. Bull Med Libr Assoc 1977 July;65:354-359.

SUBJECT HEADINGS

American Hospital Association. Hospital literature subject headings. 1977 ed. Chicago: American Hospital Association, 1977.

American Hospital Association. Hospital literature subject headings transition guide to medical subject headings. 1978 ed. Chicago: American Hospital Association, 1978.

VERTICAL FILES

Miller S. The vertical file and its satellites: a handbook of acquisition, processing, and organization. 2d ed. Littleton, CO: Libraries Unlimited, 1979.

APPENDIX A
Sources of Information for Cataloging and Classifying

American Library Association Filing Committee. ALA filing rules. Chicago: American Library Association, 1980.

Anglo-American cataloging rules. North American text. Chicago: American Library Association, 1967.

Anglo-American cataloguing rules. 2d ed. Gorman M, Winkler PW, eds. Chicago: American Library Association, 1978. Ottawa: Canadian Library Association, 1978.

Black AD. Classification for dental literature: a revision of the classification devised by Arthur D. Black. Chicago: American Dental Association Bureau of Library and Indexing Services, 1972.

Caffarel Sr. A. Classification of clinical nursing texts: a new approach. Bull Med Libr Assoc 1978 Jan;66;52-55.

Cutter-Sanborn three-figure author table. Swanson-Swift revision. Littleton, CO: Libraries Unlimited, 1969.

Immroth JP. A guide to the Library of Congress classification. 3d ed. by Lois Mai Chan. Littleton, CO: Libraries Unlimited, 1980; 83-85.

International Federation of Library Associations. ISBD (M), International Standard Bibliographical Description for Monographic Publications. 1st standard ed. London: IFLA Committee on Cataloguing, 1974.

Kamenoff L. Classification of nursing texts in a hospital library. Bull Med Libr Assoc 1979 Apr;67:247-251.

Library of Congress. Cataloging Distribution Service. R classification schedule. 4th ed, 1980.

Library of Congress. Processing Department, Catalog Publication Division. National union catalog. Washington: The Library of Congress, 1956-. Monthly. Quarterly, annual, and quinquennial cumulations.

Library of Congress. Processing Services. Cataloging service bulletin. Quarterly.

Library of Congress subject headings. 9th ed. Washington: Library of Congress, 1980. Includes headings existing through December 1978. Subsequent quarterly issues on microfiche and microfilm, 1979-.

Meyn MF, Thome MM. A new method of classifying clinical nursing monographs. Bull Med Libr Assoc 1978 Oct;66:460-461.

Monthly catalog of United States government publications. Washington, DC: Government Printing Office, 1895-. Monthly.

National Library of Medicine. Medical subject headings (MeSH). Bethesda, MD: National Library of Medicine, 1960-. Annual. Also issued as Part 2 of January *Index Medicus* and includes *Tree Structures.*

National Library of Medicine. Medical subject headings, annotated alphabetic list. Springfield, VA: National Technical Information Service. Annual.

National Library of Medicine. Medical subject headings tree structures. Springfield, VA: National Technical Information Service. Annual.

National Library of Medicine. Notes for medical catalogers. Chicago: Medical Library Association. Annual cumulations from National Technical Information Service; quarterly issues as separate sections in quarterly *Current catalog,* 1981-.

National Library of Medicine audiovisuals catalog. Bethesda, MD: National Library of Medicine, 1977-. Quarterly.

National Library of Medicine current catalog. Bethesda, MD: National Library of Medicine, 1966-. Quarterly. Annual and five-year cumulations.

National Library of Medicine current catalog proof sheets. Chicago: Medical Library Association, 1969-. Weekly.

Strauss CD. A suggested expansion of the NLM scheme for dentistry. Bull Med Libr Assoc 1973 July;61:328-332.

Westby BM, ed. Sears list of subject headings. 12th ed. New York: Wilson, 1982.

Note: Unless otherwise indicated, NLM publications are ordered through the Superintendent of Documents, Washington, DC 20402; or, National Technical Information Service, 5285 Port Royal Road, Springfield, VA 22161. LC publications are ordered from Catalog Distribution Service, Library of Congress, Washington, DC 20541.

APPENDIX B
A Partial List of Resources

BIBLIOGRAPHIC UTILITIES

OCLC, Inc. 6565 Frantz Road, Dublin OH 43221.

Research Libraries Information Network (RLIN). Research Libraries Group, Inc. Jordan Quadrangle, Stanford, CA 94305.

Washington Library Network (WLN). Washington State Library. Olympia, Washington 98504.

COMMERCIAL VENDORS

Bibliographic Retrieval Services, Inc. (BRS). 702 Corporation Park, Scotia, New York 12302.

Brodart, Inc. Book Catalog System. 500 Arch Street, Williamsport, Pennsylvania 43215. (Dewey and LC only.)

MARCIVE, Inc. P.O. Box 12408. San Antonio, Texas 78212.

CONSORTIA WITHIN OCLC MEMBERSHIP

District of Columbia Health Sciences Information Network (DOCHSIN). Georgetown University Medical Center, 3900 Reservoir Road N.W., Washington, District of Columbia 20007.

Medical Library Center of New York. 17 East 102nd Street, New York, New York 10029.

Northeastern Ohio Universities College of Medicine. Basic Medical Sciences Library. 4209 State Route 44, Rootstown, Ohio 44272.

Wayne State University School of Medicine. Shiffman Medical Library. 4325 Brush Street, Detroit, Michigan 48202.

Wright State University School of Medicine. Health Sciences Library. Colonel Glenn Highway, Dayton, Ohio 45435.

University of South Carolina School of Medicine Library. Columbia, South Carolina 29208.

COOPERATIVE LIBRARY ORGANIZATIONS

American library directory. Jaques Cattell Press, ed. New York: Bowker. See section: "Networks, consortia, and other cooperative library organizations." Annual.

Cooperative College Library Center. Suite 602, 159 Forrest Avenue, Atlanta, Georgia 30303.

Directory of library networks and cooperative library organizations, 1980. Washington, DC: National Center for Education Statistics, 1980. Available from Supt. of Docs., U.S. G.P.O., Washington, DC 20402.

Indiana Cooperative Library Services Authority (INCOLSA). 1100 West 42nd Street, Indianapolis, Indiana 46208.

State Library of Ohio. Processing Center. 65 South Front Street, Columbus, Ohio 43215.

Note: A comprehensive source book is the *Handbook of Medical Library Practice*, 4th ed. 3 vols. Darling L, ed. Chicago: Medical Library Asssociation, 1982-.

CHAPTER 6

Circulation and Maintenance of Library Materials

Judith M. Topper
Health Sciences Librarian
Lawrence Hospital
Bronxville, New York

CHAPTER 6

Circulation and Maintenance of Library Materials

Judith M. Topper
Health Sciences Librarian
Lawrence Hospital
Bronxville, New York

USER POPULATION

CIRCULATION POLICY
  Borrowing Privileges
  Circulating and Noncirculating Materials
  Loan Periods

CIRCULATION CONTROL
  Manual Systems
  Automated Systems
  Journal Routing

SECURITY AND ACCESS
  Access During Staffed Hours
  After-hours Access
  Control Systems

INVENTORIES

MATERIALS USAGE STUDIES

CURRENCY OF THE COLLECTION
  Weeding Book Collections
  Weeding Audiovisuals
  Canceling Journals

EFFECTIVE USE OF SPACE
  Determining Journal Retention Periods
  Storing Portions of the Collection
  Using Compact Shelving
  Converting to Microforms
  Participating in Cooperative Acquisitions
    Programs

PRESERVATION OF MATERIALS

BINDING

INTERDEPENDENCE OF LIBRARY
  OPERATIONS

Figures

A major function of the hospital library is to provide conditions for optimal use of library materials, both inside and outside the library. Policies and procedures which govern user groups, circulation of materials, and security of those materials are essential to effective library operation. This chapter also considers issues important to maintaining a useful and usable collection: the currency of the collection, the effective use of space, and the preservation of materials.

USER POPULATION

Defining who will use the library's services and resources is a fundamental policy decision in a hospital library. Today, most hospital libraries serve the medical and hospital staffs, although the depth and balance of service varies considerably.

In any hospital library, the user policies should reflect and advance the goals of the parent institution. Hospitals with strong teaching commitments, for example, should provide active library support for students. If a hospital wants to encourage continuing education of allied health personnel, it should include them in the library's user population. A hospital that seeks greater support from its community may wish to extend library privileges in some form to the public. The establishment of user policies most often involves collaboration among the librarian, the library committee, and the hospital administration. Decisions concerning eligible user groups and the services to which each is entitled should be included in the library's written policies and procedures. Figure 6-1 gives an outline of a circulation and use policy that includes this information.

Sometimes a librarian's decision to extend library privileges to all potential user groups within the hospital may be questioned by the medical staff. If this occurs, the librarian can usually overcome the opposition by citing the standards for professional library services of the Joint Commission on Accreditation of Hospitals (JCAH), by obtaining approval from the library committee, and by demonstrating that service to the physicians will not suffer.

Hospital librarians may not all agree on the necessity of collecting statistics on library users. The librarians who do collect statistics should balance the time required to gather them against their usefulness. Some librarians prefer to make a special, limited-time study of library users for a particular purpose, such as providing guidance for planning and budgeting, or supplying data concerning a use-related need, like increased seating space. Such studies are described by Martin (1), Port (2), and others.

Among the statistics that may be collected are a gross daily count; a count by profession or category such as doctor, nurse, or patient; a time of day count; and a count that identifies the purpose for using the library. These statistics can be used by the librarian for widely differing purposes. Figure 6-2 shows one type of form for collecting data on visitors to the library. The categories chosen for this form should reflect an individual library's clientele. Manual "counters" provide an alternative to pencil-and-paper recording. The counter is advanced for each visitor, and the total is recorded on a shorter version of the form in Figure 6-2.

Figure 6-1
Circulation and Use Policy: Topical Outline

Name of Library
Name of Hospital
Address
Circulation and Use Policy

I.   Purpose of policy

II. Use of the library
   A.   Primary clientele
     1.   Categories included
     2.   Services available
   B.   Use by nonaffiliated persons
     1.   Categories admitted
     2.   Services available
   C.   Hours
     1.   Staffed times
     2.   After-hours access
   D.   Registration of borrowers

III. Circulation policy
   A.   Circulating materials
     1.   Formats
     2.   Loan periods
   B.   Limited circulation materials
     1.   Formats
     2.   Loan periods
   C.   Noncirculating materials
   D.   Charging and discharging procedures
   E.   Policies for materials currently on loan
     1.   Reserve
     2.   Recall
   F.   Renewals
   G.   Responsibility for materials loaned
     1.   Charges for lost or damaged items
     2.   Refund policy
   H.   Overdue materials
     1.   Notices
     2.   Fines
   I.   Enforcement of regulations

IV. Review of the circulation policy
   A.   Frequency
   B.   Approval of changes

Date of adoption or latest revision

CIRCULATION POLICY

A circulation policy should balance the advantages of having an entire collection available in the library against the desire of the clientele to borrow materials for outside use. Since these two aims are in fundamental conflict, the circulation policy must provide an equitable compromise. Basically, three decisions must be made: (1) What categories of users may borrow from the library? (2) What categories of materials will circulate? and (3) What will be the loan period for each type of material?

The circulation policy should be included in the library's written policies and procedures. It should be reviewed periodically to evaluate its effectiveness in serving users' needs.

Borrowing Privileges

The nature of the relationship between the library's users and the parent institution is of paramount importance in deciding who may borrow. A library's primary clientele usually consists of the hospital's medical staff, nurses, residents, general employee population, and affiliated students. Persons who are not affiliated with the hospital, but are being served by the library, make up the secondary clientele. Borrowing privileges are often extended to the primary and not to the secondary clientele.

In some cases, primary users are further subdivided by their position in the hospital. For example, staff physicians may be given more liberal borrowing privileges than nurses, residents, or other employees. Distinctions of this sort may serve a purpose in libraries where different levels of service are appropriate for various user groups and meet specific goals of the library. These practices are harder to justify in health care institutions where achievement of optimal patient care is the goal. Pragmatically, the work of the library staff is simplified when all primary clients have the same borrowing privileges. In actual practice, however, distinctions in privileges on the basis of position sometimes exist, and librarians may have to accept them, at least for a time.

Circulating and Noncirculating Materials

Some circulation policy decisions relate to the characteristics of the materials, rather than to the categories of the users. The level of demand for particular items in a collection is an important consideration in determining whether the items will be available as circulating or noncirculating materials or whether the normal loan period will be shortened. Accordingly, a library may restrict current journal issues to use in the library, allow other

Figure 6-2
Visitor Statistics Form

WEST CENTRAL HOSPITAL LIBRARY

Visitors to Library in _____
mo./yr.

Date	Attending Physicians	Residents	Nurses	Students	Other Hospital	Public
1						
2						
3						
4						
5						
29						
30						
31						
Total						

issues of the current volume to circulate for a short time, and lend older journals for longer periods. Such considerations as the length of time required to read the material and whether all or only part of it will be read influence how long materials will circulate. Because of these factors, many libraries lend monographs for a longer time than journal issues.

The overall size of the collection may also influence circulation policy. With a very small collection, the librarian may wish to retain all materials for use in the library. Even in a larger library, basic materials such as indexes, dictionaries, and directories should be available in the library at all times. Many librarians also restrict circulation of basic texts in each subject. Finally, some types of materials are restricted to use in the library because of their format or fragile nature. Microforms, some audiovisuals, and old or rare books are examples.

If a library establishes a restrictive circulation policy, it must take other measures to make its materials available. The number of staffed hours should be extended, and arrangements should be made for after-hours access. Of equal importance is the availability of convenient photocopying equipment. Roberts has described a 135 percent increase in photocopying following institution of a restrictive journal circulation policy (3). Whatever type of circulation policy is adopted, however, a balance must be sought between the need of the library to have its materials on hand for all users and the desire of individual clients to use them elsewhere.

A reserve policy may be implemented to achieve such a balance for certain categories of high-demand materials. Items placed on reserve are usually loaned for a few hours or overnight to minimize their absence from the library. Materials that are frequently used or frequently stolen may be put permanently on reserve. They may be shelved in a separate area or left on the regular shelves and identified by special labels. Temporary reserve may be considered when students' special course assignments require the use of a limited number of specific titles. Items on temporary reserve are usually kept near or behind the circulation desk. Their customary place on the shelf should be marked with a shelf dummy and the cards in the catalog flagged to indicate reserve status.

Loan Periods

Loan periods for circulating materials vary according to the type of material and the status of the borrower. Buckland (4) and Bookstein (5) describe the effects of changes in the length of loan periods. A common-length loan period is easiest to administer, an overriding consideration in a one-person library. Variable loan periods, however, are based on differences in demand and reading time and maximize the use of the collection.

The renewal of loans should also be covered in the library circulation policy. Should the library permit loan renewals; if so, how many times? Should the library require that the item be returned for a period of time before it is borrowed again by the same person?

The library may wish to offer some special provision for long-term loans beyond the normal renewal period. Although such loans remove certain books from the library for extended periods of time, the books can be accessed through the card catalog and recalled, if needed. In addition, the librarian can telephone borrowers periodically to verify that they still need the materials they have. A major advantage of long-term loans is that they offer a compromise between departmental ownership of materials and ownership by the hospital library. When materials are primarily used by one department such as purchasing or security, long-term loans can provide an alternative to developing a departmental collection.

CIRCULATION CONTROL

Circulation control refers to the process of recording the whereabouts of materials on loan and of assuring their prompt return. The necessary attributes of a circulation control system in a special library, as detailed in a study by Fry and Associates (6), include: (1) identifying materials borrowed, (2) identifying borrowers, (3) providing means for securing the return of overdue materials, (4) providing a borrowing count, and (5) making requested books available through reserve and recall. A hospital librarian may also find it useful to be able to identify the items each borrower has on loan. In addition, the system should be simple to use and economical in relation to the total library budget.

Circulation control systems can be either manual or automated. At present nearly all hospital libraries use some type of manual system. Six activities are involved in library circulation control, whether manual or automated: (1) registration of borrowers, (2) charging, (3) discharging, (4) controlling overdues, (5) processing reserves and recalls, and (6) collecting statistics.

Manual Systems

Most hospital libraries use the conventional manual systems of circulation control. These systems are not linked to computers and employ simple methods to register borrowers, charge and discharge materials, and identify overdue materials and reserve or recall items.

Registration of Borrowers

The first activity in circulation control involves the registration of borrowers. Registration is omitted in many hospital libraries because it is time-consuming and of limited value in a small institution. Most libraries that register borrowers are large ones, often with changing user populations, that cannot know their clients personally. In such cases, registration establishes a person's right to library service and provides department and address information without requiring that it be written at every transaction. Some libraries register only unaffiliated library patrons and use other means to identify primary clientele. Alternative methods to registration may include employee identification cards or directories of the medical staff and hospital personnel.

Registration systems can be useful in supplying location information for retrieving overdues and recalls, or for providing a sample signature as a reference in deciphering names on book cards. Registration also requires users to sign a statement of responsibility for library materials, and in the case of students and residents, establishes the date of anticipated departure from the hospital. Figure 6-3 provides a sample format for a registration card.

A library that registers its users may or may not issue identification cards. These cards are subject to possible abuses and must be collected when users end their affiliation with the hospital. In general, issuance of cards is not recommended for hospital libraries except in special circumstances such as use with a charging machine.

Charging

Charging out library materials is an indispensable library function. According to Balkema the ideal charg-

ing system provides "maximum control with minimum effort at practically no cost" (7). Many small libraries use some variation of the Newark System, which was devised in the late nineteenth century.

According to the Newark System, books are provided with book pockets and cards, each card showing the call number, author, and title. If bound journals circulate, they are provided with similar pockets and cards. A borrower signs the card, which is then dated and held for reference. Sometimes a slip with the date due may be placed in the book pocket. At the end of the day, the librarian sorts the cards, records statistics, and files the cards by call number, author, or main entry. Sometimes cards are also tabbed for date due, although this is rarely done in small operations. This system is easy to use and allows materials to be borrowed even when the librarian is not present. The chief disadvantage of this system is the length of time needed for processing cards and pockets.

A similar system involves the use of individual cards that are generated for each borrowing transaction. These charge cards are especially useful for unbound journal issues, vertical file items, audiovisuals, and other materials that do not contain book pockets. In this system, the borrower or a library staff member records data about the material borrowed, the borrower's name, and the date. Charge cards can also be used for borrowing books and other hard-cover materials, if the librarian prefers, to avoid having to provide each book with a pocket and card. The major drawback of this system is that the identifying data must be recorded at each transaction and are subject to error. Also, the time involved in filling out cards is lengthened. Figure 6-4 shows a charge card for unbound materials.

Figure 6-3
Registration Card

WEST CENTRAL HOSPITAL LIBRARY

User Registration Card

Please print:
NAME (surname first) _____
HOME ADDRESS _____
_____
OFFICE ADDRESS or HOSP. DEPT. _____
OFFICE PHONE or HOSP. EXTENSION _____
POSITION:
____ Attending Physician
____ Nurse
____ Other Hosp. Employee
____ Resident
____ Student
____ Unaffil. with Hosp.

If resident or student, expected departure date _____

    I agree to comply with library rules and take full responsibility for materials charged out in my name.

SIGNATURE _____

Figure 6-4
Charge Card for Unbound Material

WEST CENTRAL HOSPITAL LIBRARY

Unbound Materials

Journal title or vertical file heading _____
_____
If journal: Volume _____
            Issue _____ Date _____

Borrower _____
Date borrowed _____

All unbound materials are due two weeks from date borrowed.

Transaction systems using sequentially numbered transaction cards and a photographic charging machine are widely used in public libraries. These systems are fast and efficient but provide no access to information about the location of individual items. They are, therefore, unsuited to use in hospital libraries.

Some larger hospital libraries use manually operated charging machines to speed the borrowing process. These machines can be used with existing book or charge cards systems, thus eliminating the problem of illegible signatures. There are some disadvantages in using charging machines, however. The most important include the cost of purchase, materials, and maintenance; the possibility of mechanical breakdowns; and the added responsibility of issuing cards to borrowers. In addition, a library staff member must be present during the charging operation. Only libraries with substantial circulations would require such machines.

Discharging

Another essential aspect of circulation control is discharging, which deals with the return of materials. Libraries should provide a convenient, well-marked place for returns and make provision for after-hours returns. If the library uses a book card system, the card for the returned item is located in the file, marked to indicate the return, and replaced in the book pocket. With charge cards, the procedure is the same, but the cards are filed or simply discarded. If the book is overdue and the library levies fines, the amount is computed and recorded. This system is designed to minimize the possibility of books being returned to the shelf without having their records removed from the circulation file. Discharging, like charging, is a time-consuming operation, but no machines exist to expedite it.

Overdue Materials

Obtaining the return of overdue materials is an ongoing problem in most libraries. Librarians wrestling with this situation may envy the policy practiced in Scotland in the early eighteenth century, which required borrowers to leave as a deposit the value of the book plus 25 percent (8). In the absence of such a powerful deterrent to overdues, librarians must develop policies and procedures for dealing with them. In a small library, it is less time-consuming to leaf through the circulation file periodically for overdue items than to flag book and charge cards or keep an additional file by date due as larger libraries do. Overdue notices may be purchased from library supply houses or developed in the hospital. One simple format, which can be imprinted on postcards, is shown in Figure 6-5. Sending multiple notices involves additional time and may encourage borrowers to ignore the first notice. In some libraries a single notice is sent, followed a short time later by a bill for replacement of the item. Some librarians feel that phone calls to borrowers are more effective and economical than sending notices.

Whatever measures are taken, a record should be made of them. The simplest method is to make a notation in pencil directly on the book card or charge card.

Fines for overdue materials are often considered to be an incentive to the user to return materials promptly. Many hospital librarians do not favor fines, feeling that they are inappropriate in a special library or that the time required to compute, record, and collect them makes them impractical. Other librarians approve of them, provided the amount charged is sufficient to serve as a deterrent. Another approach to the overdue problem is to suspend borrowing privileges for delinquent users. If all the usual methods for obtaining return of materials fail, librarians can notify the borrower's department head or supervisor or enlist the aid of members of the library committee.

The borrower is usually billed for the replacement cost of lost or seriously damaged materials, sometimes with a service charge added. Some hospitals deduct the cost of lost items from a person's paycheck. If such a policy is contemplated, however, an administrator or the personnel director must be consulted about its appropriateness. Whatever procedures are selected, it is essential that they be enforceable, that the librarian have the support of the administration and library committee, and that there be a balance between the time and effort expended and the results achieved.

Reserves and Recalls

Reserve and recall procedures assure equitable access to frequently used circulating materials. When a library user requests an item that is on loan, the librarian should

Figure 6-5
Overdue Notice

WEST CENTRAL HOSPITAL LIBRARY

A   R E M I N D E R

Please return the following overdue item(s) to the library:

Author/Title   Date Due

A fine of 50 cents a day is charged for overdue materials.

J. B. Adams
Librarian

reserve the item for use upon its return. To request an item, a user fills out a reserve slip and waits for it to be returned as notification of the book's availability. The slip is either clipped to the book card in the circulation file or filed separately. The book card is then flagged to indicate the reserve. Some librarians simply make an erasable notation directly on the book card. The simplest method that works should be adopted.

At times an item in circulation may have to be recalled. The item may be urgently needed by another person, or it may need to be placed on temporary reserve. See Figure 6-6 for a multiple-purpose recall notice. The circumstances under which materials are recalled should be described in the circulation policy in order to avoid inequities.

Circulation Statistics

Librarians should maintain statistics on the circulation of library materials. For many hospital libraries, a gross count of borrowing is sufficient. Other types of statistical counts, however, may serve a useful purpose. Statistics can be collected by format (books, journals, audiovisuals), by subject or class number, by journal title, by category of borrower, or by age of journal. Librarians collect statistics through a daily count of book or charge cards

Figure 6-6
Multipurpose Recall Card

WEST CENTRAL HOSPITAL LIBRARY

Please return the following to the library:

This material is ____ to be put on reserve
____ needed for another borrower
____ needed for binding

Your prompt cooperation will be appreciated.

J. B. Adams
Librarian

and enter the information on a form devised for that purpose. See Figure 6-7 for a sample form. If the librarian prefers to collect statistics on aspects of library activity

Figure 6-7
Circulation Statistics Form

WEST CENTRAL HOSPITAL LIBRARY

Circulation Statistics for _____
mo./yr.

Date	Books	Bound Journals	Unbound Journals	Audio-tapes	Slide Sets	Projectors
1						
2						
3						
4						
5						
29						
30						
31						
Total						

other than circulation—such as visitors, interlibrary loans, and photocopying—a single form may be designed. Statistical summaries based on the daily records should be prepared monthly and annually. Chapter 15 discusses the collecting and reporting of statistics in more detail.

Automated Systems

Manual circulation control methods are currently used in nearly all hospital libraries. Improved technology and increased networking, however, will undoubtedly make automated systems feasible for large hospital libraries in the near future.

Computerized systems perform the same functions as manual systems but offer many advantages. These advantages include increased ability to extract information from records; total inventory control; better control of reserves and delinquents; and more economical use of staff time in preparing overdue notices, placing reserves, computing fines, filing, and tabbing. In addition, the circulation control function can be integrated with control of other operations. For example, a computer currently operating in a biomedical library handles circulation, book ordering, serials check-in, accounting, cataloging, and reference assistance (9). The major disadvantage of automated systems are the purchase and maintenance costs and possible breakdown problems.

Computerized circulation control systems may soon become cost-effective for large hospital libraries because labor costs of manual systems are increasing while the costs of computer technology are declining (10). The development of new equipment, minicomputers and microcomputers, favors extension of computerized systems to smaller settings also. Librarians contemplating automated control systems may want to consider several possibilities. They have the option to use a computer already available in the hospital, share a computer being used by other libraries in a consortium or network, or acquire a free-standing or "turnkey" system for use in the library alone. Elchesen analyzes the advantages and disadvantages of each choice (11). Librarians interested in automation can keep informed by reading reviews by Bahr (12) and Scholz (13). The "New Technology" section in *Library Journal* is also informative.

Journal Routing

Hospital librarians often receive requests to route the most recent issues of journals to specific departments or staff members on a regular basis. Although journal routing is common, the practice has many disadvantages. Issues are out of the library at the time when they are most in demand; the librarian has limited control over their whereabouts; and they may not be returned promptly after use. The journals are also subject to additional wear and possible loss.

If the library chooses to route journals, several proce-dures may be followed. A routing list may accompany the journal, so that one recipient passes it along to the next. Alternatively, the journal may be returned to the library for routing to the next user. This practice prolongs the process but affords greater control.

Some libraries place conditions on journal routing such as routing only duplicate issues. Other libraries restrict routing of items to newsletters, controlled circulation journals and other non-indexed materials. When deciding whether or not to route journals, or when choosing procedures for routing, the librarian should consider the library's entire clientele and avoid favoring some groups at the expense of others.

SECURITY AND ACCESS

Library security is a subject closely related to circulation. Both involve efforts to control and regulate removal of materials and ensure fair access by all users. Without adequate security, circulation regulations can become unenforceable. As Boss points out, even in a small library, physical arrangements can promote exit control (14). When possible the library should have only one door. The charge desk should be located near the exit. In some libraries mirrors can be installed to provide a view of the door. Such security arrangements provide a psychological as well as physical deterrent to thefts.

Access During Staffed Hours

During staffed hours some libraries require that users leave briefcases and bags at the desk. As part of their effort to decrease losses, librarians should try to be flexible when enforcing circulation regulations and make exceptions when they seem justified and feasible. Undue rigidity may create an adversary situation in which users try to outwit the system. Other means of decreasing losses may involve providing duplicate copies of frequently used titles and placing photocopiers in convenient locations. When losses and replacement costs are incurred, a record should be kept to aid in budgeting for replacements and in evaluating security measures.

After-hours Access

After-hours access to the library can become a problem for security-minded librarians. In a patient care institution, it is important that essential information be available 24 hours a day. In fact, the JCAH standards require a written description of arrangements for "the provision of essential library materials when the library is closed or not staffed" (15).

Library policies concerning after-hours access vary widely, from no admission to uncontrolled access at any time. Between these extremes, however, lies a wide spectrum of possible compromises. Some libraries are locked after hours, although a key that must be signed for is available from a guard, a telephone operator, or another designated person. Some hospitals provide duplicate collections of basic texts and place them in department libraries, on-call rooms, emergency departments, or nursing stations.

Control Systems

Mechanical exit control systems are available to improve library security. Knight points out that these have become much less expensive and, therefore, applicable to smaller libraries (16). Some manufacturers now offer security systems that are integrated with automated circulation and inventory control. These systems require the insertion into each volume of a piece of electrically charged tape or other material. Before the item is checked out from the library, a staff member must deactivate the charge. Unless this is done a sensor near the exit causes an alarm to sound as the item is carried through the exit.

Security systems reduce losses substantially and usually pay for themselves in a few years. They are generally well-accepted by patrons, especially if the librarian makes the extent of any losses well-known. There are also substantial disadvantages. Installation and maintenance costs are high, and a staff member is needed near the exit at all times. Other disadvantages include false alarms, the time required to prepare the books, and a possible increase in book mutilation. Automated security systems are currently used primarily in large libraries or in those that hold important or rare collections. The use of automated security systems in hospital libraries, however, may increase with lowered costs and growing acceptance of their need.

Whatever the size of the library, the librarian should try to institute security measures that are appropriate but not extreme. A certain amount of loss is unavoidable and must be accepted. Security should never be pursued at the price of widespread antagonism of users or the erosion of good will.

INVENTORIES

The frequency with which inventories are taken in hospital libraries varies widely. Librarians often avoid or postpone inventories because they require extensive time. However, inventories provide a great deal of information about a collection and reflect the effectiveness of collection management. They also may be combined with other library operations such as usage studies or weeding. The information gathered from inventories expedites the following library procedures:

- Identifying subjects having a high rate of loss so that appropriate decisions on selection, duplicate copies, and reserves can be made
- Evaluating library security
- Discovering cataloging errors
- Locating volumes in poor physical condition that need to be repaired, replaced, or discarded

- Correcting misshelvings
- Providing more accurate statistics about the collection
- Updating the card catalog by removing cards for missing books
- Providing data for correcting and updating union lists

The process of taking inventory of a book collection involves comparing the shelf list with the materials actually on the shelves. Allowance is made for items on loan, on temporary reserve, or otherwise out of their usual positions on the shelves. Decisions to replace missing books should be weighed against the age of the book and the anticipated date of a new edition. Missing books should not be replaced immediately, since they are often returned. Returns often occur at certain times of the year, for example, when residents leave, and after specialty board or licensure examinations. A special charge card for missing material can be completed and kept in the circulation file until a replacement has been obtained or the records removed.

MATERIALS USAGE STUDIES

In a hospital library, where space and budgets are often severely limited, it is important that the collection be well-tailored to the needs of the clientele. Therefore, it may be helpful to gather information regarding the use of individual books or journals. Such a study can provide a basis for weeding, guide development of selection and retention policies, and help in making decisions on storage or conversion to microforms. It can also provide information on the effects of a change in the hospital, such as a new teaching program or termination of a residency. The JCAH encourages an ongoing effort to gather such data.

In designing a usage study, different types of use should be taken into account. One prominent type is circulation. Another is in-library use, which is usually determined by requesting users to leave materials on tables for later counting. The volume of photocopying should also be recorded. If users photocopy for themselves, they can be requested to leave the original materials on a book truck near the copier. Interlibrary loan requests may also be counted. They show the demand for titles not owned by the library. Information for the usage study is collected daily and evaluated at the end of the period of study. Descriptions of well-designed usage studies completed by hospital libraries can be found in the journal literature (17, 18).

CURRENCY OF THE COLLECTION

Maintaining the currency of the collection through weeding material that is no longer useful is a vital library activity for many reasons. It maintains the quality of the collection, eliminates outdated information, and encourages a program of replacement buying. Weeding also makes better use of space and makes the collection more attractive and usable.

Weeding Book Collections

Weeding a book collection is a task some librarians approach with reluctance. It is time-consuming, and they may worry about making a mistake. There may also be a regrettable association of a large collection with library prestige. Weeding may also be discouraged by external factors, especially opposition from the administration, the library committee or library users. In these cases, the necessity for weeding should be explained and documented. In some government-funded libraries, legal constraints against discarding materials may exist.

The weeding process should be based on written criteria. The criteria for weeding are similar to those used in the selection of new materials but also include the following: a history of the book's usage, the age and physical condition of the book, and the availability of other material on the subject.

It is desirable to weed on an ongoing basis, usually in conjunction with selection, and not just when a space crisis makes it imperative. Weeding may also be undertaken in anticipation of some special circumstance, such as moving the library or incorporating an additional collection. A question may arise about who should do the weeding—the librarian, who is familiar with the collection and users' needs; or a subject specialist, who can evaluate content. If the librarian weeds, a specialist should be consulted when there is doubt about the continued usefulness of a book. A careful approach is suggested, since weeding can be a controversial subject for library users. Evans warns, "One person's invaluable treasure is someone else's garbage" (19). Some librarians post a list of the books being considered for removal so that any objections can be registered before the material is discarded.

The amount to be weeded varies with individual circumstances. MacDonald, in an analysis of the weeding process, recommends discarding 5 percent of the book collection annually, but there are no hard and fast rules (20). If approvals for discarding are necessary or considered desirable, they should be described in the written policy. Obtaining approvals takes additional time but may prevent unnecessary conflict.

Withdrawal procedures are the reverse of procedures for new book processing. Withdrawing, or "deaccessioning" books, involves removing book pockets, cards, and date-due slips. The book is then stamped "withdrawn" or "discarded." The entry for the book is crossed out or otherwise marked in the accessions record, and the cards are removed from the shelf list and the public catalog. The number of volumes withdrawn is then subtracted from the cumulative total of the collection.

Withdrawn books, unless they are classics, rarely have any value in the secondhand book market. If they still contain useful, accurate information, they may be offered to hospital departments or to other libraries. Public libraries are often happy to have previous editions of directories or medical dictionaries. Books can be offered for exchange, sold to library users for a nominal sum, or simply given away. If the information they contain is out-of-date, or if all other disposal efforts have failed, they should be discarded.

Weeding Audiovisuals

Like books and journals, the audiovisual collection requires periodic weeding. Criteria for evaluating an audiovisual for retention or disposal are similar to those used for print but include currency and accuracy of content, relevance to the hospital's needs, effectiveness as a teaching instrument, visual and sound quality, physical condition, appropriateness of format, and use. Some libraries ask users of audiovisuals to fill out a simple evaluation form after each use. The form can be used for future reference during weeding. Because audiovisuals often form the basis of a teaching program, instructors of such programs should be involved in weeding decisions. Withdrawal and disposal procedures are similar to those used for print media.

Canceling Journals

Setting limits on the size of the journal collection is another important aspect of library management. In a description of a periodicals weeding project, Perkins points out that since the price of subscriptions is increasing, a greater proportion of the total budget will go for journals every year unless some titles are cut (21).

Library users, hospital administrators, and library committees often resist deleting journals. Therefore, the librarian should provide data to establish the need for deletion and obtain the appropriate approvals. The librarian may also make a study of the library's journal collection before making major changes so that sound choices can be made. Descriptions of such studies exist in current literature on the topic (22-24).

The most important data affecting the decision to cancel journals are those that describe the amount of use each title receives. Usage studies have been described previously. Another method, which may be combined with a usage study, is a survey to ascertain journal preferences. Perkins finds a negative correlation between actual usage and users' preferences (21), while Rosenberg notes the idiosyncratic nature of such evaluations (25). Nevertheless, in a hospital library, where users' attachment to the collection may be strong, such a survey may be valuable in clarifying users' willingness to accept change.

Significant features of journals should also be considered during evaluations: subscription cost, coverage by indexing and abstracting services, frequency of citation by other publications, and required shelf space. On the basis of such a study in a large teaching hospital, Bastille found that one-third of the journals in the library's collection satisfied 96.7 percent of the demand (26). Other significant factors for evaluation include how relevant in subject and level of content the journal is to the hospital's activities and personnel; what coverage is given by other journals in the collection; how available the journal is in microform (if this is a possible alternative); and how accessible the journal is in other libraries.

When a decision is made to cancel a journal subscription, it may prove helpful to keep the backfiles for a limited time in case a demand for the journal redevelops. It is undesirable, however, to retain indefinitely the backfiles of a title no longer received. Journal backfiles, especially of the less common titles, can be sold to dealers of secondhand periodicals. Like books, journals may also be offered to other libraries or to hospital departments, listed for exchange, or if these methods fail, simply discarded. When journal titles are deleted from the collection, library records and union lists should be updated accordingly.

EFFECTIVE USE OF SPACE

Whatever the size or configuration of the library, a practical and easily accessible arrangement of materials is essential. Books should be arranged by classification number, and journals should be alphabetized by title. Because of the importance of new material in the health sciences, journal issues of the current volume are often shelved separately from older volumes. Newly received books may be shelved temporarily in a prominent place for viewing. Audiovisuals and microforms are usually stored separately near the equipment necessary for their use. A few libraries, however, shelve them together with printed materials.

Ease of use without assistance is a paramount consideration in a hospital library, since staff is limited and the library is often used after staffed hours. If possible, the librarian should present instruction in use of the library as part of orientation programs for new nurses, residents, students, and hospital employees. Guides to the classification scheme and the journal arrangement should be prominently displayed, and the shelves should be clearly marked. In a large or complex library, diagrams can also be helpful. It may be useful to enlist the aid of a nonlibrarian who is unfamiliar with the library to evaluate the ease of locating materials unassisted.

Inadequate space is often a problem in hospital libraries. Randall cautions that if lack of space is not yet a problem in a library, available space should not be flaunted (27). The collection should be spread throughout the stacks, leaving top and bottom shelves empty for future needs. Areas where rapid growth is anticipated should be given more space to minimize future shifting of materials.

When space becomes extremely tight, corrective measures may be necessary. Klein suggests that these may include weeding books and journals, setting shorter jour-

nal retention periods, putting some material in storage, installing compact shelving, converting to microforms, and rearranging the physical setting (28). Resource-sharing with a neighboring library or within a consortium can also be helpful.

Weeding the collection has already been discussed. Consideration of other space-saving measures follows.

Determining Journal Retention Periods

Because library space is limited, it is necessary to decide how long a run should be retained of each title in the collection. Again, use is the primary consideration. Studies of retention periods for journal backfiles, such as those made by Schloman (29) and Smith (30), have indicated that collection usefulness is enhanced by variable retention periods. Libraries should retain certain titles of long-term reference value longer than the balance of the collection, and ephemeral material should be kept only a year or two. Kamenoff's report of a year-long usage study in a community hospital library provides a guide to retention periods for specific titles (31).

In general, studies such as those cited above have indicated that valuable shelf space is often wasted by storing older volumes of journals that are rarely needed. Robeson (32) and Horton (33) both recommend five-year retention periods for the majority of journal titles in small nonteaching hospitals.

Although such recommendations are useful as a general guide, the unique organization of each individual library should be considered before retention limits are set. More substantial backfiles will obviously be needed in a hospital with extensive teaching and residency programs, or one in which research is done. Other considerations include the availability of the journals elsewhere, interlibrary borrowing and cooperative collection development, and existing or anticipated clinical programs in the hospital that require journal support. Cost factors, of course, are very important. Obtaining material on interlibrary loan may entail substantial payments to the lending libraries and require valuable staff time for processing requests. However, the library may save money on binding, since titles kept for only a few years will not need to be bound.

Retention periods for all library journals should be included in a library's written policy. The library should also set a retention limit for each new title that is added to the collection.

Storing Portions of the Collection

When space problems become severe, one remedy is to store part of the collection. Decisions about what to store should be made carefully so that staff time will not be wasted in making frequent retrievals. Obvious candidates for storage include older volumes of all journals, complete runs of little-used journals, and material being held for future needs. Material may be stored in any appropriate space in the hospital or may be kept off the premises. Cooperative storage with other hospital departments or libraries may prove successful. Access to stored material should always be maintained. If material cannot remain accessible, it may be wise to consider disposing of it altogether.

Using Compact Shelving

Compact, high-density shelving slides along tracks with only a single, changeable aisle. The economical, space-saving shelving permits the storage of more volumes in a given space than conventional shelving and has the advantage of keeping the material on site. High density shelving is costly, although it is less expensive per volume shelved than conventional shelving. The added weight may also necessitate reinforcement of the floor. Another disadvantage of this type of shelving is the resistance it sometimes gets from staff and users, although resistance usually diminishes with familiarity.

Converting to Microforms

Another remedy in an overcrowded library is to convert a portion of the journal collection to microforms. Meiboom (34) and Daghita (35) describe conversion to microforms in the libraries of teaching hospitals. In a conversion project, a savings of space of about 90 percent is achieved. The collection remains intact and accessible, material does not leave the library for binding, binding costs are eliminated, and theft and mutilation practically cease. An important feature of conversion is that it can be done gradually, thus eliminating the heavy initial expense.

Microforms also have a number of disadvantages. Color is lacking, and half-tones do not reproduce well. Reader-printers must be bought and maintained, and users depend upon these machines for access to information. Material on microfilm can be read only in the library. Users often show considerable initial resistance to microforms. To gain acceptance, the librarian must explain and document the need for the conversion, provide enough reading machines, and have a liberal printing policy.

Converting a substantial portion of the collection to microform lowers the per-volume cost of the reading equipment. The usual practice is to buy back-files of some or all of the library's journals in microform, keeping paper copies of only the most current issues. Bell explains technical considerations of format, polarity, film types, and brands of reader-printers (36). Microforms may be stored separately or interfiled with bound volumes in special racks that fit on the regular shelves.

Participating in Cooperative Acquisitions Programs

Participating in a program of cooperative acquisitions with other libraries can provide access to a greater range of titles than actually occupy one library's shelves. If photocopying is anticipated, however, the projected use of the item must be analyzed in light of copyright restrictions.

PRESERVATION OF MATERIALS

Although hospital libraries do not usually collect very old books or extremely long journal runs, the proper care and preservation of materials is a concern of any library. Volumes should be shelved and unshelved carefully to avoid undue stress, and book supports should be used. Librarians should choose photocopiers with book use in mind. Avoiding extremes of temperature and humidity is also important, especially for audiovisuals and microforms. Realistically, hospital librarians often do not have a great deal of control over these matters, but they should press for conditions that are protective of library materials whenever an opportunity presents itself.

In most hospital libraries, only simple, basic repairs such as mending tears and tipping in pages should be undertaken. Some library supply companies offer useful manuals on book repairs and preservation.

BINDING

Libraries that keep their journals for more than a few years often bind all or part of their collections. Binding protects the material, reduces loss, and makes a more attractive collection. The most obvious disadvantage is the cost. In addition, bound volumes are harder to photocopy than single issues, and journals are out of the library during the binding period. Books are rarely rebound in hospital libraries, except for useful out-of-print titles. However, in maternity, pediatric, orthopedic, and other specialized hospitals, books in the subject specialty may be rebound. The retention period for journals is a major consideration when making binding decisions. In general, journals kept less than three to five years should not be bound.

In selecting a binder, the advice of other librarians in the area can be very useful. The Library Binding Institute in Boston offers a list of certified library binders who bind according to its standards. A binder usually supplies all necessary materials, such as cartons and binding slips. The binder also picks up and delivers the journals. In addition, the binder should guarantee a maximum binding time. Four to six weeks is considered reasonable service.

Sending journals out for binding immediately after completion of a volume minimizes lost issues but tends to concentrate binding activity in one or two periods a year. Binders understandably prefer a steady work flow, and better service will result if the library can accommodate them. Roberts offers a number of other suggestions for a harmonious relationship with binders, including being prepared for pickups and arranging for prompt payment (37). He also points out that frequent changing of binders to ensure acquiring the lowest bid is false economy because it involves substantial costs in terms of the librarian's time.

Before journal issues are sent to the bindery, a record should be made of their release. The simplest method is to complete one charge card for the inclusive issues and file it in the circulation file.

Additional information about the binding process can be obtained from the Library Binding Institute. The Institute offers workshops, manuals, films and filmstrips, and also maintains a laboratory at the Rochester Institute of Technology that tests bound volumes for compliance with its binding specifications.

Journals that are not bound should be stored in pamphlet boxes or Princeton files, which may be obtained from library or office supply companies.

INTERDEPENDENCE OF LIBRARY OPERATIONS

The process of maintaining a collection and making it useful to the library's clientele occupies a great deal of library staff time. When dealing with operational activities, it is essential that the librarian see their interdependence. A significant change in any one activity affects all the others, and thereby influences the functioning of the library as a whole. For example, user policies affect the hours a library remains open, the staffing patterns, and the circulation policy. Circulation policies affect the volume of photocopying and the type and extent of security arrangements that are necessary for proper circulation. Journal retention decisions affect interlibrary loan volume. All library policies affect library statistics, which must be thoughtfully interpreted if they are to provide meaningful information.

Even more significantly, all policies affect the types of users attracted to the library, the purposes for which they use the library, and the materials and services necessary to meet their needs. In this dynamic situation, it is the responsibility of the librarian to balance potentially conflicting elements and interests and provide the best possible service to the hospital and the entire user population.

REFERENCES

1. Martin LA. User studies and library planning. Libr Trends 1976 Jan;24:483-496.

2. Port JS. The Mount Sinai Medical Center Library user survey. Bull Med Libr Assoc 1977 Apr;65:289-290.

3. Roberts J. Circulation versus photocopy: quid pro quo? Bull Med Libr Assoc 1980 July;68:274-277.

4. Buckland MK. An operations research study of a variable loan and duplication policy at the University of Lancaster. Libr Q 1972 Jan;42:97-106.

5. Bookstein A. Optimal loan periods. Inf Process Manage 1975;11:235-242.

6. Fry G and Associates. Study of circulation control systems: public libraries, college and university libraries, special libraries. Chicago: Technology Project, 1961:131.

7. Balkema JB. Topics in library technology: charging systems. Bull Med Libr Assoc 1966 Jan;54:33-37.

8. Kirkwood LH. Charging systems. New Brunswick, NJ: Graduate School of Library Service, Rutgers, the State University, 1961:19.

9. Hendricks DD. Advances in medical librarianship. Adv Librarianship 1979;9:211-255.

10. Markuson BE. Granting amnesty and other fascinating aspects of automated circulation: a review of recent developments for non-experts. Am Libr 1978 Apr;9:205-211.

11. Elchesen DR. Dedicated versus resource-shared library computer systems. Spec Libr 1976 July;67:299-304.

12. Bahr AH. Automated library circulation systems, 1979-80. 2d ed. White Plains, NY: Knowledge Industry Publications, 1979.

13. Scholz WH. Computer-based circulation systems—a current review and evaluation. Libr Technol Rep 1977 May;13:231-325.

14. Boss RW. The library security myth. Libr J 1980 Mar 15;105:683.

15. Joint Commission on Accreditation of Hospitals. Accreditation manual for hospitals. 1983 ed. Chicago: Joint Commission on Accreditation of Hospitals, 1982: 147-149.

16. Knight NH. Security systems. ALA Yearbook 1980;5:280-281.

17. Kamenoff L. Journal usage at a community hospital library. Bull Med Libr Assoc 1977 Jan;65:58-61.

18. Bastille JD, Mankin CJ. Report on subsequent demand for journal titles dropped in 1975. Bull Med Libr Assoc 1978 July;66:346-349.

19. Evans GE. Limits of growth, or the need to weed. Calif Libr 1977 Apr;38:8-15.

20. MacDonald MB. Weeding the collection. Unabashed Libr 1975 Summer;no. 16:7-8.

21. Perkins D. Periodicals weeding, or weed it and reap. Calif Libr 1977 Apr;38:32-37.

22. Ash J, Morgan JE. Journal evaluation study at the University of Connecticut Health Center. Bull Med Libr Assoc 1977 Apr;65:297-299.

23. Bourne CP, Gregor D. Planning serials cancellations and cooperative collection development in the health sciences: methodology and background information. Bull Med Libr Assoc 1975 Oct;63:366-377.

24. McKeehan NC. A method for deleting selected journals. Bull Med Libr Assoc 1977 July;65:388-390.

25. Rosenberg B. Evaluation: problems of criteria and methodology. Calif Libr 1977 Apr;38:16-21.

26. Bastille JD, Mankin CJ. A simple objective method for determining a dynamic journal collection. Bull Med Libr Assoc 1980 Oct;68:357-66.

27. Randall GE. Space utilization in a special library: making do with what you get. In: Mount E, ed. Planning the special library. New York: Special Libraries Association, 1972:6-12.

28. Klein MS. Space utilization in hospital libraries with space shortages. Bull Med Libr Assoc 1977 Jan;65:63-65.

29. Schloman BF, Ahl RE. Retention periods for journals in a small academic library. Spec Libr 1979 Sept;70:377-383.

30. Smith JMB. A periodical use study at the Children's Hospital of Michigan. Bull Med Libr Assoc 1970 Jan;58:65-67.

31. Kamenoff L. Retention of journals in a community hospital library. Bull Med Libr Assoc 1977 Oct;65:446-447.

32. Robeson CA. Planning and maintenance of library facilities and resources. In: Bloomquist H, Rees AM, Stearns NS, Yast H, eds. Library practice in hospitals: a basic guide. Cleveland: The Press of Case Western Reserve University, 1972:149

33. Horton M. Acquisition of serials, free materials and government publications. In: Wender, RW, ed. Organizing and administering the small hospital library. Dallas: TALON, 1979:45.

34. Meiboom ER. Conversion of the periodical collection in a teaching hospital to microfilm format. Bull Med Libr Assoc 1976 Jan;64:36-40.

35. Daghita JM. A core collection of journals on microfilm in a community teaching hospital library. Bull Med Libr Assoc 1976 Apr;64:240-241.

36. Bell JA. Microforms: uses and potential. Bull Med Libr Assoc 1978 Apr;66:232-238.

37. Roberts S. What the library binder expects from the librarian. Libr Scene 1978 Sept/Dec;7:2-4.

READINGS

Buckland, MK. Ten years progress in quantitative research on libraries. Socioecon Plann Sci 1978;12:333-339.

Davis BB. User needs. The key to changing library services and policies. Bull Med Libr Assoc 1975 Apr;63:195-198.

Jones CL, Kasses CD. Lending services: policies, procedures and problems. In: Darling L, Bishop D, Colaianni LA, eds. Handbook of medical library practice. 4th ed. Chicago: Medical Library Association, 1982.

Lehman LJ. Circulation. In: Bloomquist H, Rees AM, Stearns NS, Yast H, eds. Library practice in hospitals: a basic guide. Cleveland: The Press of Case Western Reserve University, 1972:218-240.

Mosley IJ. Cost-effectiveness analysis of the automation of a circulation system. J Libr Automat 1977 Sept;10:240-254.

Titley J. The library and its public: identification and communications. In: Annan GL, Felter JW, eds. Handbook of medical library practice. 3d ed. Chicago: Medical Library Association, 1970:347-356.

Trochim MJ. Circulation systems. ALA Yearbook 1980;5:115-117.

Watkins C, Coker NC. Circulation policies in health science libraries. Bull Med Libr Assoc 1970 Oct;58:548-553.

Zero growth: when is NOT-enough enough? A symposium. J Acad Librarianship 1975 Nov;1:4-11.

SECTION II:

Providing Library Services

Information Services

Judith Messerle
*Director, Educational Resources
and Community Relations*
St. Joseph Hospital
Alton, Illinois

CHAPTER 7

Information Services

Judith Messerle
Director, Educational Resources and Community Relations
St. Joseph's Hospital
Alton, Illinois

Appendixes

Figures

Providing information service is the primary purpose of a hospital library. Like other specialized libraries, a hospital library must focus on meeting the specific information needs of its users. Other library functions such as the management, preservation, and organization of materials exist to facilitate the delivery of information to the user.

To be effective, information services must be designed to meet the specific needs of the user. They must be provided within the time limits defined by the user and delivered in the desired format. The information provided must also be accurate and up-to-date.

The librarian and the library staff provide information services. Their willingness to serve, skill in serving, thoroughness, professional attitude, and prompt follow-through indicate whether service is a priority.

Although hospital library users may be highly trained in their fields, they may not be well versed in using the library. Therefore, the hospital librarian must serve as the link between the specialized user and specialized resources, becoming the hospital's information specialist.

In today's changing environment, information sources are becoming increasingly abundant and complex. The need for accurate, up-to-date information for patient care, health planning, research, and education continues to grow. Quality information services provided by hospital librarians can play a distinct and valuable role in the hospital organization.

NEED FOR INFORMATION SERVICES

Hospital libraries provide information services to a diverse population. Although some libraries serve only physicians, most serve both medical staff and hospital staff. Other user groups often include students affiliated with the hospital and patients.

Assessing Information Needs

Because the library exists to meet the needs of its users, the librarian must determine those needs accurately. In planning information services, the needs of potential users as well as present users should be considered.

Needs assessments can take various forms, depending on their purpose. For example, an assessment can be done on a broad basis, covering different user groups; or on a narrow basis, targeting the needs of specific user groups. Before conducting a needs assessment, the librarian should decide what information is needed, from whom, and for what purpose. The method of needs assessment can then be designed to retrieve the information that will be useful. Although each method of needs assessment should be planned to meet the needs of a specific situation, the sample of a general survey in Figure 7-1 can serve as a starting point. Chapter 12 provides a more detailed discussion of needs assessment.

Typical Information Needs of Major User Groups

Since many diverse groups use the library, each having unique information needs, the librarian may find it helpful to define major groups and identify their typical information needs. These major groups could include the medical and nursing staff, the health care administration, allied health staff, patients, and the community at large.

Medical Staff

Medical staff members largely determine the quality of patient care in the hospital. They are responsible for the diagnosis of disease and for the prescription of treatment. Because their information needs are frequently tied to the direct care of a specific patient, physicians' requests are usually given the highest priority in the hospital library.

Physicians can be classified by privilege category, by clinical specialty, by relationship to the hospital, by educational status, or by their most common role. Primary needs for information can best be defined by categorizing physicians in specific groups: clinicians or practitioners, residents or housestaff, medical students, researchers and faculty members.

Before examining the information needs of each group, a few generalizations can be made about how most physicians usually obtain information. Most receive at least one primary medical journal, such as the *New England Journal of Medicine* or the *Journal of the American Medical Association* (JAMA), and several journals in their clinical specialty. Since most states now require continuing education for relicensure, professional meetings and seminars provide an increasingly important source of current information. Other sources of information include professional associations and fellow physicians.

Physicians who are classified as "clinicians" or "practitioners" are usually engaged in private practice. They may also be under contract to a hospital, such as pathologists or radiologists. Clinicians provide direct patient care. Their information needs often relate to specific patients and may range from a request for information, such as the recommended pediatric dosage for a particular drug, to the need for evaluating all the current literature on a specific treatment or condition. Sometimes clinicians may request assistance in locating a journal article that was read casually several months earlier. They may also request comprehensive bibliographices on a problem they are facing with a patient. Today's clinicians are requesting complex, interrelated information. For example, they may need information on the use of a specific drug in treating a particular disease or on the comparative results of treatment with different types of therapy.

Residents, or housestaff, have completed their medical school training and are practicing medicine under the supervision of faculty. Their information needs resemble those of the clinician, although they may need more basic data to support their diagnosis and treatment decisions. Since they are still learning under supervision as well as providing on-site physician coverage for the hospital, residents may require well-developed bibliographies and current information to help them formulate immediate treatment plans. Some librarians develop specialized services to meet these needs such as reprint files, which are frequently updated, or files of bibliographies for further reading.

The information needs of medical students should be considered along with those of physicians, although the students have not yet completed their degrees. Medical students perform varied tasks in hospitals, depending on the medical school's curriculum, but they are always supervised by a member of the housestaff or medical staff. Their information needs are student-oriented and focus on basic data; review articles; and thorough, topi-

cal bibliographies. These needs are related both to their responsibilities at the hospital and to the curriculum at their institutions and may include materials for required reading or viewing.

Researchers and medical school faculty members constitute another category of physician library user. Their research requests are usually much more comprehensive than those from staff providing direct patient care. A researcher tries to obtain all the information on a specific topic. Instead of focusing primarily on current information, a search may go well beyond the five-year point into a retrospective review of the literature. Often, research-related searches are not needed as quickly as patient-related searches. Research-related questions occur more frequently in hospitals with university affiliations or in hospitals having research grants.

Although these patterns of physician information needs apply in most cases, there are exceptions. At times

Figure 7-1
Needs Assessment Survey

NAME _____
                    (Optional)

JOB CLASSIFICATION _____

DEPARTMENT _____

DATE _____

1. The library offers various information services to hospital employees. Please check those you have used in the past.

   _____ Listings of magazine and journal articles on a specific subject (bibliography development)
   _____ Answers to short questions such as addresses, laboratory normals, definitions, and so forth.
   _____ Requests for specific information (such as therapy of decubiti)
   _____ Photocopy services
   _____ Ordering audiovisual programs
   _____ Computer searching (Medline)
   _____ Current awareness service
   _____ Selective Dissemination of Information (SDI)

2. Have you experienced any problems in obtaining the above services?
   _____ Yes _____ No   If yes, please explain _____
   _____
   _____

3. How often do you visit or call the library for services?
   _____ Daily   _____ Monthly
   _____ 2-3 times per week   _____ Yearly
   _____ 1 time per week   _____ Never

4. What are the ideal times for you to use the library?
   _____ 7:00 a.m.-9:00 a.m.   _____ Monday-Friday
   _____ 9:00 a.m.-12:00 Noon   _____ Saturday
   _____ 12:00 Noon-4:30 p.m.   _____ Sunday
   _____ 4:30 p.m.-( ) p.m.
   Comment: _____
   _____

5. What type of information would help you in your job performance? Please be specific.
   _____
   _____
   _____

6. What specialized areas would you like the library to consider when purchasing new materials? Please be specific to your area of specialty.
   _____
   _____
   _____

7. How can the library improve its service to provide you with the information you need?
   _____
   _____
   _____

Note: Adapted with permission from St. Joseph's Hospital Library.

primary physicians may require extensive, retrospective information, when preparing for a medical audit or case presentations, for example. Faculty physicians, too, may ask for only current information for patient care questions.

Nursing

Nursing personnel in the hospital vary greatly in educational background, job responsibilities, and interest in library use. The wide diversity of training and background of the nursing staff often makes it difficult for the librarian to determine the exact level of information needed. This problem requires the librarian's special attention.

Frequently requests from nurses are directly related to patient care. A nurse may want to review background information on a disease, check symptoms, or try to improve nursing procedures. The nursing staff rarely directs life-and-death questions to the library, but rather first seeks urgent information from the physician. Thus rapid response time for requests from nurses is often less critical than for requests from physicians.

A new interest in hospital library use has come about through the recent development of "career ladders," which encourage nursing staff to work their way through the academic process from aide to clinical specialist. Nursing shortages have generated the need for "refresher courses" to prepare RNs returning to the hospital to fill positions. These groups have information needs typical of all students: bibliographies for papers and research projects, articles from reading lists, and basic information to supplement textbooks.

Educating a nursing staff is an ongoing process. The library will be used frequently by in-service instructors in search of teaching materials, particularly audiovisuals. Patient information materials may also be sought when the nursing staff is planning new patient education programs or revising old ones.

Because health care is becoming increasingly complex, head nurses and nursing managers may find it necessary to learn or perfect management skills on the job. As nursing managers begin to seek information on staffing patterns, employee performance appraisal, and other supervisory topics, the library will become the focal point of their search. Tightening regulations will also lead to interest in improved nursing care plans, patient classification, and quality assurance.

Nurse aides may seek more information about basic nursing skills, advancing on the nursing career ladder, and communicating more effectively with patients. The nurse practitioner or nursing specialist, on the other hand, may seek clinical information directly related to patient care and to new trends in the field.

The nursing staff is deeply involved in the day-to-day care of the patient and relies heavily on quick, convenient information sources. Most RNs receive at least one professional journal at home, such as *American Journal of Nursing*, *RN*, or *Nursing*. Other means of keeping current include in-service or in-house education designed to teach new techniques and explain new equipment. Nursing staff members also frequently attend local professional or educational meetings.

Because of the demands of patient care, nurses may find it difficult to visit the library for services. As a result, their information needs often remain unidentified and unmet. To compensate, hospital librarians should work with the nursing staff to identify information needs. Convenient and prompt means of providing services to floor nurses should be developed and publicized. Such means may include encouraging telephone requests and following through on responses promptly, or taking materials to the units.

Health Care Administration

Hospital personnel involved with health care administration constitute a relatively new group of library users. Rapid change in the health care field has made information increasingly important to the hospital's management personnel. Libraries can help meet some of these information needs.

The administrative staff includes the entire management team, from the board of directors to departmental or unit supervisors. It includes administrators, financial officers, planners, public relations and personnel directors, as well as many others. Because each person or level of authority has different information needs, a brief synopsis of areas of specific interest follows.

The administrator, associate and assistant administrators, and administrative assistants are in the business of running a highly complex institution. They interact with physicians; hospital employees; patients; the community at large; and federal, state, and local government organizations. This complex network of relationships and needs requires accurate information for effective decision-making.

Daily information needs can be met by the newsletters and journals that flood the hospital administrative offices. These publications, often part of membership benefits in specific hospital organizations, may be routed among the administrative group. Information on community activities may be provided by routing the Chamber of Commerce newsletter, local newspapers, or clippings from those papers. Newsletters from organizations and publications of neighboring hospitals will also come to administrative offices, and the library may be able to help with distribution, access, or storage.

Keeping up-to-date with legislation and regulations is difficult and yet critical for the administrative staff. The *Federal Register*—along with the state register, if one exists—is a must for any hospital today. Many hospital libraries have taken on the responsibility for collecting, scanning, and routing this important document. Pertinent sections of the *Federal Register*, identified by the

American Hospital Association, are indexed in the *Health Planning* database.

Other library services needed by the administrative staff include information searches, bibliographies, and current awareness services to assist in planning new programs, studying problem areas, or preparing presentations. If administrators are not aware of these library services, it is the librarian's responsibility to find creative ways of demonstrating how library services can benefit the hospital's administration.

The governing body of the hospital has the responsibility for setting overall direction and policy for the institution. This group may be composed of community leaders who are knowledgeable of the community but may have little direct information about hospital practices and problems. Although they can get much of this information from administrative staff, the governing body may need more information on health care in general. To meet this need, the hospital can provide subscriptions to journals and newsletters in the health care field. If more in-depth information is required by board committees as they work to prepare plans for full board review, a hospital administrative staff member can work with the committee to gather information. Alternatively, board members themselves may use the library directly.

Needs for information arise naturally in the course of managing any department, although department heads may not automatically turn to the library as a source for this information. The director of physical therapy may need information on the charges allowed by Medicare for outpatient therapy, for example, or the business office director may want to see the Medicare forms used by other institutions. Most departments in the hospital represent professions or specialized occupations and have their own special associations, journals, newsletters, and standard texts. If the librarian knows the information sources of each discipline, those sources can either be added to the collection or made available from other libraries, when needed.

Allied Health

The allied health fields include a broad spectrum of health professionals, such as respiratory therapists, laboratory technologists, and radiation therapists. These users have become important members of the health care team since specialization and sophisticated equipment have become a necessary part of current health care. To furnish adequate information services, the librarian should develop a basic understanding of the services that each allied health group provides.

Allied health users generally approach the library seeking information on new technology or clarification of procedures. Depending on the level of the users' training, their requests may range from basic to very complex. Because "career ladders" within the specialized fields provide for career mobility and professional growth, the allied health user may also be seeking information that

supplements a formal or informal educational program.

Each specialty group of allied health has its own journal, newsletter, and organizations to provide current information. The librarian should consider purchasing the best specialty publications for the library.

Patients

Although some libraries have provided recreational and health education materials to patients for many years, patients are only recently being identified as a separate category of library users in hospitals. Their use of library resources requires acquisition of materials that are less clinically and technically oriented. For some libraries, providing information services to patients may also require a change in library policy and increased interaction with other hospital departments, as well as with the public library. Chapter 21 discusses library services for patients in greater depth.

The Community

The community may also benefit from information services provided by the library. Services may be dispensed directly to the community or indirectly through librarians' participation in organizations or hospital departments that offer community health education programs. Librarians may also work with public libraries who support efforts to provide health information. Chapter 22 provides more information on community health information services.

Dealing with Reluctant User Groups

Results of needs assessment and knowledge of the library's user population should reveal the identity of groups using the library infrequently, or not at all. Once groups of nonusers have been identified, the librarian can begin planning to increase their awareness of library services. Outreach to new user groups should be done at a carefully planned pace. Attempts to increase services in all areas at once may result in overextension and seriously affect the librarian's ability to provide all the services promised. Service to all groups is a long range goal, not one that can be achieved instantly without budget increases and additional support staff.

After targeting a specific group for attention, the librarian should focus on the needs of that group. Interviewing selected members of the group can be very valuable in discovering needs. Scanning literature appropriate to that particular group is also worthwhile. By scanning newsletters the librarian may identify legislative issues that can be meaningful to the group. To identify useful points in the literature, the librarian should question each item's relevance to the current hospital situation. For example, what is the hospital doing in a particular area now? How will this affect its present financial picture? Is the hospital considering day surgery? By combining this questioning approach with the information received through needs analysis, the librarian can identify items of potential interest to nonusers.

The pediatrics staff, for example, might be targeted as a nonuser group. If a needs analysis reveals that the pediatrics department is debating the pros and cons of a specific procedure for newborn infants, the librarian might flag current items in the literature that deal with the topic and route them to the department with a note, "thought this might be of interest." Forwarding current, unsolicited material identifies the library as an information source and establishes the librarian as a key information person.

In addition to flagging current information, the librarian may also send bibliographies relevant to activities in a targeted department. These unsolicited bibliographies may encourage previous nonusers to recognize the value of the service, and help them to identify their needs. Once an unsolicited bibliography is sent, a follow-up phone call or personal visit can verify that the references are helpful. This is also an opportune time to suggest further search for specific materials.

Timing is critical when providing an unsolicited bibliography to nonuser groups. Bibliographies are most effective when sent at the time a new hospital program is being developed or an existing one is being updated. If the personnel department, for example, is reviewing a wage and salary program, access to a bibliography on such a topic would be very useful. The personnel staff may also be receptive to additional information in other areas that are causing difficulty. If the unsolicited bibliography arrives after the draft is on its way to the administrator for review, however, the bibliography will probably not be used.

Another method for dealing with reluctant user groups is to determine how these groups receive their information: through formal sources such as journals or newsletters, or through informal sources such as associations, colleagues, or meetings. By knowing the information chain for each user group, the librarian can suggest available resources to fill in the gaps. For example, if the nursing director attends only a few meetings per year and receives one nursing administrative journal, the librarian can easily identify alternate information resources that may prove helpful. This technique is particularly effective with nonusers who have been on the job for a number of years but may not be aware of current resources and services. Most hospital staff members will not be reluctant users if they can be shown that the library is a hospital-wide service provided by a staff that is capable of meeting each user's individual needs.

TYPES OF INFORMATION SERVICES

If the library is to be viewed as an information service center rather than an information storage unit, the librarian must provide users with the precise information they need, in the form they need, and within the time limits that it is needed. Although this statement sounds straightforward and uncomplicated, it describes a librarian's most difficult responsibility. The reference interview provides the opportunity for the librarian to work with the user to define the precise characteristics of the information request.

The Reference Interview

The reference interview gives the librarian the opportunity to clarify what the user is requesting and determine which library services and materials are available to meet the request. Sometimes clients make requests that reflect their perception of what the library can provide, rather than what they actually need. Some clients feel they must bring a specific citation to get information. Others fear that the librarian will not understand their requests if they become too specific. Finally, some simply fail to realize that their request for general information on diabetes may not produce the specific information on diabetic foot care that they really wanted.

During the reference interview, it is important that the librarian asks questions if he or she does not fully understand the information given by the user. Of equal importance is requesting the spelling of words that are unfamiliar but important to the search. Most health care practitioners are willing to answer relevant questions if the librarian shows interest. As the librarian learns more about the terminology, it becomes easier to explore search questions with users.

Some librarians new to the health care field express doubt about understanding the user's request without formal study of medical terminology. Although formal study can be useful, the alert librarian who asks questions, learns pronunciation, and consults a medical dictionary when in doubt about the meaning of words can acquire the proficiency he or she needs for medical reference work.

The Reference Interview Setting

The reference interview is, in many ways, a personal exchange of information. The setting in which that exchange occurs influences the quality of the interaction between the librarian and the user.

With a little planning, the library can be arranged to provide a private area for the reference interview. That area can be established by placing the librarian's desk away from tables and stack areas where others might be working. The use of a screen can add to the sense of privacy.

Since the goal of the interview is to establish a personal exchange of information, the interview area should be comfortable for both the user and the librarian. It should be designed so that both can sit down or stand at a counter to discuss the request. Whatever the setting, the user and the librarian should be at equal height. If one person is sitting and the other standing, superior and inferior positions may be established, thus inhibiting the exchange of information. If approached by a user who chooses not to sit, the librarian should stand also.

Once the place of the interview is established and both parties are comfortable, the librarian should give the user undivided attention. If the library has several staff members, someone can be designated to take messages or to help other users while the librarian is involved in the interview. If the librarian works alone, he or she can develop ways of minimizing interruptions. The librarian can put callers on hold, ask other users in the library to wait, or simply use a smile and a raised hand to avoid interruptions.

These interview preparations may seem contrived. However, they require little effort, and the results are satisfying and productive.

Reference Interviewing Techniques

During the reference interview it is essential that the librarian and the client refine the client's initial request for service. Client queries can be incomplete, misleading, or unclear and as such will usually elicit inadequate responses. In these cases, the user often attributes the unacceptable response to the inadequacy of the librarian rather than to the incompleteness of the request.

Refining the question is a process of negotiation. The librarian asks questions to increase understanding and to encourage the user to be more open in expressing specific needs.

Jahoda and Braunagel offer a series of clues to help identify questions that need refinement. One such clue involves being alert for a request for a specific reference tool; another involves looking for questions that can be answered on a variety of levels (1).

Good reference interviewing requires good communication skills, tact, and empathy for the user. Some of these skills are easily learned; others take time and effort to master.

During the reference interview, the following techniques may be useful:

- Maintain eye contact when talking with the user.
- Reinforce communication by responding verbally or by nodding.
- Use questions that require the user to expand on the point.
- Rephrase the user's comments to indicate that you understand what he or she is saying.
- Use slight facial expressions to question and to show interest.
- Stand still. If you are nervous and impatient, the user will not be at ease.
- Avoid making early conclusions or conclusions that may prejudice the issue. Let the user do most of the talking.
- Never ask directly why the user wants something. Obtain that information through indirect questioning.
- Avoid emphasizing the elements of the request at the expense of missing the message.

- Avoid lines of questioning that make a client uncomfortable. Shift emphasis if that occurs.
- Pay attention to the inflection and tone of your voice. The librarian who did not hear the question and responds, "You want *what*?", may lose a user forever.

In addition to refining a client's request for information or literature search, other details are required.

- *Basic data.* What is the user's name, department, phone number, and date of request?
- *Subject.* What information is the user seeking?
- *Desired product or format for response.* Does the client want journal articles, a book, a bibliography, a statistical table, a one-word answer, or a definition?
- *Amount of material.* Does the client want one review article, several relevant articles, or as much as possible?
- *Level.* What is the educational background of the ultimate user?
- *Acceptable language.* Is English preferred?
- *Time period to be searched.* Will the search cover one year, five years, ten years?
- *Time requirements.* How urgent is the request? What is the final deadline?
- *Delivery of materials.* Will the materials be picked up or mailed?

Use of a search request form, such as the sample in Figure 7-2, guarantees that all the necessary information is gathered and documented. Most hospital librarians prefer asking questions and completing the form themselves rather than having the user fill out the form. This procedure increases the opportunity for interaction. Such a form records information for the search and for statistical records. The statistical data depends on what is useful in a particular library. The same form can be used for information searches that do not involve bibliographies.

After obtaining all the necessary information for beginning the search, the librarian should restate the problem to the user for final feedback and analysis before identifying a plan of action. A plan of action should include the following:

- Probable direction
- Anticipated time for response
- If search is involved, an interim plan for feedback
- Plan for delivery of documents—mail to office, deliver, hold for pick-up

The Literature Search

The actual search strategy is determined largely by the elements defined by the user, the tools available to the librarian, and the librarian's previous experience with that particular type of request. For years hospital librarians have provided manual searches, relying heavily on a few major indexes and basic in-house texts. Although

Figure 7-2
Information and Literature Search Request

Today's Date: _____

Requester: _____

Request For (Name): _____

Department: _____

Address: _____

User:

Staff Physician ____	Administration ____	Medical Student ____
Post Doc / Fellow ____	Nursing Service ____	Other Student ____
Housestaff ____	Support Services ____	Other _____

First time user: Yes ____   No ____

Time Requirements: Rush ____   24 Hours ____   1-2 Days ____   Other ____

How do you intend to use this information?

Patient Care ____	Job-related Problem ____	General Information ____
Rounds / Reports ____	Teaching ____	School Course ____
Administrative Problem ____	Prepare Talk / Paper / Book ____	

How do you want to receive this search?   Pick up in Library ____   Mail ____

What kind of search do you want?

____ A few very relevant articles   ____ A general overview of subject   ____ Comprehensive search
(review articles)

SEARCH REQUEST: (BE AS SPECIFIC AS POSSIBLE)

Specifications relevant to search request:

    Languages: All ____   English Only ____   English Abstract ____ Other _____

    Human Only ____   Animals: All ____   Specify _____

    Male ____   Female ____   Age Groups _____

How many years do you want to cover?   1 2 3 4 5 6 7 8 9 10 Years
(Circle)

To your knowledge, how many articles have been written on this subject:

    ____ Few (10)   ____ Some (25)   ____ Many (50)

LIBRARY USE:

Librarian's Initials: _____   Check when complete: _____

Search Tools: _____   Time Taken: _____

active reference service can be provided manually, today more and more hospital libraries are obtaining access to online databases, either through a terminal in the library itself or through cooperative arrangements. Because online searching is a complex subject, no overview of searching techniques will be attempted here. The *Handbook of Medical Library Practice,* fourth edition, volume one, contains an excellent chapter on searching and search techniques (2). Management aspects of providing online services are considered later in this chapter.

Manual searching is the backbone of reference service in many hospital libraries. Although it is time-consuming, a few basic guidelines can make the job easier and less frustrating.

First, if the index is accompanied by a thesaurus, the librarian should look for the appropriate subject heading in the thesaurus before going to the index. This preliminary step allows the librarian to see all the related subject headings and choose the appropriate one. Also, it is easier to check cross references in a thesaurus.

The National Library of Medicine's *Medical Subject Headings (MeSH)* is the thesaurus used for *Index Medicus* and other NLM indexes. *MeSH* has two parts: an alphabetical list of subject headings and a hierarchical list of those same headings divided into broad classes of related terms. This latter section is called the "tree structures."

By looking up a term alphabetically and then tracing it by means of the assigned class number to its place in the tree structure, the searcher can see at a glance which terms are more general and which are more specific than the given heading. This advantage allows the searcher to choose which term is best for the specific situation. Figures 7-3 and 7-4 show examples of the two parts of *MeSH.*

A second principle of searching is that an article is usually indexed under the most specific subject heading available. Thus, an article on "bundle-branch block" will not be indexed under "heart block" since the more specific term is available.

A third concept that applies to many indexes is called the "precoordinated" indexing term. The subject heading "Heart Surgery" is an example of this concept. Since "surgery" is a standard subheading in *MeSH,* it seems logical to search for general articles on surgery of the heart by checking the subheading "Surgery" under the heading "Heart." However, because of the large volume of literature on this subject, *MeSH* provides the precoordinated subject heading "Heart Surgery." Another example is the heading "Lung Neoplasms." Instead of searching under "Neoplasms" and "Lung Diseases," the searcher can go directly to the precoordinated form "Lung Neoplasms."

A novice librarian or an experienced librarian who is using a specific index for the first time will benefit from reading the instructions in the front of an index. William Beatty has written a brief guide to searching the literature of medicine (3). Although intended for clinicians, it is a useful summary for librarians.

Figure 7-3
From the Alphabetical Section of *MeSH*

```
HEART, ARTIFICIAL
E7.450.470              E7.858.82.374
E7.858.565.458
67


HEART ATRIUM
A7.541.358
68


HEART AUSCULTATION
E1.145.569.499+         E1.706.110.458
XU   HEART MURMURS
XU   HEART SOUNDS


HEART BLOCK
C14.280.67.558+
X    ATRIOVENTRICULAR BLOCK
X    AURICULO-VENTRICULAR DISSOCIATION
XU   SINOATRIAL BLOCK


HEART CATHETERIZATION
E1.145.569.540
see related
     PULMONARY WEDGE PRESSURE
X    CATHETERIZATION, HEART
```

During the literature search itself, the librarian should continually refer to the mutually defined reference question, evaluating the responses in terms of the request. Is the product of the search really what the user is looking for? If the search reveals incidental concepts that might be relevant, the librarian can contact the user to see if expansion or refinement of the original question is in order. If problems occur during the search, the user should also be contacted.

The librarian should analyze the final product of the literature search in terms of anticipated response. Is the result what the user expects? Is it within the desired time frame, and is it in the format requested?

If the librarian cannot respond satisfactorily in the time span agreed upon in the reference interview, the user should be told what has been done to date and why there is a problem. Often, a new time can be negotiated. Letting the user wait longer than expected reflects negatively on library service.

Depending on the guidelines identified in the reference interview, the librarian can present the results of a literature search to the user in a number of ways. These include a bibliography, the document itself, an abstract, or a highlighted document.

A Bibliography

A bibliography presents the user with a broad spectrum of materials from which to choose. Prior to compi-

Figure 7-4
From the Tree Structures of *MeSH*

CARDIOVASCULAR DISEASES	C14
HEART DISEASES	C14.280
ARRHYTHMIA	C14.280.67
ARRHYTHMIA, SINUS	C14.280.67.93
ASYSTOLE*	C14.280.67.146
AURICULAR FIBRILLATION	C14.280.67.198
AURICULAR FLUTTER	C14.280.67.248
BRADYCARDIA	C14.280.67.319
EXTRASYSTOLE	C14.280.67.470
HEART BLOCK	C14.280.67.558
ADAMS-STOKES SYNDROME	C14.280.67.558.137
BUNDLE-BRANCH BLOCK	C14.280.67.558.323
SINOATRIAL BLOCK*	C14.280.67.558.750
WOLFF-PARKINSON-WHITE SYNDROME	C14.280.67.558.865
SICK SINUS SYNDROME	C14.280.67.829
TACHYCARDIA	C14.280.67.845
TACHYCARDIA, PAROXYSMAL	C14.280.67.845.695
VENTRICULAR FIBRILLATION	C14.280.67.932
CARCINOID HEART DISEASE*	C14.280.129 C4.557.112
CARDIAC OUTPUT, LOW	C14.280.148
CARDIAC TAMPONADE	C14.280.155

lation, the librarian should determine the comprehensiveness or depth of the bibliography and the expected length. Most users will not require that a bibliography be typed. A handwritten list will usually suffice. The librarian should determine the amount of time to be spent on a compilation and should retain a dated copy for the library files. In searches that can be easily converted to existing index terms, a comprehensive bibliography of journal articles can be pulled together by photocopying relevant areas of *Index Medicus* or other indexes. In cases that require more selectivity or involve several terms, it may be more expedient to write out the citations or supply a computer search.

A bibliography prepared by hand or typed, should be carefully proofread. Further, it is useful to list the sources of the citations. This will save reverification if it becomes necessary to request the material from another library. It may also be helpful to divide the bibliography into monographic and serial sources, starring or otherwise indicating the material available within the library.

Some members of hospital library consortia share bibliographies with one another. The National Library of Medicine (NLM) also provides literature searches on topics of wide appeal. A complete list of these topics appears each month in *Index Medicus* and *Abridged Index Medicus*.

The Document

Another common response to information requests is to provide the document identified in the search. The document may come from the library's own collection or from another library, agency, or other lending source.

Again, the librarian should review the user's request. If the user has requested three or four articles discussing pros and cons of lithium therapy for psychotic patients, and the search has produced 40 citations, the librarian may contact the user again to discuss the results. Alternatively, three or four articles that cover the issue best can be sent, along with the complete bibliography and an offer to supply other articles if needed. The key point is to determine in the reference interview how much information the user wants and how much selection and evaluation is expected from the librarian. As a general rule, the librarian will probably evaluate and select less material for medical and technical searches and more for searches in nursing, management, and health care administration.

The Abstract

Another possible format for delivery of the search information is the abstract. Some online databases include abstracts along with citations, and these can be printed directly for the user.

Original abstracting, on the other hand, requires analytical skill and some subject knowledge on the part of the librarian and demands time and objectivity. An abstract summarizes the main points of an article, usually in 150-300 words. If a librarian does original abstracting, it is usually in nonmedical areas and for a highly restricted user group. In some libraries, the librarian may provide abstracting with searches for the administrative staff. Because of the time involved in this process and the potential room for bias, it is recommended that such a highly specialized service be offered with great caution, if offered at all.

A Highlighted Document

One final method of formating or packaging information is highlighting. This method requires that the librarian review, analyze, and select the relevant points of an article, marking them with a highlighting pen. Pink or blue highlighters are preferable to yellow, since yellow reproduces as a black streak if photocopied. Also, highlighting should never be done in the original source.

This technique is highly effective as an alternative to abstracting, since it allows easy review and also makes the entire document accessible. It can be used very effectively when sending unsolicited "relevant information," or when a specific piece of information requires background for interpretation.

The Information Search

Although many requests for information lead to the indexes, not every request is best answered by a journal article. When a requester is seeking basic information about a disease process or a therapeutic protocol, a textbook is often the best place to look first. If more current or more specific information is then needed, the librarian will have the historical perspective needed to assess the articles found in the indexes. In many instances, the references at the end of a book chapter suggest the best articles on the subject. The book collection is also useful when searching for facts or statistics. Many books have excellent charts, illustrations, and appendixes that can supplement the ready reference collection.

In general, looking up key words and phrases in a dictionary or medical textbook prior to a search provides a better understanding of the concept involved. Skimming a review article on a given topic is another way of learning more about the subject and locating further references. Usually, these reviews of the literature include very lengthy bibliographies. Review articles are also useful in determining the amount of material published on a subject or on one specific aspect of a subject, such as diagnosis or drug therapy. This type of information helps the librarian decide whether to narrow or broaden the focus of the search.

Ready Reference Service

Although literature and information searches may be highly rewarding, ready reference or "quick answer" reference work can make up a significant part of the library's workload and be very valuable to the hospital staff. Ready reference questions are short questions that can be answered quickly by facts. Most such questions come to the library by telephone and grow in number as the library establishes its reputation for prompt, accurate

responses. In some hospital libraries, this service is called "fast answer" service to make the name meaningful to hospital users.

Fast answer services in the hospital library may include the following:

- *Addresses.* The library is a source for addresses located in a variety of directories. Typical requests include addresses of state licensing agencies, medical schools, national foundations, federal agencies, and other types of organizations.
- *Zip codes.* The library may be asked to provide zip code information to secretaries throughout the hospital.
- *Information from physician directories.* Addresses for physicians in other cities are frequently needed by a wide range of hospital departments and medical services.
- *Telephone numbers.* The library can maintain both white and yellow pages for nearby communities and urban centers or cities where regional branches of federal agencies are located, as well as phone books for the state capital. Administration and management personnel use this service frequently if well publicized.
- *Information from directories of area social service agencies and health associations.* By quick access to such directories, the library can provide addresses, phone numbers, and contacts for patient referral.
- *Definitions.* Frequently a clinical unit calls to get a definition for an unusual syndrome or clinical term.
- *Normals.* Nurses may request specific information on normal values or ranges for lab tests to help them understand patient test results.
- *Supplies.* Access to the *Thomas Register*, perhaps through another library, provides prompt answers about suppliers.
- *Plane schedules.* Hospital libraries can make airline schedule information available to medical and hospital staff traveling for continuing education opportunities. If the schedule updating service is too expensive, a local travel agency may be willing to supply such information on a routine basis.
- *Information from motel directories.* Access to the *Hotel/Motel Red Book,* or a public library that has the tool, can save money for the seminar attendee and hospital.

Librarians should answer ready reference questions with the same care that the more complex questions receive and provide the name of the reference source. Inappropriate responses to questions may cause delay, chaos, or hardship and can ultimately discredit the library's services.

Outreach Service

A number of hospital librarians actually take their services out into the hospital, rather than wait for the user to request the service in the library. One of the most innovative of these outreach services began during the mid-sixties, when an innovative library staff member, later appropriately called a "clinical medical librarian" (CML), took reference service out to the user on wards and units (4).

Today, most CML programs function in hospitals with medical school affiliations. In these hospitals, a medical librarian participates in rounds with assigned teams of students and faculty and notes clinical questions as they arise. Responses to the questions and backup literature on specific clinical conditions can be quickly provided to the members of the team.

Among the effects documented by such a CML program are the following:

- Communication between the librarian and the health professionals and students is greatly facilitated. Information needs are clearer because the librarian is present as the questions arise.
- Information services are more personal and can be tailored to individual patient-care problems. Also, CMLs provide answers to questions more quickly, often before a question is actually asked.
- CMLs tend to improve the study habits and library skills of the students and faculty with whom they work.
- CMLs can review the current literature quickly and help faculty and students select and evaluate good up-to-date articles for patient-care problems. Subjectively at least, CMLs and their users feel that their services contribute to improved patient care and medical education (5).

Obviously, clinical librarians can be extremely valuable to clinical students and faculty. The service is costly in terms of staff time, however, and requires extensive investigation and full administrative support before initiation.

There are other ways to implement the concept behind the clinical librarian program—having the librarian participate in the user's problem-defining activities. For example, the librarian can attend selected medical, nursing, or hospital committee meetings and prepare a relevant package of material. Attendance at selected committee meetings or conferences need not be a daily activity. It can be scheduled as needed.

Other outreach services reported in the literature include LATCh, literature attached to charts (6); and LASS, literature attached to staff studies (7). Variations of LATCh occur in response to hospital functions and procedures. Ordinarily, as the medical staff or housestaff conduct rounds, they request clinical information from the library on a patient's condition. After a search, the librarian attaches the requested materials to the patient's chart. Materials may be for the medical staff, the residents, the nursing staff, or perhaps even for the patient. LASS operates on the same basis but provides literature for members of the administrative staff.

Current Awareness Service

A fourth type of information service provided by the library is current awareness service. Current awareness services furnish users with up-to-date information on selected topics. Once the user identifies the need, the library supplies the material on a routine basis.

Routing

One type of current awareness service common to health care institutions is routing. This activity is undoubtedly already going on in many institutions but may not be handled by the library. Systematizing and organizing the routing procedures can increase the library's visibility and indirectly enhance the library's image as an information center. On the other hand, routing materials is time-consuming and involves carefully designing procedures to balance the interest of specific users with the needs of all groups.

If the decision is made to initiate a routing service for a specific user group, the librarian should work with that group to define what information is needed regularly. Routed items may include relevant association newsletters, house organs from other health care institutions, tables of contents from the *Federal Register*, or health care bills pending in the state legislature. After materials are organized into a packet, the librarian should make sure the packet is routed systematically. A two-day holding limit should be urged so that the materials continue to move among group members. Preprinted routing slips, including the names and the procedure, speed the process. A list of all materials in each packet should be kept and the contents checked when the packet is returned. Once established, routing services should be evaluated periodically to ensure their relevance to the target groups.

Tables of Contents

A second type of current awareness service is supplied by *Current Contents* and other publications that consist of the content pages of journals. These monthly publications cover journals in life sciences, clinical practice, and behavior and social sciences. They can be circulated to specific user groups to permit a quick review of the current literature. Because of the volume of materials, however, some users feel this service does not meet their specific need. Before investing in the commercial service, the librarian may wish to request sample issues and test their value.

Selective Dissemination of Information

Still another type of current awareness service is "selective dissemination of information" (SDI) service. This service matches specialized topics or profiles against the current literature. A user might request, for example, all the literature available on chemotherapy for lung neoplasms. The librarian would manually check the indexes as they arrive for all such articles and forward the bibliographic citations for these articles to the user.

SDI services are available from the major vendors of bibliographic searching systems. SDI searches can be run on the NLM computerized databases by using the latest update tags. The current month of MEDLINE can be accessed through a separate file called SDILINE. SDI searches on the NLM databases can also be performed automatically. The forms used to request this service are available to all MEDLINE centers. Hospital libraries that do not have access to MEDLINE can request SDI searches from a local MEDLINE center. Instructions for using SDI services or systems other than NLMs are included in the appropriate users' manual.

SDI users should define their needs in specific terms to avoid being overwhelmed by the sheer volume of material. Periodic reviews of the SDI profile with the user are important to evaluate the performance of the service and to update the search terms. The librarian may want to maintain a file of all SDI profiles, a listing of review dates, and perhaps even a copy of the bibliographies sent.

News Clipping Service

Most hospital administrations are interested in up-to-date information about health care institutions and their activities in the local area. A newspaper clipping service is an excellent way for the librarian to help supply this information.

Articles dealing with local hospitals, health care advances in the community or neighboring cities, and information on technological advances can be photocopied and routed to the administrative staff. Librarians can also place copies of articles in the medical staff lounge for physicians who are interested in keeping up-to-date with local health care news. This procedure, however, should be approved by the hospital's administration since the clippings may contain articles about competing hospitals.

If clippings are to be effective, they should be received the day of publication or the day after. This may place pressure on the librarian who has to review and clip the papers. An alternative procedure is to use volunteers or hospital staff with periodic work loans, such as the PBX operator on the midnight shift.

All clipped articles should carry the date of publication and newspaper title. To assure permanence, articles can be mounted on 8½" x 11" paper and photocopied. If clipping services are provided by the public relations department, the librarian might arrange to retain and index a file of relevant articles.

ONLINE SERVICES

Availability of online services has created another important area of management decision making for the hospital librarian. During the seventies, some remarkable changes took place in the area of literature searching. New systems that combined the capabilities of computers with communications technology emerged. Librarians acquired the ability to search the files of literature indexes and abstracting services stored in computers at remote locations.

Computerized files of information, or databases, have been used for some time to produce printed periodical indexes such as *Index Medicus* and *Hospital Literature Index* as well as catalogs such as the *NLM Current Catalog*. Today, with online searching, the librarian uses a computer terminal linked by telephone to those same information files. This enables the librarian to select citations by author, subject, publication date, or a combination of these elements and create individualized bibliographies.

Advantages of Online Searching

Using MEDLINE, the online version of *Index Medicus*, as an example, the advantages of online searching over conventional manual searching can be outlined as follows:

- *Time-saving*. Searching MEDLINE is faster than searching *Index Medicus* manually.
- *More access points*. Citations in the MEDLINE database can be retrieved by author, journal title, date of publication, and single words and phrases in the title and abstract, as well as by the MeSH index terms.
- *Depth of indexing*. In NLM databases, an article is assigned more index terms (subject headings) than appear in the printed index. This allows access to both major and minor points of an article.
- *Hierarchical searching*. Online searching in NLM databases provides the ability to search for all subjects included in a specific segment of the hierarchical arrangement of terms (trees) relatively simply by "exploding" the numerical code for that subject area.
- *Multiple concept searching*. Two or more subjects or other access points can be searched at the same time. Using logical connectors "AND" and "OR" to link access points increases the flexibility and precision of online searching.
- *Currency*. Computerized databases are usually updated before the printed equivalent is available. They are automatically cumulated on line. Therefore, it is not necessary to search monthly or annual volumes individually.
- *Printed bibliographies*. A tailored bibliography, often with abstracts, is usually the product of the online search.

Planning

Planning for any new service, including online searching, involves gathering information, determining the current and projected need, and estimating the costs. Information about online services is available from the NLM, regional medical libraries, state library networks, experienced searchers, vendors of online services and databases, as well as from the literature.

A librarian should also evaluate the current reference services against the perceived advantages of online services. Particularly in the initial phases, a librarian should record statistics for computerized services in categories that can be compared to previous manual search services. In this way, the benefits of online searching can be demonstrated.

In addition, a librarian needs to explore options on several aspects of online searching: staffing; budgeting; selecting databases, vendors, and equipment; and developing policies. Decisions in each area should take into account both the projected initial volume of searching and the desired volume after the service is established.

Staffing

Whether the library has one staff member or several, online searching affects staffing patterns, and plans to accommodate the changes should be considered in advance. Hospital libraries rarely add a staff position to provide online searching. More frequently, a staff member with the interest and the aptitude must be trained.

Online searching requires staff time for interviewing users, formulating search strategies, and operating the computer terminal. In addition, time is needed for training, promoting the service, orienting users and staff to changes, keeping statistics, participating in user groups, and keeping abreast of changes in databases and search systems.

A searcher must be able to fit these activities into the current workload, or else arrangements must be made to reduce or reassign current responsibilities. The searcher's usual duties may be affected particularly when he or she is actually using the terminal. Interruptions while searching are expensive. Therefore, procedures should be developed to provide uninterrupted search time. Since many libraries report increased use of other services, particularly journal circulation and interlibrary loan, librarians should consider ways of adapting to these changes.

Finally, plans should be made to provide searching in the event that the searcher is absent. Training a backup searcher is ideal, but in many hospital libraries that is not feasible. Agreements with other local searchers to provide backup for each other usually offer the most practical solution, but such agreements involve time in providing reciprocal backup. Procedures should specify how requests are handled during the times search service is unavailable.

Budgeting

A librarian should compare the costs of providing the advantages of online searching to the ongoing costs of offering the present level of reference services. Ongoing costs for manual reference services include personnel time and searching tools. Expenses for online searching services are more extensive, involving start-up and ongoing costs. Start-up costs for online services include the terminal, phone installation, training (including travel), searching tools, office supplies, and equipment. Ongoing expenses for online services include terminal maintenance, local or long distance phone service, online and page charges, personnel time, supplies, and training and continuing education.

By projecting these expenses over several years, a librarian may be able to demonstrate the cost effectiveness of adding online services, particularly in light of improved and expanded services. Equipment prices and connecting charges change frequently, so the librarian should obtain information on current prices from specific vendors.

Along with estimating costs, a librarian should consider options for supporting the cost of online searching. Many hospital libraries choose to incorporate these costs into the library budget and provide free online searches as part of the overall reference function. Other systems exist, however.

The library could charge users for searches to recover costs. This system involves total or partial cost recovery and can be handled as a flat charge or a charge based on the actual cost of the search. Another alternative is to add a profit factor to user charges.

Fees could also be charged back to the user's department, thus relieving the library staff of the problems surrounding the handling of money. It is important that the librarian work with the administration and the accounting department to establish a satisfactory arrangement for all parties involved.

Selecting Databases

Librarians should select databases that can answer the most frequent subject requests. Usually, MEDLINE and the Health Planning and Administration databases satisfy most hospital library requests. Cancerlit, CATLINE, and AVLINE are also useful.

Databases in peripheral areas such as management, business, psychology, and education can increase the library's ability to meet less frequent needs. Even if only a small number of databases are used at the time online service is implemented, the librarian should plan for future service areas. Appendixes A and B following Chapter 8 provide a list of the most useful databases and a list of major vendors of computerized databases. Because databases are constantly changing, current information should be requested from vendors during the planning phase.

Selecting Vendors

Bibliographic databases created by indexing agencies such as NLM are made available by vendors of computer search services. Four major vendors are the NLM; Bibliographic Retrieval Services, Inc. (BRS); DIALOG Information Services, Inc.; and System Development Corporation (SDC). In selecting a vendor, the librarian should look at the databases and the price charged for access to the system and for other services.

The most important factor in selecting a vendor is whether it currently offers access to the essential databases. Because only NLM provides online searching of all of its 17 databases, hospital libraries most frequently select NLM services. However, BRS and DIALOG offer MEDLINE and Health Planning and Administration along with dozens of other databases.

Based on knowledge of information needs in the institution, a librarian should identify which additional databases would be used if available. Once a librarian has signed an agreement with a vendor, the librarian has access to all the vendor's databases, although charges may vary from database to database.

Vendors of online search services determine fees in various ways. The following list of possible charges can help the librarian compare the costs of services from each vendor.

Subscription Fee

Some vendors charge an annual fee for access to the system. A discount or the ability to share a single membership (password) may be available to certain library groups, such as consortia or state library networks.

Online Charges

The vendor may charge a flat hourly rate or break charges down as follows:

- *Telecommunications charges.* Rates are set by Telenet or Tymnet and others at an hourly rate for a "bargain" long distance data transmission phone connection. In areas without local access, the telephone company will bill libraries separately for long distance charges to the telecommunications node.
- *Connect charge.* Libraries are billed by the hour for all time connected to the system. Discounts are available to some users based on total usage, group membership, or both.
- *Database royalties.* Libraries are charged by the hour or by citation. The database producer charges the fee for the right to use the information. Royalties vary with the database and on a given database from vendor to vendor.

Offline Charges

The vendor may assess fees for searching or printing offline plus mailing costs. Stored searches incur a monthly fee plus printing and mailing charges.

Training

The cost and the duration of training offered by vendors varies. NLM offers training courses in Washington, D.C., and at regional locations. Library networks and professional organizations, as well as database and system vendors also offer training. Travel to training sites is at the expense of the user, so location and duration as well as the course fee affects the total cost.

Searching Tools

Manuals on the vendor's system and on individual databases are tools for librarians. They can be purchased from the vendor or the database producer. Newsletters that update procedures and offer searching tips are usually provided free of charge by vendors and database producers.

Equipment

Access to databases for bibliographic searching requires a telephone-compatible data terminal. Factors involving size, speed, type of print, and cost influence the selection of a computer terminal. Because of constant changes in the field of databases, the librarians should read the current literature on this subject and talk to other searchers about their preferences. Useful information and references appear in Chapter 6 of the *Handbook of Medical Library Practice* (2). If compatible equipment is available elsewhere in the hospital, using it could significantly reduce the initial costs.

Librarians usually prefer a printing terminal to a cathode ray terminal (CRT). A standard data terminal purchased for online searching may also serve as a printer for a CRT model or home computer already in the hospital. If a librarian wants to become familiar with equipment before purchasing, it is possible to lease a terminal with the option to buy.

A phone coupler, or modem, connects the data terminal to the phone line. Some portable terminals have a built-in modem. An additional phone line reserved for searching is advised if the library currently has only one line. Space and furniture that will allow uninterrupted searching as well as security for the terminal are other considerations when selecting equipment for computer services.

Policies

During the planning stages, a librarian should attempt to develop general policies governing search services. The policies should outline who will use the service; when and if fees will be paid, and by whom; who will select databases; and how backup service will be provided.

Policies related to changes in other services should also be considered. After the service has operated for some time, the librarian should evaluate and modify policies based on experience.

Proposals for Online Searching

A librarian should submit a proposal to the administration for the addition of online services only after well-defined plans have been made and information has been secured. Time spent in careful preparation of the proposal is usually repaid in administrative understanding and approval.

The format for proposals may vary but most include the following:

- *Summary.* Documentation ordinarily begins with a brief summary of the proposal.
- *Description of online searching.* A brief definition and description of the process should include information on the purpose of searching, the use of computer terminals to access remote files via phone connection, and the products of the search. A brochure supplied by a user group, regional medical library, or vendor may be included with the proposal.
- *Advantages to the hospital.* A statement about the advantages of adding online services, tailored to the individual needs of the hospital may include:
  - Use of information retrieved through searches to improve patient care and decision making in the hospital
  - Improved quality of online searches over manual searches—more thorough and current information translated more quickly into a convenient printed bibliography
  - Availability of searching to more user groups, such as students or support services staff, who can be served without adding staff or purchasing tools in additional subject areas
- *Cost estimates.* An estimate of service costs should include:
  - Comparison of initial and ongoing costs for online and manual searching
  - Presentation of options for recovering all or part of service costs
  - Budget for succeeding years
  - Comparison of cost of providing searches with the cost of searches provided by other libraries
- *Advantages to the library.* A description of the advantages of online searching in terms of providing library services may include statements on:
  - More effective use of staff reference time
  - Ability to provide more searches because of reduced time for each search
  - Ability to produce more current, relevant, and thorough searches from more data than library can access manually
  - Access to more information without purchasing indexes in less frequently needed subject areas
  - Use of databases for interlibrary loan verification, for acquisitions and cataloging information, and for ready reference (verifications for users, author's names, addresses)
  - Ability to provide bibliographies with reduced clerical time, or ability to add this service if not presently provided
- *Policies and procedures.* Suggested policies and procedures may be summarized for the administration with the original proposal if these require approval before implementation of online services.
- *Implementation.* An outline of the steps necessary to implement online searching should include a chronol-

ogy and any deadlines or suspense times (budget request deadlines, time to process contracts, training dates).
- *Sample searches.* Sample searches on subjects of interest to major user groups and to the recipient of the proposal illustrate the advantages of online searching.

Sections of a proposal can be documented with appropriate statistics, cost estimates, testimonials of need from medical staff and other library users, and articles from the literature.

Implementation Schedule

To begin online bibliographic searching, the librarian must arrange for a number of activities to begin simultaneously. Each of these activities is described below.

Contracts

Once databases and vendors are selected, the library must sign contracts or agreements with the vendor or library network to authorize access to the search service. This process should be timed so that the period covered by the subscription fee begins as close as possible to the actual date of service, thus avoiding any unnecessary expense.

Equipment

The library should order the terminal and modem for delivery just before service is to begin. Phone installation should take place first so that equipment can be tested immediately upon delivery. Service agreements should start just prior to the beginning date of service to avoid being charged for coverage when the equipment is not in use.

Training

New searchers should be trained before the first date of actual use so that practice reinforces formal training. The library must have a trained searcher before NLM grants access to its system. Although other vendors do not require training, it is a prerequisite for cost-effective searching. The new searcher may schedule a brief practice period to sharpen skills before the official service begins. If vendors offer free or reduced connect time to new users or trainees, the time can be most effectively used right after training.

Searching Aids

The searcher should have access to manuals for each vendor's system and for each database. These manuals should be available from the start of service.

Forms and Procedures

User request forms, evaluation forms, logs, and statistical report forms should be ready for the first day of service. Although the librarian may revise these after some experience, usable drafts are needed from the beginning. The librarian should determine procedures for handling requests and assessing and collecting any fees in advance of the service.

Staff Orientation

All library staff, even those not directly involved in providing the service, should receive information about the capabilities of online searching and its impact on library service. The staff needs guidelines for handling new user request forms, statistical records, and questions that accompany the addition of online services. Staff should be aware, as much as possible, of progress in implementing the service. Intensive, specific orientation should immediately precede the beginning of service.

User Education

The library can provide user education on a one-to-one basis or in structured group presentations, as soon as the search service is inaugurated. In either case, the librarian should consider having explanatory materials, such as sample request forms and sample searches, available for independent study. Introduction to search services should become part of any orientation to library services. The librarian may target particular user groups for specific education once the service is established.

Promotion of Services

The librarian should develop promotional materials to present to the medical staff, administrators, key managers, and other professionals for their use at orientation sessions. Demonstrations and open houses, as well as other ideas suggested in Chapter 17, may be useful in making users aware of the new service.

Monitoring

The complexity of the record-keeping system depends on the ultimate use of the data being recorded. A librarian should keep a record of the name of the requester, the name of the database being used, the subject of the search, and the online time. See Appendix A for a sample online services log. This information is useful for the annual report as well as the verification of the monthly bill for online charges.

Additional data may be included to help determine who pays for the search and to review the search strategy for quality assurance purposes. Periodically, the librarian may wish to compare usage and cost figures for manual and computer searching in order to determine the benefits of continuing the service. Evaluation forms completed by users after each search can help in developing the searcher's skills to meet users' needs. These forms are most effective when designed by the searcher with the individual situation in mind. A sample form is provided in Appendix B as a starting point.

Hospital librarians who currently have online services available report numerous changes in the library since the addition of that service. Use patterns change, interlibrary loan volume increases, journal holdings may need to expand, and the library often enjoys a new prestige.

MANAGING INFORMATION SERVICES

Sound management of information services is necessary in order to provide the variety of services needed by a multi-faceted user population. Types and levels of services, service priorities, tools, and available budget must be wisely balanced and then documented. The purpose of this management is not to impose restrictions or reduce use but to make realistic allocations of limited resources, based on needs and use.

Management decisions concerning information services have not become easier over the last few years. Expanded user groups, increasing costs of library materials, the availability of online services, and the emergence of cooperative services all compete for limited resources. Today's decisions affect the library's future, its image, and its potential for services.

Policies and Procedures

Library policies determine service and, therefore, deserve careful formulation. Information services policies should be approved by the library committee and the hospital administration. They should be consistent with the goals and objectives of the library and the hospital. The elements common to most information service policies include definitions of users, services provided, levels of service for each category of user, hours of service, and evaluation methods. Procedures for providing information services should also be documented to provide consistency.

Definition of Users

An effective service policy defines the major groups the library serves. It can define groups by listing those who are served or by listing those who are not served. In most cases, the better approach identifies groups that are served by broad category such as medical or hospital staff and specific groups of affiliated students. The definition of users could also include or exclude the local public library, library consortia members, health care professionals not affiliated with the hospital, community members at large, or attorneys.

Decisions about clientele may have a major impact on allocation of resources for information services. Further, these decisions must be made in accordance with the hospital's general philosophy and policy. If the hospital has a strong investment in community outreach or has made a major commitment to area health education programs, the library may be expected to have a similar commitment. The definition of user groups should be approved by the hospital library committee and the hospital administration.

Definition of Services

The hospital library's information services policies should also define the kinds of services provided, such as bibliography development, ready reference, clinical medical librarian services, photocopying, routing, abstracting, and orientations. A brief explanation of each service should be given, along with any limitations or exceptions.

Hours of Service

The information services policy should also spell out hours of service. These hours should conform to user needs as much as possible within the confines of staff and budget. For greatest utilization, the library should be open and staffed during the hours of physician rounds, nursing staff breaks, and mealtimes. Librarians should also consider maintaining evening hours, depending on user need.

The policy should also identify methods for gaining access to the library during those hours when it is closed. Many libraries provide a key that can be checked out at the hospital's switchboard or arrange for the hospital's security department for access. The librarian may also want to establish a plan whereby he or she can be called at home if an emergency arises.

Service Evaluation

Because of the increasing emphasis on quality assurance and on the standards for professional library services issued by the JCAH, the information services policy should include a section on evaluation. This section should define the library's plan for needs analysis and follow-up reference evaluation.

Evaluation of User Satisfaction

Developing a mechanism for evaluating all information services is another important management task. Evaluation of library services in general is discussed in Chapter 12. Only the evaluation of information services will be considered here.

Meaningful evaluation of user satisfaction is sometimes difficult because users may respond based on their perception of what the library can do rather than whether the information they received was genuinely useful. Users may be satisfied if their expectations are minimal. On the other hand, they may be dissatisfied if their expectations are high. The librarian will have to construct the evaluations carefully to obtain the most useful responses.

The two most common techniques for evaluating information services are informal interviews and written surveys. Both should take place with the user immediately following the service transaction. A survey sent to known users, independent of a specific request, is usually less helpful. Users generally complete such a survey from general impressions rather than from memory of specific instances.

In a personal interview, the librarian can tailor the questions to the situation and follow up on responses. The search can also be redone immediately if problems are uncovered. The evaluation also appears to users as one more phase in the total process and often makes them feel that the service is responsive to their needs.

The major disadvantages of interviewing are the time involved, the lack of quantifiable results, and the possibility of lack of candor from the respondent. Because most interviews are informal, they are usually evaluated individually rather than collectively. As a result, patterns in responses may be overlooked.

A survey completed after the transaction quantifies and records responses. The user, however, may feel that it takes more time and is less personal than an interview. Unless the librarian reads the results immediately, the opportunity to correct problems on the spot may be lost.

Regardless of the format of the evaluation, the librarian will probably be looking for information in the following areas:

- *Response time.* Was the response prompt enough to satisfy the user's perceived needs?
- *Amount of material.* Was the material provided in sufficient quantity? Too much quantity?
- *Depth.* Did the material provided cover what the user needed to know?
- *Format.* Would the response have been more helpful if it had been in a different format?
- *Applicability.* Was the response helpful? Could it have been more helpful?

Record-Keeping

A hospital library should maintain several types of information services records. Typically, the two main categories of records are counts and records of the actual transactions.

Counts

Measuring service levels continuously documents the use of service and shows patterns in that use. Because statistics take time to maintain, a librarian should determine intended use of each measurement in advance. Categories should be clearly defined so that they fill the intended purpose.

Typically, libraries keep several kinds of statistics relating to information services.

- *User count.* Users can be counted as they enter the library or at a specified interval, such as every hour. Both methods involve some inaccuracy, and the most convenient method should be chosen. A manual counter saves a great deal of time in counting users.
- *Numbers and types of information requests.* Typical categories for information requests are directional, fast answer or ready reference, information searches, and computer and manual literature searches.
- *User groups.* This information helps document who uses library services and at what levels.

• *Purpose of use.* Some libraries find it helpful to document the reasons for library use, often to substantiate the claim that library services support patient care.

• *Miscellaneous.* In specific situations, librarians may want to keep track of subjects of use, photocopies, telephone requests, and the amount of time per request.

Information Service Records

Depending on the kinds of services the library provides, it may be necessary to keep a second kind of record to document the information provided. For example, all literature searches may be kept on file for future reference. Librarians can maintain records on ready reference questions, perhaps using a log of phone calls received. The need for such records should be weighed against the time required to maintain them or to acquire them again.

REFERENCES

1. Jahoda G, Braunagel JS. The librarian and reference queries: a systematic approach. New York: Academic Press, 1980.

2. Egeland J, Foreman GE. Reference services: searching and searching techniques. In: Darling L, Bishop D, Colaianni LA, eds. Handbook of medical library practice, 4th ed. Vol. I. Chicago: Medical Library Association, 1982.

3. Beatty WK. Searching the literature and computerized services in medicine: guides and methods for the clinician. Ann Intern Med 1979 Aug;91:326-332.

4. Algermissen V. Biomedical librarians in a patient care setting at the University of Missouri-Kansas City. Bull Med Libr Assoc 1974 Oct;62:354-358.

5. Byrd GD. Outreach, innovation, service, and cooperation: the UMKC Health Sciences Library. Show Me Libraries. 1980 Dec; 31:26-28.

6. Sowell SL. Latch at the Washington Hospital Center, 1967-1975. Bull Med Libr Assoc 1978 Apr;66:218-222.

7. Doyle FM. LASS: A new library service for hospital managers. Hosp Libr 1978 Jan;3:8.

READINGS

Atherton P, Christian RW. Librarians and online services. White Plains, NY: Knowledge Industry Publications, 1977.

Bunge CA. Professional education and reference efficiency. Springfield, IL: Illinois State Library, 1967. (Illinois State Library, Research series no. 11).

Byrd GD, Arnold L. Medical school graduates' retrospective evaluation of a clinical medical librarian program. Bull Med Libr Assoc 1979 Jul;67:308-312.

Chen CC, ed. Quantitative measurement and dynamic library service. Phoenix: Oryx Press, 1978.

Evans E, Borko H, Ferguson P. Review of criteria to measure library effectiveness. Bull Med Libr Assoc 1972 Jan;60:102-110.

Hahn RC. The library in a small hospital with an active research component. Mo Med 1971 Dec;68:924-927.

Hamberg M, Clelland RC, Bommer MR, Romist LE, Whitfield, RM. Library planning and decision making systems. Cambridge, MA: MIT Press, 1978.

Hawkins DT. Impact of on-line systems on a literature searching service. Spec Libr 1976 Dec;67:559-567.

Holst R. Stephens M, Welch E, Goldberg K. The reference interview: preparation for positive results. Chicago: Midwest Health Science Library Network, 1982.

King DW, Bryant EC. Evaluation of information services and products. Washington, DC: Information Resources Press, 1971.

Kramer J. How to survive in industry: cost justified library services. Spec Libr 1971 Nov;62:487-489.

Lancaster FW. The cost-effectiveness analysis of information retrieval and dissemination systems. J Am Soc Inf Sci 1971 Jan-Feb;22:12-27.

Lancaster FW. The measurement and evaluation of library services. Washington, DC: Information Resources Press, 1977.

Lopez M, Rubacher R. Interpersonal psychology: librarians and patrons. Cath Lib World 1969 Apr;40:483-487.

Martin L. User studies and library planning. Libr Trends 1976 Jan;24: 483-496.

McCarn DB. MEDLINE: an introduction to online searching. J Am Soc Inf Sci 1980 May;31:181-192.

McCarthy SE, Maccabee SS, Feng CCH. Evaluation of Medline service by user survey. Bull Med Libr Assoc 1974 Oct; 62:367-373.

Oliphant, CA. Handling information successfully—one of management's most difficult problems. Hospital Management Communications 1979 Sprint;3:4-7.

Orr, RH. Measuring the goodness of library services: a general framework for considering quantitative measures. J of Documentation 1973 Sep;29:315-332.

Rothstein S. The measurement and evaluation of reference service. Libr Trends 1964 Jan;12:456-472.

Van Gieson WR. The hospital library in transition. Hosp Prog 1978 June;59:66-69.

APPENDIX A
Sample Online Services Log

SYSTEM NAME _____

DATE	SEARCHER	DATA-BASE	PRIME TIME*	LOG-ON	LOG-OFF	TOTAL ONLINE TIME	SEARCH FORMU-LATION TIME	OFFLINE SEARCHING OR PRINTING	USER NAME/ DEPT.	SUBJECT	COMMENT

*This column is for NLM, only. For BRS and DIALOG, this column could refer to total cost, supplied online by the system for each search.

Note: A separate log designed for each system can simplify verifying bills.

APPENDIX B
Computer Search Evaluation

Name: (optional)   Department: (optional)

USER GROUP:

Staff physician _____   Administration _____   Medical student _____
Post Doc/Fellow _____   Nursing service _____   Other library _____
Housestaff _____   Support service _____   Other _____

Was this your first computerized bibliographic search?

   Yes ____   No ____

What was the overall level of satisfaction with your search?

   Excellent ____   Good ____   Fair ____   Poor ____

If satisfaction was fair or poor, check the appropriate reason:

   Too few citations retrieved ____   No relevant citations retrieved ____
   Too many irrelevant citations retrieved ____   Other _____

What percentage of the total citations retrieved were relevant to your needs?

   0% ____   25% ____   50% ____   75% ____   100% ____

Did the search miss references that you found through other sources?

   Yes ____   No ____   If yes, how did you find the sources?

How helpful was the librarian in planning your search?

   Very helpful ____   Helpful ____   Not very helpful ____   Not at all helpful ____

How could the librarian have been more helpful?

   More thorough interview ____   Offering of alternatives other than search ____
   Explanation of search process ____   Other _____
   More feedback before search was completed ____

If you were not satisfied, did you discuss the results with the librarian?

   Yes ____   No ____

If no, why not?

   My time was limited ____   Librarian was not available ____
   Search was picked up after regular hours ____   Other _____

Would you request another computer search from this library?

   Yes ____   No ____

If this service were not free, would you be willing to pay for the service?

   Yes ____   up to $2.00 ____ $2.00-$5.00 ____ $6.00-$10.00 ____   over $10.00 ____
   No ____

Note: This sample is based on a form designed by Christine Foster, Wishard Memorial Hospital, Indianapolis, Indiana.

Information Resources

Ruth Holst
Director of Library Services
Columbia Hospital
Milwaukee, Wisconsin

CHAPTER 8

Information Resources

Ruth Holst
Director of Library Services
Columbia Hospital
Milwaukee, Wisconsin

GUIDES TO REFERENCE SOURCES

SOURCES OF FACTUAL INFORMATION
Directories
Dictionaries
Standard Textbooks
Drug Information Sources
Statistical Sources
Legal Sources
Accreditation Sources
Other Types of Information

SOURCES OF BIBLIOGRAPHIC INFORMATION
Book and Periodical Sources
Lists of Recommended Publications
Indexes
Abstracting Services
Government Publications
Proceedings
Current Awareness Sources
Online Sources of Information

SOURCES OF INFORMATION ON
AUDIOVISUALS
Printed Sources
Online Sources

USING RESOURCES EFFECTIVELY

USING COMMUNITY RESOURCES
Information and Referral
Information Clearinghouses
Using the Telephone

CREATING A RESOURCE FILE

Appendixes

Hospital personnel use information for patient care, continuing education, and hospital-based research. Information is needed to plan, operate, and evaluate hospital programs. It can be obtained through a variety of sources, including the hospital library. Whether individuals come to the hospital library for the information they need usually depends on their past experience with the library and on the library's reputation for being helpful.

This chapter will deal with the resources that the librarian needs to locate facts and information. Although the size of the collection and the amount of money spent on library resources are both important, the key to good library service is the librarian's knowledge of information resources and the ability to use them effectively.

The creative librarian views all library resources as potential reference tools. The reference sources discussed in this chapter, however, are those that concentrate many facts into one source or those that provide lists of sources to consult for needed information. These resources, usually called "the reference collection," often do not circulate and are shelved separately from the rest of the collection.

In building the reference collection, the librarian should use lists of recommended reference sources as guides. Using such lists can prevent expensive mistakes. Also, the librarian should learn about the programs and subject specialties that are emphasized in the hospital and the new activities that are being planned. This type of data is helpful in anticipating information needs. Records should be kept of questions that cannot be answered using the library's resources. These records can be useful in deciding which new resources the library should acquire. Policies and techniques for selecting library resources are discussed in more detail in Chapter 3.

The four types of information resources usually required in hospital libraries will be discussed below. They include guides to reference sources, sources of factual information, souces of bibligrahic information, and sources of information on audiovisuals. The use of community resources and suggestions for creating a resource file are also discussed.

GUIDES TO REFERENCE SOURCES

All hospital libraries should have basic reference sources such as dictionaries and directories to answer questions commonly asked in hospitals. The individual librarian must decide which additional resources are necessary to fill the information needs of doctors and other professionals in the hospital.

Several books and lists identify reference works that the librarian may wish to purchase or consult. The most comprehensive retrospective source is *Medical Reference Works 1679-1966: A Selected Bibliography*, edited by Blake and Roos and published by the Medical Library Association (MLA).* Supplements to this work were published in 1970, 1973, and 1975.

Another MLA publication, Roper and Boorkman's *Introduction to Reference Sources in the Health Sciences*, provides an excellent review of reference sources that should be available in all large medical libraries. The *Handbook of Medical Library Practice*, 4th edition, includes a discussion of reference resources commonly found in health science libraries. A more general work, *Health Sciences Information Sources*, serves as a guide to the literature of the health sciences. Most hospital libraries can afford to purchase only a fraction of the sources listed in these books. However, the annotations they contain can be very useful during the selection process.

Additional guides to reference sources in specific subject areas are also available to aid the hospital librarian in building the reference collection. This chapter will identify only a small number of the hundreds of reference works in the health sciences. The librarian may wish to use the guides mentioned above and in Appendix A to learn more about specific subject areas.

SOURCES OF FACTUAL INFORMATION

The hospital librarian is frequently asked to locate facts and figures on a variety of subjects. Finding answers to these inquiries requires a familiarity with the entire library collection, since the answer to a question may be buried in the appendix of a textbook. Some of the more common sources of factual information are discussed below.

Directories

Directories are valuable reference tools. Some provide biographical information. Others contain information on educational programs, organizations and institutions, or government agencies and officials. Health care directories described as "comprehensive" are also available. Each of these types of directories will be discussed below.

Biographical Information

Information about physicians can be found in a number of sources. The two sources used most frequently are the *American Medical Directory* and the *Directory of Medical Specialists*. The *American Medical Directory* lists all the medical doctors in the United States. It is arranged geographically by state and city. The following information about each physician is included: name, address, medical school attended, year of licensure, and type of practice. An alphabetical index of names is also included. The *Directory of Medical Specialists* lists only physicians from the United States and Canada who are certified by the American Board of Medical Specialties. It is arranged into sections by specialty, with geographical divisions within each section. It contains more biographical information than the *American Medical Directory*.

*For more information on sources cited throughout the chapter, see Appendix A.

Included are the physician's date of birth, postgraduate training, hospital and teaching affiliations, military record, and professional memberships. Telephone numbers are also included.

Most professional associations for nurses and allied health professionals also publish directories. *American Men and Women of Science* and *Who's Who in America* provide biographical information on a wide range of professionals. Professional associations at the state and local level may also publish directories of their members. Directories are usually sold to members at a reduced price. The librarian may wish to ask hospital staff members who belong to an association to donate a copy of the association's directory to the library.

Educational Programs

There are several useful sources of information about medical education and training programs. *Medical School Admission Requirements* provides prospective students with information on preparing for medical school and applying for admission. The *AAMC Directory of American Medical Education* contains information about medical programs in the United States and Canada. It also lists names and addresses of key people at these schools. *The World Directory of Medical Schools* lists medical schools in more than 100 countries. Senior medical school students may find the American Medical Association's (AMA) *Directory of Residency Training Programs* helpful for selecting postgraduate training opportunities. Information about other health science occupations can be found in the *Allied Health Education Directory*. This publication describes each occupation and its accreditation process. It also contains a listing of educational programs by state.

Another source of information about educational programs is the *Journal of the American Medical Association* (*JAMA*). It publishes two education issues annually. One is called *Medical Education* and contains facts about undergraduate, graduate, allied health, and continuing education. The other is entitled *Continuing Education Courses for Physicians* and lists courses for physicians by specialty. In addition, five directories are continuously updated and published in rotating order in alternating issues of JAMA. These include (1) organizations of medical interest; (2) upcoming meetings in the United States; (3) foreign meetings; (4) state medical associations, examinations, and licensure; and (5) a semiannual listing of AMA officials.

The National League for Nursing (NLN) publishes many directories of nursing education programs. Some appear in *Nursing Outlook* but all are issued as separate publications of the NLN.

Organizations and Institutions

The *American Hospital Association Guide to the Health Care Field* is an important source of information about hospitals. Entries include address and telephone number, number of beds, type of facilities, classification and control information, type of accreditation, occupancy rate, budget, and number of personnel. The *AHA Guide* also lists addresses for a wide range of state, regional, national, and international health organizations and agencies. These include health systems agencies (HSAs), professional health associations, state licensing boards, government agencies, Blue Cross-Blue Shield plans, professional standards review organizations (PSROs), and hospital associations. The *Canadian Hospital Directory* provides information about hospitals and other health organizations, institutions, and programs in Canada. A buyer's guide to medical products is also included.

The American Journal of Nursing and *Nursing Outlook* both include annual directories of nursing and related organizations on the state, national, and international levels. Although both journals are published by the same company, the two lists are not the same.

The most comprehensive guide to health science libraries is the *Directory of Health Sciences Libraries in the United States, 1979*. Published by the MLA, it is arranged geographically and has an alphabetical index of libraries.

Additional information may be found in *Health Organizations of the United States, Canada and the World*. It lists a large number of groups that are involved in health care and related fields. The following information is given for each organization: address, purpose, financial situation, awards, publications, affiliations, meetings, and key officials. The *Encyclopedia of Associations* can also be consulted for information about associations.

Government Agencies and Officials

The *United States Government Manual* is an annual publication that describes the purposes and programs of government agencies and lists the top officials of each. Briefer descriptions are included for quasi-official agencies and certain international organizations. Name, subject, and agency indexes are also provided.

The *National Health Directory* is an annually updated list of key health personnel at national, state, and local levels. The names of health committee members, health agency personnel, state agency officials, and local health officials are included. Local lists are incomplete and information may no longer be accurate because of changes in personnel. However, this directory may be a useful resource for doctors and administrators who contact key health officials frequently.

"Comprehensive" Directories

A comprehensive directory for the health care field does not exist. The two directories discussed below each contain a great deal of information. They may be useful resources, especially in larger hospital libraries.

Medical and Health Information Directory lists the same organizations that appear in the *AHA Guide* but includes only a fraction of the hospitals. Information is also given regarding grants, honors and awards, health maintenance organizations (HMOs), area health education centers (AHECs), consultants, poison control centers, research centers, drug companies, biomedical publications, audiovisual producers, libraries, and foreign medical schools. However, most of the lists are incomplete.

Health Care Directory 77-78 is a guide to institutions, publications, organizations, and services in the health care field. It also includes information on adoption, organ transplant registries, and medical illustrators. However, it is very expensive and does not have an index.

Dictionaries

Every hospital library should have at least one good medical dictionary. Two of the best available are *Dorland's Illustrated Medical Dictionary* and *Stedman's Medical Dictionary*. The *Illustrated Dictionary of Eponymic Syndromes and Diseases and their Synonyms* and the *Dictionary of Medical Syndromes* are excellent sources of information on diseases and syndromes that are named for specific people. *A Psychiatric Glossary* contains definitions of more than 1,000 terms. These definitions are authorized by the American Psychiatric Association. The *Diagnostic and Statistical Manual of Mental Disorders* offers diagnostic classifications as well as definitions of mental disorders. The *Encyclopedia and Dictionary of Medicine and Nursing and Allied Health* defines medical and nursing terms in simplified language. It may be appropriate for libraries that need a less technical dictionary.

Standard Textbooks

Standard textbooks in medicine, nursing, and other health care fields are important sources of factual information. Some textbooks also contain lists of references that may be helpful. See Appendix A for lists of recommended texts, such as those published by Brandon and Hill. Some of these lists will be discussed later in the chapter.

Drug Information Sources

Questions about drugs arise frequently. Although the pharmacy department can answer many of these questions, the hospital library should have some basic reference works dealing with drugs. The *Physician's Desk Reference (PDR)* is a commonly used source. It contains the same information that appears on drug package inserts, including actions, administration and dosage, side effects and precautions. *PDRs* are also available in several specialized subject fields. Two sources of information about over-the-counter drugs are the *PDR for Nonprescription Drugs* and the *Handbook of Nonprescription Drugs*.

Selected drugs are evaluated in the *AMA Drug Evaluations*. These evaluations are based on published and unpublished scientific data and on the opinions of expert reviewers. Drugs are organized into therapeutic categories and are evaluated individually within each category. The *American Hospital Formulary Service* is a subscription service in two loose-leaf volumes. It is arranged by classification of drugs. Each entry describes the drug's chemistry, actions, absorption, uses, cautions, interactions, and dosages. An index of names and synonyms appears at the end of the work.

Goodman and Gilman's Pharmacological Basis of Therapeutics contains more information on the history and chemistry of drugs than some of the other sources. It is organized into broad categories of drugs. Conn's *Current Therapy* discusses drugs and also presents an annual update for all methods of therapy. It is arranged by body systems and diseases.

In addition to the basic reference works discussed above, there are two specialized books that the librarian should be aware of. Hansten's *Drug Interactions* discusses how drugs interact with foods, laboratory tests, and other drugs. *Clinical Toxicology of Commercial Products* lists the toxic ingredients of commercially available products often involved in accidents in the home. Sewell's *Guide to Drug Information* is a useful addition to any hospital library collection. It discusses techniques and sources for locating drug information.

Statistical Sources

Locating statistics can be very time-consuming. However, there are two guides to help the hospital librarian locate statistics more efficiently. *Facts at Your Fingertips* is arranged alphabetically by subject and gives names, addresses, and telephone numbers of people, agencies, and organizations that supply statistics. It is available free from the National Center for Health Statistics (NCHS). *Health Statistics: A Guide to Information Sources* arranges sources of data by category and includes several useful appendixes. Both of these publications refer mainly to government sources of statistics.

Statistics also appear in periodical literature. When searching indexes that use the *Medical Subject Headings* (MeSH) vocabulary, certain subheadings may be used with the applicable subject heading. These subheadings include etiology, manpower, mortality, occurrence, statistics, supply and distribution, and utilization.

The federal government and various health organizations and associations are also good sources of statistics. They will be discussed below.

Government

The federal government is the best source of free and inexpensive statistical publications covering a variety of health topics. The NCHS publishes many reports using data from its surveys and studies. Reports from NCHS include data on health and disease, mortality, manpower, facilities, resource utilization, population, births, deaths, marriages, and divorces.

NCHS's major publication is *Vital and Health Statistics*. It includes more than 500 individual reports grouped into subseries, many of which are indexed in *Index Medicus*. *Series 10: Data from the Health Interview Survey* and *Series 11: Data from the Health Examination Survey and the Health and Nutrition Examination Survey* are probably the most useful to hospital librarians. Since 1976, *Advance Data from Vital and Health Statistics* has provided early release of selected data. Most of this information is later included in *Vital and Health Statistics*.

The *Catalog of Publications of the National Center for Health Statistics* is a cumulative listing of the *Vital and Health Statistics* series from 1962 to 1980. It also lists most other NCHS reports from 1976 to 1980. Future catalogs will cover five-year periods.

The Center for Disease Control (CDC) also publishes valuable data. The two most widely used publications are *MMWR Morbidity and Mortality Weekly Report* and the *Annual Summary*. The weekly *MMWR* publishes data on diseases reported to state health departments. The *Annual Summary* condenses the weekly *MMWR* publications and also includes data from the National Surveillance Program and the NCHS.

A good general source of data is the annual *Statistical Abstract of the United States*, which contains several sections on health. The hospital library may not need to purchase this publication every year. The World Health Organization publishes *World Health Statistics Annual*. It contains information on births, causes of death, infectious diseases, health personnel, and hospitals. This information is supplied by the governments of participating countries.

Organizations and Associations

Many health organizations and associations publish statistics. The American Hospital Association (AHA) publishes *Hospital Statistics*, which gives the results of an annual survey sent to all hospitals in the United States. Statistics are given for hospital utilization, personnel, finances, facilities, and services.

Two nurses' organizations publish statistics. The American Nurses Association's (ANA *Facts about Nursing* includes information on the education, wages, and distribution of nurses. The National League for Nursing (NLN) publishes the *NLN Nursing Data Book*, which focuses on statistical data related to nursing education.

Many health organizations distribute free materials on request. For example, the American Cancer Society publishes *Cancer Facts and Figures*. Many other reports and pamphlets are also available. Local chapters of many of these organizations may be contacted by telephone.

Legal Sources

Hospitals are subject to a variety of laws and regulations. It is important for the hospital librarian to know which staff members handle legal issues and to work closely with those individuals when selecting legal information resources. In some hospitals, it may be the administrator or one of the assistant administrators. Larger hospitals may have an attorney on staff to manage legal affairs. In any case, the library is likely to be only one of several sources of legal information. Also, many reference tools dealing with the law may be kept in the departments that use them frequently.

The librarian should be familiar with basic legal resources. The *Hospital Law Manual* interprets laws pertaining to hospitals and medical personnel. This annually updated loose-leaf manual has a three-volume attorney's set and a three-volume administrator's set. Most hospitals need to purchase only the administrator's set.

Laws are published in the U.S. Code. Hospitals may wish to purchase only the single titles containing laws that concern them. The *Code of Federal Regulations* (*CFR*) is updated daily by the *Federal Register*. These publications include the regulations that are issued by government agencies under the authority of public law. The hospital may wish to purchase only those titles of the *CFR* that relate to its concerns.

The Health Care Financing Administration (HCFA) publishes a series of health insurance manuals (HIM). Some of these manuals may be used by the hospital's accounting department. The two manuals that most hospitals need to refer to are *Medicare: Hospital Manual* (HIM 10) and *Medicare: Provider Reimbursement Manual* (HIM 15). These loose-leaf manuals are updated regularly as new laws and regulations are passed. A more detailed analysis of Medicare laws is given in the *Medicare and Medicaid Guide*, published by Commerce Clearing House. Its companion set is the *Medicare and Medicaid Guide: New Developments*. Both of these guides provide annotations and interpretations of the material covered in the HCFA manuals.

The hospital librarian should also be aware of state and local laws and regulations. Each state has its own statutes and administrative codes. Most states publish guides relating to Medicaid funds.

Two secondary sources of legal information are well suited to the hospital library. The *Handbook of Legal Medicine* summarizes the physician's responsibility with regard to such issues as informed consent, abortion, and cases of violent death. *Law Every Nurse Should Know* deals with nurses' rights, duties, and liabilities under the law.

Many of the primary sources of legal information may be too expensive for most hospitals to purchase. Thus, the librarian should find out which local public and academic libraries own these materials. The hospital's law firm may also own these resources and may even have staff available to help find needed information.

Accreditation Sources

Hospitals may be subject to standards set by accrediting agencies such as the Joint Commission on Accreditation of Hospitals (JCAH). Compliance with these standards is usually voluntary. However, accreditation by recognized agencies implies that a hospital provides a certain quality of patient care. The quality of a hospital's educational programs may also be evaluated by such agencies.

Several JCAH publications can help hospitals meet minimum standards. The *Accreditation Manual for Hospitals* is published annually and includes standards that must be met by each department or service to achieve quality care. The *Hospital Survey Profile*, a companion document, asks specific questions relating to the JCAH standards. These questions are to be answered a few months before the surveyors visit the hospital. *JCAH Perspectives* announces policy changes and new standards before the next edition of the *Accreditation Manual for Hospitals* is published.

The Canadian Council on Hospital Accreditation publishes the *Guide to Hospital Accreditation*. This guide assists Canadian hospitals in meeting standards of quality patient care.

Many programs in the hospital must comply with standards that are specific to individual disciplines. For example, the NLN uses *Criteria for the Evaluation of Diploma Programs in Nursing* as the basis for its accreditation process for these programs. The American College of Surgeons accredits cancer programs using the criteria outlined in *Cancer Program Manual*. The major source of psychiatric standards is *Consolidated Standards Manual for Child, Adolescent and Adult Psychiatric, Alcoholism and Drug Abuse Facilities*, published by the JCAH. Although primarily intended for psychiatric facilities, it also applies to certain types of outreach programs associated with acute care hospitals. Hospital laboratories may be evaluated using the College of American Pathologists' *Standards for Accreditation of Medical Laboratories*. For information about hospital library standards, see Chapter 2.

Many additional publications list standards for hospital programs. Hospital personnel involved in various programs are usually good sources of information on these publications.

Other Types of Information

In addition to health science resources, a hospital library should have a general reference collection. Records of information requests may be helpful in deciding which resources to acquire. Basic reference works such as an unabridged dictionary, a thesaurus, and an encyclopedia are essential. Even an old encyclopedia is better than none, since the historical information remains unchanged. A zip code directory, a secretary's manual, and an almanac are useful and inexpensive additions to the collection. *Bartlett's Familiar Quotations* and *Familiar Medical Quotations* are good sources for verifying quotations.

Travel Aids

The hospital library should own or have access to some basic references on travel. A good road atlas is useful and inexpensive. The *Traveler's Toll Free Directory* lists toll free numbers for hotels and motels across the United States. *Health Information for International Travel* is essential for travel abroad. It is published by the CDC as part of *MMWR* and lists immunizations required for travel in various countries. The *Official Airline Guide* can save travelers time and money.

Writing Guides

Writing and publishing guides may be needed by professional staff members or students. Most scientific journals provide information on style and format for prospective contributors. In 1979 the International Steering Committee of Medical Editors published *Uniform Requirements for Manuscripts Submitted to Biomedical Journals*. At that time, the requirements were endorsed by the editors of 20 major medical journals. Many other journal editors have subsequently endorsed them. The requirements include guidelines for the title page, abstract, key words, text, acknowledgements, references, tables, and illustrations.

Various specialized style guides are also available. These include the AMA *Stylebook/Editorial Manual*, the *Council of Biology Editors Style Manual*, and a *Manual for Writers of Term Papers, Theses and Dissertations*. Two comprehensive style manuals that also include information about the printing process are *Chicago Manual of Style*, published by the University of Chicago Press, and the United States Government Printing Office *Style Manual*.

Guides on effective writing may also be helpful, particularly those intended for health professionals. Such guides include *Dx and Rx: A Physicians' Guide to Medical Writing* and *Professional Writing for Nurses in Education, Practice, and Research*.

Grants and Foundations

Many hospitals seek grants as a source of additional funding for new programs and projects. *The Foundation Directory* provides information about foundations whose assets exceed $1,000,000 or whose annual grants total $100,000 or more. Entries include application information, donors and key officers, financial data, and the types of programs that interest the foundation. The annual *Foundation Grants Index* provides a subject guide to individual grants of $5,000 or more awarded during the past year. It also lists previously awarded grants. These two resources are published by the Foundation Center and should be used together for best results. The Foundation Center also has a national network of more than 80 libraries. Free access to publications and professional assistance are available through the network.

Another source of information about grants is the *Annual Register of Grant Support*. This publication describes grant support programs offered by government agencies, foundations, corporations, community trusts, and other organizations. Entries include the grant program's purpose, duration, dollar amount, eligibility requirements, and application instructions. Grant programs are organized by category. Subject, organization, geographic, and personnel indexes are also included.

Information about library grants from the federal government is available from the nearest regional medical library or the National Library of Medicine (NLM). Announcements concerning all types of federal grants are published in the *Federal Register* under the name of the sponsoring agency.

Several books are recommended for the novice grant seeker. They include *The New How to Raise Funds from Foundations, the Art of Winning Foundation Grants, Foundation Fundamentals: A Guide for Grantseekers,* and *Grants: How to Find Out About Them and What to Do Next.*

SOURCES OF BIBLIOGRAPHIC INFORMATION

Much of the hospital librarian's time is devoted to locating bibliographic information about books, journals, and other publications. This information is needed to verify interlibrary loan requests, to select and acquire library materials, and to compile bibliographies on various topics.

Book and Periodical Sources

There are many sources of bibliographic information for books and periodicals in the health sciences. Sources for current publications will be discussed below. For a discussion of retrospective sources, refer to *Introduction to Reference Sources in the Health Sciences.*

One of the most useful sources for current publications is Bowker's *Medical Books and Serials in Print.* It includes an annual list of books arranged by subject, author, and title. Since 1978 it has also contained a listing of serials arranged by subject. A title index to the serials is included as well. Complete ordering information is given, including publisher, price, and international standard book and serial numbers (ISBN and ISSN). A directory of publishers completes the volume.

Bowker also publishes the comprehensive *Books in Print* in four volumes. Its two-volume companion is *Subject Guide to Books in Print.* Hospital libraries that purchase or borrow a large number of books in nonmedical as well as medical fields may find these two titles worth the additional cost.

Larger hospital libraries may wish to purchase *Ulrich's International Periodicals Directory.* It lists currently available serials in all subjects. The serials section of *Medical Books and Serials in Print* is taken from the database used to produce *Ulrich's.*

Another source of bibliographic information is the NLM. The CATLINE database is available online to MEDLARS centers and in printed form as the *NLM Current Catalog.* CATLINE includes books and serials cataloged by the NLM. The *NLM Current Catalog* is a quarterly publication with annual cumulations. It includes bibliographic information that can be accessed by subject and main entry. It also includes classification information based on the NLM classification scheme. Other sources of information are *Health Science Serials,* available only on microfiche, and the *Index of NLM Serial Titles.* These are both products of SERLINE.

Lists of Recommended Publications

Numerous lists of recommended books and journals for health science libraries have appeared since 1970. Although these lists are primarily intended as selection tools, they can also help users who are looking for recommended books or journals to borrow or purchase. Some of the more up-to-date lists are discussed below.

The two Brandon/Hill lists are the most widely acclaimed of the so-called core lists. *Selected List of Books and Journals for the Small Medical Library* covers all subject areas and is published every two years in the April issue of the *Bulletin of the Medical Library Association.* Its companion, *Selected List of Nursing Books and Journals* was part of the original Brandon/Hill list until 1979. Other sources of recommended nursing publications include *Books of the Year,* published every January in the *American Journal of Nursing; Lippincott's Guide to Nursing Literature;* and *Guide to Library Resources for Nursing.*

A Library for Internists IV is the fourth revised list published by the American College of Physicians. It represents the choices of authorities in the field of internal medicine and contains a separate section for each subspecialty.

The librarian who wishes to acquire additional resources in the field of health care administration will find two publications particularly useful. These publications are the AHA's *Administrator's Collection* and *A Selected Bibliography for the Well-Read Health Services Manager,* published by the American College of Hospital Administrators.

Many of the MLA's continuing education courses cover specialized areas of health science literature, such as mental health and health care administration. The outlines that accompany these courses frequently include lists of recommended publications. Several other lists in specific areas such as dentistry and emergency medicine are also available. Additional lists appear in Chapter 3.

The librarian can search *Index Medicus, Hospital Literature Index,* or their online equivalents to locate recommended materials and lists of materials in specialized subject areas. Subject headings such as "book reviews," "bibliography," "reference books," and "periodicals" can be used. Another alternative is to contact the professional association or volunteer organization for a particular field to find out if a list of recommended publications is available. Many of these organizations have bibliographies that have never been published but are available free or at a reasonable price.

Public and academic libraries are often good sources for bibliographies in general subject areas. For example, lists of materials on writing resumes or on various business topics may be available.

Indexes

Indexes form the backbone of the hospital reference collection. The foremost index to health science literature is the NLM's monthly *Index Medicus*. It provides subject and title access to approximately 2,600 medical journals each year. The NLM also publishes the *Abridged Index Medicus*, which covers approximately 120 of the most widely used medical journals. Annual cumulations for these two indexes are published separately.

MeSH is the subject thesaurus for all NLM indexes. *MeSH* is available as part of a subscription to *Index Medicus* and as a separate publication. *Index Medicus* also provides a section of review articles. They are compiled in the *Bibliography of Medical Reviews*, which appears in *Cumulated Index Medicus*.

The *International Nursing Index* is a quarterly NLM publication that uses MeSH vocabulary. It provides complete coverage of 300 nursing journals. It also indexes articles on nursing from 2,000 other journals. The bimonthly *Cumulative Index to Nursing and Allied Health Literature (CINAHL)* indexes more than 300 nursing periodicals. Also included are publications of the ANA, the NLN, and the Department of Health and Human Services, as well as 150 selected journals in ten allied health fields. *CINAHL* also lists the audiovisuals, book reviews, and pamphlets that appear in the journals indexed.

The AHA's *Hospital Literature Index* is now produced in conjunction with the NLM's computerized indexing system and uses MeSH vocabulary. This quarterly index provides excellent coverage of all hospital journals. It also indexes hospital-related articles from other journals.

Index to Dental Literature offers a quarterly index to journal articles, dissertations, and theses in the field of dentistry. Although it uses MeSH vocabulary, there are additional subject headings for areas in which MeSH is not specific enough. These quarterly indexes are also available in cumulations.

Although it may be impractical for hospital libraries to own the more general periodical indexes, it is important to know how to access them. It may even be possible to arrange a reciprocal agreement with a local public or academic library to do occasional searches for each other. Indexes that the hospital librarian may wish to search are listed below.

- *Readers' Guide to Periodical Literature*
- *Business Periodicals Index*
- *The Education Index*
- *Applied Science and Technology Index*
- *General Science Index*
- *The Engineering Index*
- *Humanities Index*
- *Library Literature*
- *Science Citation Index*
- *Social Science Citation Index*

Abstracting Services

Abstracting services are used mostly in larger hospital libraries. *Abstracts of Health Care Management Studies* annually published 1,800 abstracts of journal articles. It also contains abstracts of unpublished material, such as research reports and theses.

Excerpta Medica provides abstracts of articles from 3,500 biomedical and chemical journals. It is available in 45 separate sections, making it possible to purchase only those sections that are needed.

Psychological Abstracts, *Chemical Abstracts*, and *Biological Abstracts* are too expensive for most hospital libraries. However, the librarian should know where to locate these resources in response to a user's request.

Most abstracting services are available online. If a particular source is used infrequently, paying for each access to its online equivalent is usually more economical than owning the printed version of the source. Shared online access through a consortium is a possibility if direct access is not feasible. Online sources of information are discussed later in this chapter.

Government Publications

The best source of information about government publications is the *Monthly Catalog of United States Government Publications*. Four indexes in each issue provide access by subject, title, author, and series. *MEDOC* is a quarterly index to United States government documents in the health sciences and is arranged by Superintendent of Documents (SuDOC) numbers. It includes indexes by subject, title, and series. *MEDOC* is available in both printed form and online.

Document depository libraries can provide access to government documents. They also serve as a backup source for information about such documents. Out-of-print documents can sometimes be obtained directly from the issuing agency.

Proceedings

It is sometimes difficult to gain access to the published proceedings of symposia, association meetings, and seminars. A list of sources for locating conference proceedings appears in *Introduction to Reference Sources in the Health Sciences*. The *NLM Current Catalog* provides subject and title access to a large number of proceedings cataloged by the NLM. The proceedings of seminars and meetings sponsored by a professional association are sometimes published in the association's official journal. CATLINE, the online version of *Current Catalog*, enables the librarian to search for conference names by text word.

Current Awareness Sources

A major alerting publication is the Institute for Scientific Information's *Current Contents* series, which reproduces the contents pages of journals. *Current Contents: Social and Behavioral Sciences*, *Current Contents: Clinical Practice*, and *Current Contents: Life Sciences* are the most useful titles for the hospital library. The series provides copies of the tables of contents of selected journals soon after they are published. Author and key word subject indexes are also included.

Online Sources of Information

Searching periodical indexes for references to journal articles can be very time-consuming. A thorough search requires scanning titles under all potential subject headings in the hope that titles of key articles accurately express their content. Online searching can greatly simplify certain aspects of the searching process.

Computer databases are produced from the records of various periodical indexes in all subject fields. They are accessible through vendors who make databases available online. Databases make it possible to do literature searches quickly and efficiently without actually owning the printed editions of indexes.

The NLM provides access to 17 databases in the health sciences. Twelve of these contain citations to books, journals, audiovisuals, or miscellaneous printed materials. The five nonbibliographic databases contain factual information that can be retrieved directly using a variety of search techniques. Most NLM catalogs and indexes are produced from these 17 databases. Thus, most information is available both online and in printed formats.

The databases that hospital librarians use most often are MEDLINE, Health Planning and Administration, Cancerlit, and CATLINE. MEDLINE covers clinical aspects of health care. The Health Planning and Administration database covers nonclinical aspects of health care such as economics, personnel, facilities, planning, and utilization. Cancerlit deals with cancer research as well as clinical treatment of the disease. CATLINE, which covers serials and monographs cataloged by the NLM, is useful for identifying books published on a given topic.

Lists of databases are usually out-of-date as soon as they are published due to the rapid growth of the online industry. The *Directory of On-Line Information Resources* is a reasonably complete list that includes a description of the database, the supplier, and the content of a unit record. Appendix B describes databases of interest to hospital librarians. Appendix C lists vendors who make these databases available.

SOURCES OF INFORMATION ON AUDIOVISUALS

The number of requests for help in locating audiovisuals has recently increased in most hospital libraries. Some hospitals may have a separate audiovisual department

that provides production services and handles equipment checkout. However, these departments do not always provide reference services. Suggestions on how to develop and index a collection of catalogs from audiovisual producers and distributors are given in Chapter 10. The *AV Source Directory* provides a list of audiovisual companies as well as a subject index to these companies.

Printed Sources

There is no source comparable to *Books in Print* in the field of audiovisuals. However, there are catalogs and indexes to audiovisuals in the health sciences.

The NLM publishes the *National Library of Medicine Audiovisuals Catalog* and the *National Medical Audiovisual Center Catalog* as by-products of its AVLINE database. AVLINE is available online to all MEDLARS centers. The *NLM Audiovisuals Catalog* is a quarterly index to health science audiovisuals. The fourth issue is an annual cumulation. Motion pictures and videocassettes available on loan from the National Medical Audiovisual Center (NMAC) are listed in the *National Medical Audiovisual Center Catalog*. Most audiovisuals listed in the NLM and the NMAC catalogs are professionally reviewed programs with "recommended" or "highly recommended" ratings. Both sources provide access by title and subject.

Several other reference tools provide subject access to bibliographic information on audiovisuals in the health sciences. The *Health Sciences Videolog* covers video programs only. The *HERC Catalog* is an annual publication that lists inexpensive audiovisuals used by hospital educators. *Medical Audiovisuals: A Comprehensive Catalog* and *Health Sciences AV Resources List: 1978-1979* are both fairly comprehensive lists that cover a broad range of formats and subjects.

Index to Audiovisual Serials in the Health Sciences is a quarterly MLA publication that indexes serials such as Audio Digest tapes and Network of Continuing Education videotapes. The *Audiovisual Equipment Directory* is a useful source of information on audiovisual hardware.

Online Sources

Two databases are especially useful for online access to information about audiovisuals. AVLINE, the NLM database, covers health science audiovisuals from 1970 to the present. Each month, 100 to 200 entries are added. The National Information Center for Educational Media (NICEM) includes all subjects but is most useful to hospital libraries in the areas of health and safety, psychology, and the social sciences. See Chapter 10 for a table listing online databases that include citations for audiovisuals.

USING RESOURCES EFFECTIVELY

Effective use of resources involves more than knowing what resources exist and how to use them. The hospital librarian must also make decisions about which resources to acquire and which to share or access from other sources. For example, an expensive directory may be referred to infrequently or may contain the type of data that does not change substantially in each edition. In this case the librarian may decide to buy the directory every two years rather than every year.

The library may be part of a consortium, or there may be other local libraries that cooperate informally. If so, it may be possible to share the cost of expensive items. The purchase of new editions of certain titles might be rotated among several hospital libraries so that one library always has the latest edition. Or a list of expensive sources might be divided among several libraries so that each is responsible for purchasing the latest editions of specific titles.

USING COMMUNITY RESOURCES

The hospital librarian should become familiar with the many resources available in the community. Health and social service agencies exist in almost every community, and many have a wealth of information within easy reach. The personnel associated with these agencies are also a valuable resource.

Information and Referral

Every state has information and referral centers. To locate the nearest one, consult the *I and R Workers Handy Directory: The Directory of Information and Referral Services in the United States and Canada*.

In addition, most large cities have directories of community resources that include agencies, associations, hot lines, and other public service entities. Most of these service organizations accept telephone requests. Many will even take requests from callers outside the service area if the caller's area lacks the needed service. The librarian should become aware of toll free numbers and hot lines within the state. Many government agencies provide these numbers for state residents. It is also a good idea to record consumer information telephone numbers that appear in various newsletters from time to time.

Information Clearinghouses

As of 1980 the federal government sponsored 76 bureaus, centers, clearinghouses, and services that provided health information to consumers, professionals, researchers, and organizations. *Health Information Resources* is a directory of these resources. It is arranged by topic and has a subject index. Annual updates keep the information current. Entries include name, address, sponsor, authorizing legislation, audience, description, publications, automated database, and conditions. Appendix D lists agencies that are classified as information clearinghouses.

Using the Telephone

Use of the telephone is often the most efficient and cost-effective way to get information. A direct telephone request is faster than a letter and allows for immediate interaction between the source and the person requesting information. It may also be less expensive to call a resource library or agency long-distance than to purchase the reference source that contains the needed information.

Whether calling an individual, a service organization, or a government agency, the rules of common courtesy should always be observed when requesting information over the telephone. The caller should always state his or her name, location, and the purpose of the call. Such information is especially important to the many agencies and government units that keep records of calls and use such records to justify their existence. The information obtained should be recorded along with the name of the person who gave the information. It may sometimes be necessary to ask for the name of a person who may be contacted for further information.

CREATING A RESOURCE FILE

The hospital librarian becomes aware of new sources of information almost every day. This type of information may come from materials received by mail, professional reading, conversations with other librarians or hospital staff members, or as the result of an information search. The librarian can develop a resource file to organize this information in a central location. A vertical file is suggested for this purpose, since it can hold materials of varying shapes and sizes. A loose-leaf notebook or a card file can also be used in conjunction with the vertical file.

A resource file can contain various types of information. Examples include:

- Notes about people in the hospital or community who have expertise in a particular area
- Records of reference materials stored in other hospital departments
- Advertisements for expensive reference books that the librarian may wish to access from another library
- Brochures or news clippings that describe public information services, hot lines, or information clearinghouses
- Fact sheets about government agencies and private organizations, outlining location, hours, names of key personnel, publications, and types of services
- Lists of names, addresses, and telephone numbers of key state and local health officials
- Notes about resources in the library that contain useful illustrations

Whatever the content of the resource file, it should be organized according to the library's needs. If it is arranged in broad categories by type of resource, a subject index is suggested to make it more accessible.

APPENDIX A
Information Resources

GUIDES TO REFERENCE SOURCES

American Dental Association. Basic dental reference works. 4th ed. Chicago: American Dental Association, 1980.

Binger JL, Jensen LM. Lippincott's guide to nursing literature: a handbook for students, writers and researchers. Philadelphia: Lippincott, 1980.

Blake JB, Roos C, eds. Medical reference works 1679-1966: a selected bibliography. Chicago: Medical Library Association, 1967. Three supplements 1970, 1973, 1975.

Chen C-C. Health sciences information sources. Cambridge, MA: MIT Press, 1981.

Cohon MS, Rice BS, Noble V. Information sources in pharmacy and pharmacology. Kalamazoo, MI: Upjohn, 1980.

Interagency Council on Library Resources for Nursing. Reference sources for nursing. Nurs Outlook 1982 June;30:363-367.

Kirz HL, Turner KA. A sample reference library for the emergency department. JACEP 1976 Mar;5:200-204.

McClure LW. Reference services: policies and practices. In: Darling L, Bishop D, Colaianni LA. Handbook of medical library practice, 4th ed. Vol. I. Chicago: Medical Library Association, 1982.

Rees AM, Young BA. The consumer health information source book. New York: Bowker, 1981.

Roper FW, Boorkman JA. Introduction to reference sources in the health sciences. Chicago: Medical Library Association, 1980.

Rubinton P, Sacks MH, Frosch WA. On searching the literature: an annotated bibliography of selected psychiatric sources. J Psychiatr Educ 1980 Spring;4:57-75.

Sewell W. Guide to drug information. Hamilton, IL: Drug Intelligence Publications, 1976.

Strauch KP, Brundage DJ. Guide to library resources for nursing. New York: Appleton-Century-Crofts, 1980.

Twenty excellent psychiatric reference books. Behav Med 1978 Apr;5: 29-33.

DIRECTORIES, BIOGRAPHICAL

American medical directory. 28th ed. Chicago: American Medical Association, 1982.

American men and women of science: physical and biological sciences. 14th ed. New York: Bowker, 1979.

American men and women of science: social and behavioral sciences. 13th ed. New York: Bowker, 1978.

Directory of medical specialists. 20th ed. Chicago: Marquis Who's Who, 1981.

Who's who in America 42d ed. Chicago: Marquis Who's Who, 1982.

DIRECTORIES, EDUCATIONAL

AAMC directory of American medical education 1980-81. Washington, DC: Association of American Medical Colleges, 1980.

Allied health education directory 10th ed. Chicago: American Medical Association, 1981.

Directory of residency training programs 82/83, accredited by the Accreditation Council for Graduate Medical Education. Chicago: American Medical Association, 1982.

Journal of the American Medical Association. Vol. 1-. Chicago: American Medical Association, 1883-. Weekly.

Medical school admission requirements, United States and Canada 1983-84. Washington, DC: Association of American Medical Colleges, 1983.

National League for Nursing. Associate degree education for nursing 1981-82. New York: National League for Nursing, 1981. (NLN Publication No. 23-1309).

National League for Nursing. Baccalaureate and master's degree programs in nursing accredited by the National League for Nursing 1981-82. New York: National League for Nursing, 1981. (NLN Publication No. 15-1310).

National League for Nursing. Baccalaureate programs accredited for public health nursing preparation, 1981-82. New York: National League for Nursing, 1981. (NLN Publication No. 15-1313).

National League for Nursing. Diploma programs in nursing accredited by the National League for Nursing, 1981-82. New York: National League for Nursing, 1981. (NLN Publication No. 16-1542).

National League for Nursing. Doctoral programs in nursing, 1981-82. New York: National League for Nursing, 1981. (NLN Publication No. 15-1448).

National League for Nursing. State-approved schools of nursing— L.P.N./L.V.N. 1981. New York: National League for Nursing, 1981. (NLN Publication No. 19-1854).

National League for Nursing. State-approved schools of nursing— R.N. 1981. New York: National League for Nursing, 1981. (NLN Publication No. 19-1853).

World directory of medical schools. 5th ed. Geneva: World Health Organization, 1979.

DIRECTORIES, ORGANIZATIONS AND INSTITUTIONS

American Hospital Association guide to the health care field. Chicago: American Hospital Association, 1972-. Annual.

Canadian hospital directory. Vol. 1-. Toronto: Canadian Hospital Council, 1953-. Annual.

Directory. Amer J Nurs 1981 Apr;81:847-860.

Encyclopedia of associations. 17th ed. Detroit: Gale Research, 1982.

Official directory. Nurs. Outlook 1981 Oct;29:610-612.

Rees AM, Crawford S, eds. Directory of health sciences libraries in the United States, 1979. Chicago: Medical Library Association, 1980.

Wasserman P, Kaszubski M, eds. Health organizations of the United States, Canada and the world: a directory of voluntary associations, professional societies and other groups concerned with health and related fields. 5th ed. Detroit: Anthony T. Kruzas Associates, 1981.

DIRECTORIES, GOVERNMENT

National health directory. 6th ed. Rockville, MD: Aspen, 1982.

United States government manual 1981/82. Washington, DC: Government Printing Office, 1981.

DIRECTORIES, COMPREHENSIVE

Kruzas AT, ed. Medical and health information directory. 2d ed. Detroit: Gale Research, 1980.

Norback CT, Norback PG. The health care directory 77-78. Oradell, NJ: Medical Economics, 1977.

DICTIONARIES

Diagnostic and statistical manual of mental disorders. 3d ed. Washington, DC: American Psychiatric Association, 1980.

Dorland's illustrated medical dictionary. 26th ed. Philadelphia: Saunders, 1981.

Magalini S, Scrascia E. Dictionary of medical syndromes. 2d ed. Philadelphia: Lippincott, 1981.

Miller BF, Keane CB. Encyclopedia and dictionary of medicine and nursing and allied health. 3d ed. Philadelphia: Saunders, 1983.

A psychiatric glossary. 5th ed. Washington: American Psychiatric Association, 1980.

Stedman's medical dictionary. 24th ed. Baltimore: Williams & Wilkins, 1982.

DRUG INFORMATION SOURCES

AMA drug evaluations. 5th ed. Chicago: American Medical Association, 1983.

American hospital formulary service. Washington, DC: American Society of Hospital Pharmacists, 1959-. Loose-leaf.

Current therapy. Philadelphia: Saunders, 1949-. Annual.

Gilman AG, Goodman LS, Gilman A, eds. Goodman and Gilman's the pharmacological basis of therapeutics. 6th ed. New York: Macmillan, 1980.

Gosselin RE, et al. Clinical toxicology of commercial products. 4th ed. Baltimore: Williams & Wilkins, 1976.

Handbook of non-prescription drugs. 7th ed. Washington, DC: American Pharmaceutical Association, 1982.

Hansten PD. Drug interactions. 4th ed. Philadelphia: Lea & Febiger, 1979.

Physician's desk reference. Oradell, NJ: Medical Economics, 1947-. Annual.

Physician's desk reference for nonprescription drugs. Oradell, NJ: Medical Economics, 1980-. Annual.

Sewell W. Guide to drug information. Hamilton, IL: Drug Intelligence Publications, 1976.

STATISTICAL SOURCES

Advance data from vital and health statistics of the National Center for Health Statistics. Hyattsville, MD: National Center for Health Statistics. Irregular.

American Cancer Society. Cancer facts and figures. New York: American Cancer Society, 1978-. Annual.

Annual summary 1980. Atlanta: Center for Disease Control, 1981. (MMWR Morbidity and Mortality Weekly Report 1981 Sept;29[54]). (HHS Publication no. [CDC] 81-8241).

Catalog of publications of the National Center for Health Statistics. Hyattsville, MD: National Center for Health Statistics, 1981. (DHHS Publication No. [PHS] 81-1301).

Facts about nursing. New York: American Nurses' Association, 1935-.

Facts at your fingertips: a guide to sources of statistical information on major health topics. 5th ed. Hyattsville, MD: National Center for Health Statistics, 1981. (DHHS Publication No. [PHS] 81-1246).

Hospital statistics. Chicago: American Hospital Association, 1972-.

MMWR morbidity and mortality weekly report. Vol. 1. Atlanta: Center for Disease Control, 1952-. Weekly.

NLN nursing data book 1981: statistical information on nursing education and newly licensed nurses. New York: National League for Nursing, 1982.

Statistical abstract of the United States. Washington: Bureau of the Census, 1878-. Annual.

Vital and health statistics. Hyattsville, MD: National Center for Health Statistics, 1963-. Irregular.

Weise FO. Health statistics: a guide to information sources. Detroit: Gale Research, 1980.

World health statistics annual. Geneva: World Health Organization, 1962-. Annual.

LEGAL SOURCES

Creighton H. Law every nurse should know. 4th ed. Philadelphia: Saunders, 1981.

Federal Register. Washington, DC: Government Printing Office, 1936-. Daily.

Hirsch CS, Morris RC, Mortiz AR. Handbook of legal medicine. 5th ed. St. Louis: Mosby, 1979.

Hospital law manual. Germantown, MD: Aspen Systems Corporation, 1974-. Quarterly.

Medicare and medicaid guide. Chicago: Commerce Clearing House, 1966-. Loose-leaf.

Medicare and medicaid guide: new developments. Chicago: Commerce Clearing House, 1967-. Loose-leaf.

Medicare: hospital manual. Washington, DC: Health Care Financing Administration, 1966-. Loose-leaf. (HEW Publication No. [HCFA] 16).

Medicare: provider reimbursement manual. Washington, DC: Health Care Financing Administration, 1966-. Loose-leaf. (HEW Publication No. [HCFA] 15).

ACCREDITATION SOURCES

American College of Surgeons. Cancer program manual. Chicago: American College of Surgeons, 1980.

Canadian Council on Hospital Accreditation. Guide to hospital accreditation. Toronto: Canadian Council on Hospital Accreditation, 1977.

Commission on Laboratory Inspection and Accreditation. Standards for accreditation of medical laboratories. Skokie, IL: College of American Pathologists, 1974.

JCAH Perspectives. Chicago: Joint Commission on Accreditation of Hospitals, 1981-. Bimonthly.

Joint Commission on Accreditation of Hospitals. Accreditation manual for hospitals. 1983 ed. Chicago: Joint Commission on Accreditation of Hospitals, 1982.

Joint Commission on Accreditation of Hospitals. Consolidated standards manual for child, adolescent and adult psychiatric, alcoholism and drug abuse facilities. 1981 ed. Chicago: Joint Commission on the Accreditation of Hospitals, 1981.

Joint Commission on Accreditation of Hospitals. Hospital survey profile. 1982 ed. Chicago: Joint Commission on Accreditation of Hospitals, 1982.

National League for Nursing. Criteria for the evaluation of diploma programs in nursing. 4th ed. New York: National League for Nursing, 1975.

GENERAL SOURCES

Bartlett's familiar quotations. 14th ed. Boston: Little, Brown, 1968.

Strauss MB, ed. Familiar medical quotations. Boston: Little, Brown, 1968.

TRAVEL AIDS

Health information for international travel. Atlanta: Center for Disease Control, 1974-. Annual.

Official airline guide. North American edition. Oakbrook, IL: Frank M. Lobach, 1943-. Semimonthly.

Traveler's toll free telephone directory, 1980. Burlington, VT: Landmark Publishing, 1980.

WRITING AIDS

American Medical Association. Stylebook/editorial manual. 6th ed. Littleton, MA: PSG 1976.

CBE Style Manual Committee. Council of Biology Editors style manual: a guide for authors, editors and publishers in the biological sciences. 4th ed. Arlington, VA: Council of Biology Editors, 1978.

Dirck JH. Dx and Rx: a physician's guide to medical writing. Boston: GK Hall, 1977.

Kolin PC, Kolin JL. Professional writing for nurses in education, practice, and research. St. Louis: Mosby, 1980.

Chicago manual of style. 13th ed. Chicago: University of Chicago Press, 1982.

Turabian KL. A manual for writers of term papers, theses and dissertations. 4th ed. Chicago: University of Chicago Press, 1973.

Uniform requirements for manuscripts submitted to biomedical journals. Ann Intern Med 1979 Jan;90:95-99.

U.S. Government Printing Office. Style manual. rev. ed. Washington, DC: Government Printing Office, 1973.

SOURCES OF GRANT INFORMATION

Annual register of grant support 1982-83. 16th ed. Chicago: Marquis Who's Who, Inc, 1982.

Dermer J. The new how to raise funds from foundations. 2d ed. New York: Public Service Materials Center, 1979.

The Foundation directory. 8th ed. New York: The Foundation Center, 1981.

Foundation grants index, 1980. New York: The Foundation Center, 1981.

Hillman H, Abarbanel K. The art of winning foundation grants. New York: Vanguard Press, 1975.

Kurzig C. Foundation fundamentals: a guide for grantseekers. Rev. ed. New York: The Foundation Center, 1981.

White VP. Grants: how to find out about them and what to do next. New York: Plenum Press, 1976.

BOOK AND PERIODICAL SOURCES

Books in print. New York: Bowker, 1948-. Annual.

Health science serials. Microfiche. Bethesda, MD: National Library of Medicine, 1979-. Quarterly.

Index of NLM serial titles. Bethesda, MD: National Library of Medicine, 1972-.

Medical books and serials in print: an index to literature in the health sciences. New York: Bowker, 1978-. Annual.

National Library of Medicine current catalog. Bethesda, MD: National Library of Medicine, 1966-. Quarterly.

Subject guide to books in print. New York: Bowker, 1948-. Annual.

Ulrich's international periodicals directory. 19th ed. New York: Bowker, 1981.

LISTS OF RECOMMENDED MATERIAL

Allyn R. A library for internists IV: recommended by the American College of Physicians. Ann Intern Med 1982 Mar;96:385-401.

American College of Hospital Administrators. A selected bibliography for the well-read health services manager. Chicago: American College of Hospital Administrators, 1979.

American Hospital Association. Administrator's collection. 1978 ed. Chicago: American Hospital Association, 1978.

Binger JL, Jensen LM. Lippincott's guide to nursing literature: a handbook for students, writers and researchers. Philadelphia: Lippincott, 1980.

Books of the year. Amer J Nurs 1983 Jan;83:94-104.

Brandon AN, Hill DR. Selected list of books and journals for the small medical library. Bull Med Libr Assoc 1981 Apr;69:185-215.

Brandon AN, Hill DR. Selected list of nursing books and journals. Nurs Outlook 1982 Mar;30:186-199.

Horton MA, Hammon WE, Curtis T, Horton F. A suggested current literature and reference library for respiratory and chest physical therapists. RC 1979 Feb;24:138-141.

Moseley JL. Selected list of family medicine books and journals for the small medical library. Bull Med Libr Assoc 1980 July;68:297-298.

Raskin RB, Hathorn IV. Selected list of books and journals for a small dental library. Bull Med Libr Assoc 1980 July;68:263-270.

Strauch KP, Brundage DJ. Guide to library resources for nursing. New York: Appleton-Century-Crofts, 1980.

Taub A. Understanding the legislative process: an annotated bibliography of selected references. Health Educ 1980 July-Aug;11:13-14.

INDEXES

Abridged index medicus. Vol. 1- . Bethesda, MD: National Library of Medicine, 1970- . Monthly.

Cumulated abridged index medicus. Vol. 1- . Bethesda, MD: National Library of Medicine, 1970- . Annual.

Cumulated index medicus. Vol. 1- . Bethesda, MD: National Library of Medicine, 1960- . Annual.

Cumulative index to nursing and allied health literature. Vol. 22-. Glendale, CA: The Seventh-Day Adventist Hospital Association, 1977-. Bimonthly.

Hospital literature index. Vol. 13-. Chicago: American Hospital Association, 1957-. Quarterly.

Index medicus. Vol. 1-. Bethesda, MD: National Library of Medicine, 1960-. Monthly.

Index to dental literature. Vol. 1- . Chicago: American Dental Association, 1962- . Quarterly.

International nursing index. Vol. 1- . New York: American Journal of Nursing, 1966- . Quarterly.

Medical subject headings. Bethesda, MD: National Library of Medicine, 1960- . Annual.

ABSTRACTING SERVICES

Abstracts of health care management studies. Vol. 15- . Ann Arbor, MI: Health Administration Press, 1979-. Annual.

Excerpta medica. Amsterdam: Excerpta Medica Foundation, 1947- . Monthly.

GOVERNMENT PUBLICATIONS

MEDOC. Salt Lake City, UT: Eccles Health Sciences Library, University of Utah, 1974- . Quarterly.

Monthly catalog of United States government publications. Washington, DC: Government Printing Office, 1895- . Monthly.

CURRENT AWARENESS SOURCES

Current contents: clinical practice. Vol. 1- . Philadelphia: Institute for Scientific Information, 1973- . Monthly.

Current contents: life sciences. Vol. 1- . Philadelphia: Institute for Scientific Information, 1958- . Monthly.

Current contents: social and behavioral sciences. Vol. 1- . Philadelphia: Institute for Scientific Information, 1969- . Monthly.

SOURCES OF INFORMATION ON AUDIOVISUALS

AV source directory: a subject index to health science AV producer/distributor catalogs. 2d ed. Chicago: Midwest Health Science Library Network, 1982.

Health sciences AV resource list: 1978-1979. 2d ed. Farmington, CT: University of Connecticut Health Center Library, 1978.

The health sciences videolog. 1981 ed. New York: Video-Forum, 1981.

HERC: free film reference, 1981. 5th ed. Lincoln, NE: Hospital Educators Resource Catalog, Inc., 1981.

Index to audiovisual serials in the health sciences. Vol. 1-. Chicago: Medical Library Association, 1977-. Quarterly.

Medical audiovisuals: a comprehensive catalog. Baltimore: Welch Medical Library, Johns Hopkins University, 1977.

National Library of Medicine audiovisuals catalog. Bethesda, MD: National Library of Medicine, 1977- . Quarterly.

National Medical Audiovisual Center Catalog. Bethesda, MD: National Medical Audiovisual Center, 1981.

Stevens M, ed. Audio-visual equipment directory. 28th ed. Fairfax, VA: National Audio-Visual Association, 1982.

ONLINE SOURCES OF INFORMATION

Directory of on-line information resources. 6th ed. Rockville, MD: Capitol Systems Group, 1981.

INFORMATION AND REFERRAL RESOURCES

The I and R handy directory: the directory of information and referral services in the United States and Canada. Phoenix: AIRS Publications, n.d.

National Health Information Clearinghouse. Health information resources in the Department of Health and Human Services 1980. Washington, DC: National Health Information Clearinghouse, 1980. (HHS Publication No. (PHS)80-50146).

APPENDIX B
Databases of Interest to Hospital Librarians

Databases of interest to hospital librarians can be divided into three categories: primary, specialized, and related. Primary databases are generally most used in the hospital library. Specialized databases are useful in specific subject areas. The specialized category also includes special-purpose databases like SDILINE. Related databases cover areas outside the health sciences. These databases are often useful in serving the hospital's diverse user groups.

DATABASE	PRODUCER	VENDOR	DESCRIPTION
PRIMARY			
AVLINE	National Library of Medicine	NLM	Citations for audiovisual teaching materials in the health sciences.
CATLINE	National Library of Medicine	NLM	Citations for the same health-related monographs, proceedings, and theses included in its printed equivalent, the *NLM Current Catalog*.
HEALTH PLANNING AND ADMINISTRATION	National Library of Medicine	BRS DIALOG NLM	Citations for journal articles dealing with the non-clinical aspects of health care delivery. *Hospital Literature Index* is produced from this database.
MEDLINE	National Library of Medicine	BRS DIALOG NLM	Citations for English and foreign-language journal articles in the biomedical fields, corresponding to *Index Medicus*, *Index to Dental Literature*, and the *International Nursing Index*.
SPECIALIZED			
AGRICOLA	National Agricultural Library	BRS DIALOG	Citations for English and foreign-language journal articles and monographs in the field of agriculture, including food and nutrition.
BIOETHICS	Kennedy Institute of Ethics	NLM	Citations for English-language journal articles, monographs, court decisions, bills, laws, and audiovisuals in the fields of medicine, nursing, philosophy and religion.
BIOSIS	BioSciences Information Service	BRS DIALOG SDC	Citations for journal articles, government documents, monographs, proceedings, and theses in the life sciences from two printed sources, *Biological Abstracts* and *Bioresearch Index*.
CANCERLIT	National Cancer Institute	NLM	Citations for articles, monographs, government documents, proceedings, and theses dealing with all aspects of cancer.
CANCERPROJ	National Cancer Institute	NLM	Summaries of ongoing cancer research projects.
CAS	Chemical Abstracts Service	BRS DIALOG SDC	Citations for monographs, articles, documents, patents, theses, dissertations, and proceedings taken from *Chemical Abstracts*.
CHEMLINE	Toxicity Information Program	NLM	A dictionary file of information on chemical compounds, formulas, synonyms, and nomenclature.
CHILD ABUSE & NEGLECT	National Center for Child Abuse & Neglect	DIALOG	Citations for a variety of English-language materials covering research in the field of child abuse and neglect.
CLINPROT	National Cancer Institute	NLM	Descriptions of clinical investigations of anticancer agents and treatment modalities.
DRUG INFO/ ALCOHOL USE/ ABUSE	University of Minnesota College of Pharmacy	BRS	Citations for journal articles, monographs, conference papers, audiovisuals, and unpublished works in the field of drug and alcohol abuse.

DATABASE	PRODUCER	VENDOR	DESCRIPTION
SPECIALIZED			
EPILEPSYLINE	National Institutes of Health	BRS	Citations and abstracts of English and foreign-language journal articles taken from *Epilepsy Abstracts*.
ERIC	National Institute of Education	BRS DIALOG SDC	Citations for journal articles, research reports, dissertations, congressional hearings and reports, and curriculum guides in the field of education. Includes counseling and library science.
EXCERPTA MEDICA	Excerpta Medica Foundation	DIALOG	Abstracts of English and foreign-language journal articles in the biomedical fields.
FSTA	International Food Information Service	DIALOG	Citations and abstracts of journal articles, monographs, patents, research reports, and proceedings in the field of food science. Taken from *Food Science and Technology Abstracts*.
INTERNATIONAL PHARMACEUTICAL ABSTRACTS	American Society of Hospital Pharmacists	DIALOG BRS	Information on all phases of the development and use of drugs and on professional pharmaceutical practice.
MEDOC	University of Utah	BRS	Citations to government publications in the health sciences.
NIMH	National Institute of Mental Health	BRS	Citations to journal articles, monographs, technical reports, conference papers, and audiovisuals in the general area of mental health.
POPLINE	Population Information Program	NLM	Citations and abstracts to journal articles, monographs, technical reports, and unpublished works in the areas of family planning, population, and reproduction.
PSYCINFO	American Psychological Association	BRS DIALOG SDC	Citations and abstracts for English and foreign-language journal articles, monographs, government reports, proceedings, theses, and preprints in the fields of psychology and behavioral science.
RTECS	National Institute for Occupational Health and Safety	NLM	Toxicity data on more than 40,000 chemical substances. Taken from the *Registry of Toxic Effects of Chemical Substances*.
SCISEARCH	Institute for Scientific Information	DIALOG	Citations for journal articles in the fields of science and technology. Taken from several ISI publications including *Science Citation Index*.
SDILINE	National Library of Medicine	NLM	Citations from the current month of the MEDLINE database.
SERLINE	National Library of Medicine	NLM	Citations for journals in the biomedical fields. Taken from *Index Medicus* and many other sources, including *Excerpta Medica* and *Chemical Abstracts*.
SOCIOLOGICAL ABSTRACTS	Sociological Abstracts, Inc.	DIALOG BRS	Citations and abstracts of journal articles, monographs, conference papers, theses, and preprints taken from *Sociology*.
TDB	Toxicology Data Bank	NLM	Information file on chemistry, pharmacology, and toxicology. Extracted from 61 standard textbooks, handbooks, and monographs.
TOXLINE	Toxicology Information Program	NLM	Citations for journal articles drawn from 11 subfiles covering animal and human toxicology, chemicals, pollutants, and pharmacology.

DATABASE	PRODUCER	VENDOR	DESCRIPTION
RELATED			
American Men and Women of Science	R.R. Bowker Company	BRS DIALOG	Biographical data on more than 130,000 scientists in the physical and biological sciences.
Books in Print	R.R. Bowker Company	BRS DIALOG	Citations for books in all subject areas published or distributed in the U.S.
Compendex	Engineering Information Inc.	BRS DIALOG SDC	Citations for engineering and technological literature, including biomedical and genetic engineering.
Federal Register	Capitol Services International	DIALOG	Comprehensive coverage of federal regulatory agency actions as published in the *Federal Register*.
ABI/Inform	Data Courier, Inc.	BRS DIALOG SDC	Citations for all phases of business management and administration.
LISA	Learned Information Ltd.	DIALOG SDC	Citations for journal articles, book reports, and conference papers in 20 languages in the field of library and information science.
Magazine Index	Information Access Corporation	DIALOG	Citations from more than 370 popular magazines, including some major library journals.
Management Contents	Management Contents Inc.	BRS DIALOG SDC	Citations for business and management-related topics.
GPO Monthly Catalog	U.S. Government Printing Office	BRS DIALOG	Machine-readable equivalent of the *Monthly Catalog*.
NICEM	National Information Center for Educational Media	DIALOG	Citations for audiovisuals in all subject fields.

APPENDIX C
Major Vendors of Online Databases

Bibligraphic Retrieval Services, Inc. (BRS)
1200 Route 7
Latham, New York 12110

Dialog Information Services, Inc. (DIALOG)
3460 Hillview Avenue
Palo Alto, California 94304

National Library of Medicine (NLM)
8600 Rockville Pike
Bethesda, Maryland 20014

System Development Corporation (SDC)
2500 Colorado Avenue
Santa Monica, California 90406

APPENDIX D
Information Clearinghouses

Arthritis Information Clearinghouse
P.O. Box 34427
Bethesda, Maryland 20034

Cancer Information Clearinghouse (CIC)
National Cancer Institute
Office of Cancer Communications
9000 Rockville Pike, Building 31, Room 10A18
Bethesda, Maryland 20205

Clearinghouse for Occupational Safety and Health
   Information
National Institute for Occupational Safety and Health
Robert A. Taft Laboratories
4676 Columbia Parkway
Cincinnati, Ohio 45226

Clearinghouse on Child Abuse and Neglect Information
P.O. Box 1182
Washington, D.C. 20013

Clearinghouse on Health Indexes
National Center for Health Statistics
Division of Analysis
3700 East-West Highway
Hyattsville, Maryland 20782

Clearinghouse on the Handicapped
Office for Handicapped Individuals
Office of Human Development Services
200 Independence Avenue SW, Room 338D
Washington, D.C. 20201

Division of Poison Control
Food and Drug Administration
5600 Fishers Lane, Room 1345
Rockville, Maryland 20857

High Blood Pressure Information Center
Landau Building
120/80 National Institutes for Health
Bethesda, Maryland 20205

National Clearinghouse for Alcohol Information
   (NCALI)
National Institute on Alcohol Abuse and Alcoholism
P.O. Box 2345
Rockville, Maryland 20852

National Clearinghouse for Drug Abuse Information
   (NCDAI)
National Institute on Drug Abuse Information
P.O. Box 416
Kensington, Maryland 20795

National Clearinghouse for Emergency Medical Services
P.O. Box 911
Rockville, Maryland 20852

National Clearinghouse for Family Planning Information
Office for Family Planning
Bureau of Community Health Services
P.O. Box 2225
Rockville, Maryland 20852

National Clearinghouse for Human Genetic Diseases
1776 East Jefferson Street
Rockville, Maryland 20852

National Clearinghouse for Mental Health Information
   (NCMHI)
Public Inquiries Section
5600 Fishers Lane, Room 11A-21
Rockville, Maryland 20857

National Clearinghouse on Aging
Office of Human Development
Administration on Aging
330 Independence Avenue SW
Washington, D.C. 20201

National Clearinghouse on Domestic Violence (NCDV)
P.O. Box 2309
Rockville, Maryland 20852

National Diabetes Information and Education
   Clearinghouse (NDIC)
805 15th Street NW, Suite 500
Washington, D.C. 20005

National Health Information Clearinghouse (NHIC)
P.O. Box 1133
Washington, D.C. 20013

National Health Standards and Quality Information
   Clearinghouse (NHSQIC)
11301 Rockville Pike
Kensington, Maryland 20795

National Injury Information Clearinghouse
Consumer Product Safety Commission
5401 Westbard Avenue, Room 625
Washington, D.C. 20207

National Rape Information Clearinghouse (NRIC)
National Center for the Prevention and Control of Rape
5600 Fischers Lane, Room 11A-22
Rockville, Maryland 20857

National Rehabilitation Information Center
Catholic University of America
4407 Eighth Street, NE
Washington, D.C. 20017

Office on Smoking and Health
Technical Information Center
Park Building, Room I-16
5600 Fishers Lane
Rockville, Maryland 20857

Venereal Disease Clearinghouse (VD Interchange)
Center for Disease Control
Bureau of State Services
Technical Information Services
Atlanta, Georgia 30333

CHAPTER 9

Interlibrary Loan

Patricia Jones Wakeley
*Program Coordinator: Communication and
   Administration*
Midwest Health Science Library Network
Management Office/Library of the Health Sciences
University of Illinois at Chicago
Chicago, Illinois

and

Mary Bayorgeon
Director of Library Services
Health Science Library
St. Elizabeth Hospital
Appleton, Wisconsin

*Currently:
Manager, Information Services Department
Library of the American Hospital Association,
   Asa S. Bacon Memorial
American Hospital Association
Chicago, Illinois

CHAPTER 9

Interlibrary Loan

Patricia Jones Wakeley
Program Coordinator: Communication and Administration
Midwest Health Science Library Network
Management Office/Library of the Health Sciences
University of Illinois at Chicago   Chicago, Illinois
and
Mary Bayorgeon
Director of Library Services
Health Science Library, St. Elizabeth Hospital
Appleton, Wisconsin

Figures

In a typical working day, a hospital library may provide information and materials to physicians, nurses, an X-ray technician, the head of the laundry service, an assistant administrator, the in-service education director, and members of the counseling staff. If a library has a good collection development program, it will already have acquired a solid core collection in anticipation of the basic needs of its users. Given the diverse and rapidly changing needs of a hospital staff, however, a comprehensive collection that meets every possible need is neither feasible nor cost-effective. A hospital librarian must develop alternative ways of obtaining materials that are infrequently needed, such as sharing resources with other libraries, and participating in networks.

Interlibrary loan is a form of resource sharing that provides access to materials owned by other libraries. Through interlibrary loan, materials in a variety of formats can be shared and more fully used by the larger health care community. This chapter discusses the policies, procedures, and responsibilities involved in transferring materials between libraries.

RESPONSIBILITIES OF PARTICIPATING LIBRARIES

Resource sharing is essentially a voluntary activity. But because interlibrary loan transactions involve certain responsibilities on the part of participating libraries, formal agreements and funding arrangements are becoming more common. The American Library Association (ALA) National Interlibrary Loan Code clearly states that recourse to interlibrary loan should not be considered a substitute for collection development (1). As a general rule, a library should borrow only those materials which are not part of its own collection development program and for which there is no recurring need. The librarian making the request should be familiar with standard interlibrary loan procedures and the copyright law, and should attempt to verify the location of the material before initiating a request. Courtesy, as well as professional practice, dictates that the borrowing library should complete the forms properly, assume responsibility for the safety of the material, and comply with all the loan conditions established by the lending library. The lending library, on the other hand, should develop a generous interlibrary loan policy consistent with the interests of its primary clientele. A library's interlibrary loan policy should be available on request, and a lending library should process applications for loans promptly.

The responsibilities that apply to loans between libraries with no specific agreements are more fully described in the ALA National Interlibrary Loan Code. Libraries participating in special networks must also conform to specific network policies and procedures.

INTERLIBRARY LOAN POLICIES

Since access to the collections of other libraries is essential in order to maintain effective hospital library service, each hospital library should adopt an interlibrary loan policy statement. Such a statement must necessarily differ for each institution, in order to meet the library's own particular needs and commitments. The Joint Commission on Accreditation of Hospitals (JCAH), in its standard for Professional Library Services, recognizes the importance of resource sharing and requires that interlibrary loan and other sharing arrangements be documented (2).

A comprehensive interlibrary loan statement of policy should describe any resource sharing agreements, and thus will meet the JCAH documentation requirements. A loan policy should also establish a balance between interlibrary loan and collection development and should identify the library's responsibilities as a lender and as a borrower. The policy statement should define acceptable levels of cost and staff-time for both borrowing and lending. Because requirements and responsibilities differ for borrowing and for lending, separate policy statements may be advisable. Such policy statements should be approved by appropriate administrative units within the hospital and should be reviewed regularly.

Developing a Borrowing Policy

A policy statement for interlibrary loan borrowing should include:

- Objectives of the hospital library's interlibrary loan borrowing program
- Relationship to collection development
- Types of library users eligible for interlibrary loan service
- Network participation and borrowing channels
- Relevant provisions of the Copyright Act of 1976
- Responsibility for costs

Each of these topics is discussed below.

Objectives

A statement of objectives should define the role of interlibrary loan borrowing in the context of the hospital library's service goals and briefly describe any restrictions. For example, a library may have adopted as its general service goal the JCAH Principle for Professional Library Services: "The hospital shall provide library services to meet the informational, educational, and, when appropriate, the research-related needs of the medical and hospital staffs" (2:147). With this as a general service goal, a library might state as its general objective for interlibrary loan borrowing: To provide a means of access to work-related materials not available in the hospital library.

A library may wish to have measurable service objectives in addition to a general objective. For example, user satisfaction with interlibrary loan service is often measured in terms of delivery speed and cost, so specific service objectives might be determined, such as:

- X percent of all requests initiated will be supplied to the requester within one week of the date of the request.
- X percent of all requests supplied will be supplied at a cost of not more than X dollars per request.

Specific objectives such as these will vary according to the size of the library's collection, its location, its access to bibliographic tools, and its participation in resource sharing cooperatives and networks. Measurable objectives will not only determine the way an interlibrary loan borrowing program is carried out, but will also be useful for evaluation of the program.

Relationship to Collection Development

Although interlibrary loan may be heavily relied upon during a library's developmental period, it should be regarded as a supplement to, not a substitute for, a vigorous collection development policy. The interlibrary loan policy statement must clearly define the relationship between interlibrary loan and collection development. Guidelines must be developed so that interlibrary loan borrowing records can be used for collection analysis and for deciding whether to buy specific items. In developing these guidelines, a librarian should consider the nature of the library's primary clientele, its programs, and its teaching functions. Attention must be given to the Copyright Act of 1976, which prohibits libraries from borrowing multiple copies in lieu of subscription or purchase. Guidelines should specify the frequency with which borrowing records will be analyzed and give a general indication of the criteria that will be used to determine when purchases should be made.

The decision to purchase a title might be indicated if interlibrary loan requests are generated because of:

- A new department or service
- A new user group previously unserved
- A new program or emphasis in the hospital
- An unmet need now identified

Borrowing, instead of purchasing, might be the most appropriate action, even though fees are involved, if:

- A title is requested primarily for work on a project that is nearing completion.
- There is heavy use of a title by only one staff member.
- A title is so expensive that continued borrowing, even with royalties and borrowing charges, is more cost-effective.
- A title is requested primarily by staff who have direct access to this title through a medical school, or other, library.

If the library is involved in a formal cooperative acquisition or retention program with other libraries, analysis of interlibrary loan records for joint collection development may form part of the cooperative agreement. Such agreements should be included in any interlibrary loan policy statement.

Service Limitations

Any service limitations should be identified in the policy statement so that the library's clientele clearly understands what services are and are not available. Will all hospital employees be able to request materials through interlibrary loan, or will the service be limited to particular groups, such as staff physicians or management personnel? Ideally all employees should be able to use the service. If the library also permits use of its facilities by patients, employees or students from other institutions, or the general public, their access to interlibrary loan service should be specified.

Network Participation and Borrowing Channels

The policy statement should describe the channels for interlibrary loan borrowing, such as local cooperative groups, agreements among groups of libraries, the Regional Medical Library (RML) network, state networks, and non-network sources. The policy should also indicate the circumstances in which it is appropriate to bypass those channels. In addition, the policy statement should indicate compliance with policies and procedures of local cooperative groups, the RML program and other networks, and the ALA National Interlibrary Loan Code.

Copyright Law

Any statement of policy must acknowledge the library's responsibilities as a borrower under the copyright law. These responsibilities include posting appropriate notices of the law, determining whether copy requests comply with the law, and maintaining appropriate records. The policy statement should also describe the library's interpretation of its rights to make copies under the law. A librarian may wish to have this section of the policy statement reviewed by the hospital's legal counsel. The copyright law is discussed in detail later in this chapter.

Responsibility for Costs

Since many libraries now charge for interlibrary loan, it is important to state how these charges will be met. Will they be covered in the library budget, charged back to appropriate departments, charged to the individual borrower, or paid from a special fund? Or will the library choose not to borrow from those libraries that charge for interlibrary loans? How charges will be met, the extent to which the library will try to avoid loan charges (which in turn will affect borrowing patterns), and how unexpected charges will be handled should all be covered in the policy statement.

Developing a Lending Policy

The decision to lend materials to another library has potential impact on the hospital library's primary clientele. Materials may be on loan to another library when needed by a hospital staff member. The library must maintain a balance between its commitment to resource sharing and its responsibilities to its primary users. A lending policy statement must define and maintain this balance. Such a statement should include:

- Objectives of the hospital library's interlibrary loan lending program
- Network participation and lending channels
- Types of material eligible for loan
- Relevant provisions of the copyright law
- Responsibility for costs
  Each of these topics is discussed below.

Objectives

As was the case with the policy statement on borrowing, a statement of objectives for interlibrary lending should relate to the library's overall service goal. An interlibrary lending policy might have as a general objective: To encourage resource sharing by making materials available to other libraries through loan or copy. The policy statement should identify any constraints necessary to maintain an appropriate balance between the needs of the library's primary clientele and the needs of other libraries. The policy statement might include measurable criteria, such as:

- X percent of all interlibrary loan requests received by the library will be processed within two days of receipt.
- No more than X percent of the material on loan will be material simultaneously requested by the hospital library's primary clientele.

Network Participation and Lending Channels

The description of network participation and lending patterns in the lending policy statement should resemble that in the borrowing policy statement. In each case, the policy statement should list cooperative groups, agreements among groups, and networks whose participants may borrow from the hospital library. The statement should note any categories of libraries that may not borrow and any inappropriate network channels. It should affirm the library's agreement to conform to appropriate network policies and to the ALA National Interlibrary Loan Code.

Material Eligible for Loan

In order to minimize the impact of lending on primary clientele, many libraries place some limitation on the type, format, and quantities of material eligible for loan. For example, most libraries will not lend standard reference tools such as the *American Medical Directory*, the *Physicians' Desk Reference* (PDR), or *Grant's Atlas of Anatomy*. Most libraries prefer to photocopy requested journal articles rather than to lend complete issues, although some libraries lend single issues or bound volumes of journals. Some libraries will provide photocopies only; no books are loaned. The high replacement cost of audiovisuals, the greater likelihood of their being damaged, and the more frequent in-house demand for this type of material must be considered. A comprehensive policy statement should list the types of material that will be available for loan; whether photocopy service will be provided; and any conditions of loan or copy, including in-house use, loan period, acceptance of renewals, and responsibility for any damages that might occur.

Copyright Law

The policy statement must acknowledge the library's responsibilities as a lender under the copyright law. These responsibilities include determining whether requests for copies received from other libraries comply with the law and affixing appropriate notice to any copies made. A librarian may wish to have this section of the policy statement be reviewed by the hospital's legal counsel. The copyright law is discussed more fully later on in this chapter.

Responsibility for Costs

At present, most hospital libraries do not charge for interlibrary loan service. Increases in the volume of loans and in costs associated with both borrowing and lending may require, however, that charging for this service be considered. Costs associated with providing interlibrary loan service include labor; materials and supplies; equipment use and maintenance; postage or shipping charges; replacement of lost or damaged materials; an appropriate proportion of indirect costs such as heating and lighting; and the cost of depreciation of the collection. Billing is itself an additional cost.

A library with a low lending volume can usually absorb the costs of interlibrary loan service. But the volume of loan transactions may increase to a point where it is not possible to provide effective service without allotting additional funds for staff, supplies, or equipment. One source of additional funds is the service charge. In evaluating this option, the librarian must carefully review both the hospital's policy with respect to fee-for-service and the potential impact on relationships with other libraries. A helpful overview is provided in *User Fees: A Practical Perspective*, edited by Miriam Drake (3).

Questions that must be asked include whether it is possible for the library to charge for services. If so, will the fee structure be based on full cost recovery or will it be partially subsidized? Will any revenue be available for use by the library? How will hospital policy and procedures affect plans for billing and receipt of payment? To what extent must the library staff become involved in billing and collection?

Once possibilities within the hospital have been identified, the impact on relationships with other libraries must be assessed. Does the library borrow more than it lends? Does it wish to charge libraries that are not charging it? Do cooperative agreements stipulate that members may or may not charge one another? Will volume drop if fees are initiated?

If a library decides to charge for services after assessing these internal and external factors, an appropriate fee structure must be developed. As a basis for this decision, the library should conduct a cost study. Then the library can consider other factors, such as hospital policy, the established charges of other libraries, and relationships with other libraries. All decisions about charging for interlibrary loans should be documented in the library policy.

COPYRIGHT RESTRICTIONS

The Copyright Act of 1976 (Title 17 of the United States Code) became effective in January 1978. It establishes certain requirements of libraries that participate in interlibrary loans involving photocopying or some other form of duplication. Some of the requirements, such as the posting of various notices and warnings, are straightforward. Other provisions of the law are more difficult to interpret and remain open to judicial review. Every hospital librarian should become thoroughly familiar with the copyright law. Each of the national library associations has prepared publications that provide valuable assistance in explaining the provisions of the law, stressing the rights and responsibilities of libraries and library users and discussing common practice in interpreting the law. These publications, which are listed at the conclusion of this chapter, should be available in every hospital library, along with the text of the law and relevant guidelines. They should be used to develop the hospital library's lending and borrowing policies and procedures for compliance with the law, in consultation with the hospital's legal counsel.

Three sections of the copyright law have particular significance for librarians. Section 106 defines the exclusive rights of copyright owners, and Section 107 recognizes the doctrine of "fair use" and limits the exclusive rights of copyright owners granted in Section 106. Section 108 further limits the exclusive rights of copyright owners, and authorizes the reproduction of copies by libraries in certain situations that may not be covered under "fair use."

Also of importance to librarians involved in interlibrary loan transactions are the Commission on New Technological Uses of Copyrighted Works (CONTU) Guidelines for the Proviso of Subsection 108(g)(2). These guidelines are an attempt to define how many copies constitute substitution by a borrowing library for subscription to or purchase of a title. These guidelines are not part of the law but will certainly be considered in any judicial interpretation.

Under the Copyright Act of 1976 and CONTU Guidelines, a borrowing library must:

- Post a "Display Warning of Copyright" at locations where interlibrary loan requests are accepted
- Include an "Order Warning of Copyright" on application forms used to request copies
- Evaluate each photocopy request in light of the requirements of Sections 107 and 108 and determine whether the request falls within the requirements of the law or the CONTU Guidelines
- Maintain records as required by the law

Lending libraries also have certain obligations. A lending library must:

- Accept only those copy requests that indicate that the borrowing library is in compliance with the law or the CONTU Guidelines
- Include a notice of copyright on all photocopies supplied

Posting Notices and Warnings

As noted above, the copyright law Section 108 (d) requires a library to post a Display Warning of Copyright at all locations where requests for copies are accepted. The text of the warning appears in Figure 9-1. Section 108

Figure 9-1
Notice of Copyright Restrictions

Notice
Warning Concerning
Copyright Restrictions

The copyright law of the United States (Title 17, United States Code) governs the making of photocopies or other reproductions of copyrighted material.

Under certain conditions specified in the law, libraries and archives are authorized to furnish a photocopy or other reproduction. One of these specified conditions is that the photocopy or reproduction is not to be "used for any purpose other than private study, scholarship, or research." If a user makes a request for, or later uses, a photocopy or reproduction for purposes in excess of "fair use," that user may be liable for copyright infringement.

This institution reserves the right to refuse to accept a copying order if, in its judgment, fulfillment of the order would involve violation of the copyright law.

(e) requires that an Order of Warning of Copyright appear on all photocopy application forms. The text of both notices is the same. Requirements for wording, type, size, and location of these notices are prescribed by the Register of Copyrights and may be found in *The Copyright Law and the Health Sciences Librarian*, published by the Medical Library Association (4).

Section 108(a)(3) requires that any photocopy supplied by a library must include a notice of copyright. The Council of National Library Associations recommends this language: "Notice: This material may be protected by copyright law (Title 17, U.S. Code)" (4). Many libraries tape this notice to the glass plate of the copier so that it automatically appears on each photocopy produced. Other alternatives are to stamp each copy with the notice or to attach the notice to each photocopy.

Determining Compliance with the Law

When requesting an interlibrary loan that will be filled by a photocopy, the requesting librarian must determine whether that request complies with the copyright law or the CONTU Guidelines. For these purposes, the key portions of the law are those that deal with "fair use" (Section 107) and with specific applications of the law to library photocopying (Section 108). Full discussion of these provisions is found in the publications of the national library associations and in *Applying the New Copyright Law: A Guide for Educators and Librarians*, by Jerome K. Miller (5).

The judicial concept of fair use has been in existence since 1802, but it has proved difficult to define, either in the courts or statutes. The Copyright Act of 1976 states that the factors to be considered in determining fair use should include:

- The purpose and character of the copy's use
- The nature of the work being copied
- The amount of material being copied
- The effect of making the copy on the potential market for, or value of, the work.

As a general rule, a single copy of an article or portion of a book such as a chapter, made at the request of a library user for private use, may be considered a fair use. Miller's book includes a "Fair Use Checklist" that is helpful in determining whether a particular instance of photocopying is a fair use (5).

Section 108 of the law addresses certain rights of reproduction specific to libraries and archives not discussed under the concept of fair use as defined in Section 107. For interlibrary loan, the key subsection is 108(g)(2) which states:

> *...Provided*, That nothing in this clause prevents a library or archives from participating in interlibrary arrangements that do not have, as their purpose or effect, that the library or archives receiving such copies or phonorecords for distribution does so in such aggregate quantities as to substitute for a subscription to or purchase of such work.

The law does not specifically define how many copies constitute substitution. This issue is addressed in the CONTU Guidelines for the Proviso of Subsection 108(g)(2). Basically, these guidelines state that a library may not receive more than five photocopies in a single calendar year from a copyrighted journal title published in the last five years. The five copies may be of the same article for five different people or may be of five different articles; copying from the same title is the determining factor. The CONTU Guidelines also address the question of receipt of copies of portions of copyrighted works other than periodicals. In this instance, the guidelines suggest, libraries may receive no more than five photocopies per year per title as long as the copyright on the material is in effect.

There are exceptions to the CONTU Guidelines. If the library owns the material but is unable to supply a copy because the item is damaged or lost, the "rule of five" is waived. The rule is also waived if the library has entered a subscription for the title. These are logical exceptions, since the intent of the law is to prevent libraries from requesting photocopies in lieu of purchase. The CONTU Guidelines are important but are not law. Nor do they address photocopying of journal articles more than five years old. The guidelines must be considered as a significant aid in interpreting the law, but they are not a substitute for sound understanding and good judgment on the part of the librarian. Further, it should be pointed out that neither Section 108 nor the CONTU Guidelines eliminate the possibility of applying fair use.

Once the librarian has determined that a request falls within the requirements of the law or the CONTU Guidelines, this must be noted on the interlibrary loan request form. The ALA form provides two boxes: CCG is checked if the request falls within the CONTU Guidelines; CCL is checked if the request conforms to other provisions of the law (for example, fair use).

If a request falls outside the requirements of the law or the guidelines, the librarian may:

- Attempt to borrow the original
- Obtain a reprint from the author or publisher
- Obtain permission to copy from the publisher and pay any royalty fee imposed
- Investigate use of the Copyright Clearance Center and payment of royalties
- Enter a subscription for the title or purchase the book
- Refuse to fill the request

Certain publications permit copying freely or waive their rights to collect royalties. Such publications usually include statements to this effect in the preliminary pages of the journal. Publications in the public domain (such as United States government publications which are not eligible for copyright protection) may also be copied without restriction. In addition, the policies of both the United States Public Health Service (PHS) and the National Institutes of Health (NIH) state that communications in primary scientific journals publishing initial reports of original research supported in whole or in part by PHS or NIH grant funds may be copyrighted by the journal. The journal does so with the understanding that individuals are authorized to make, or have made by any means available to them, without regard to the copyright of the journal, and without royalty, a single copy of any such article for their own use. The indication of grant support is usually in the form of a footnote on the first page of the article. Where PHS or NIH support is noted, the article may be copied without inclusion in the "rule of five."

Because the responsibility for determining compliance lies with the requesting library, the lending library need only determine that one of the two copyright compliance boxes on the ALA form has been checked. If ALA forms are not used, some other means should be used to inform the lending library that the request is in compliance with the copyright law.

PROCEDURES FOR BORROWING PRINT MATERIALS

Failure to fill out a request form properly or to route it through appropriate channels is a disservice to the library's users since it inevitably delays the receipt of needed materials. Thorough familiarity and compliance with interlibrary policies and procedures can significantly reduce the time between initiation of a request and receipt of the requested material.

The procedures described below are basic and apply to any interlibrary loan borrowing transaction. Individual cooperatives and networks, however, may have developed protocols which eliminate or alter some of these

Figure 9-2
In-house Interlibrary Loan Application Form: Book Request

Note: Based on a form developed by Nancy Stump, Interlibrary Loan Department, Sangamon State University, Springfield, Illinois.

procedures, or require the use of special forms and abbreviations. It is important to follow network protocols when borrowing from those sources. Procedures for borrowing audiovisual materials are discussed in Chapter 10.

Initiating the Request

In order to process and transmit an interlibrary loan request, the hospital librarian needs certain information from the person making the request. This information includes:

- Identification of the material the user needs (citation)
- The source where the user found out about the material (source of reference)
- Name, position, department, and telephone number of the requester
- Latest date the material requested will be useful
- Charges the requester is willing to accept

To expedite this information-gathering, in-house interlibrary loan application forms can be developed, which can be used by both library staff members and clients. Good forms encourage requesters to provide necessary information and serve as a checklist for library staff. Forms should be easy for the user to understand, quick to fill out, highly visible, and in abundant supply. Colored card or paper stock makes the forms easy to see and easy to use. Multiple part forms simplify records management. A supply of forms might be kept available in various hospital departments and staff lounges and distributed in batches to heavy users. An ample supply should be available in the library, not only at library staff desks but also on tables near the indexes and in reading areas.

Figures 9-2 and 9-3 show examples of application forms for book and journal article requests. Some librarians prefer to use a single combined form. The article request

Figure 9-3
In-house Interlibrary Loan Application Form: Article Request

APPLICATION FOR INTERLIBRARY LOAN
ARTICLE REQUEST

TODAY'S DATE _____/_____/_____   NO LONGER NEEDED AFTER _____/_____/_____

JOURNAL TITLE _____

VOLUME _____ MONTH AND YEAR _____ PAGES _____

AUTHOR OF ARTICLE _____

WHERE DID YOU FIND REFERENCE TO THIS ITEM? (GIVE COMPLETE CITATION)

_____

WEST CENTRAL HOSPITAL LIBRARY
PLEASE FILL OUT THIS FORM COMPLETELY

PLEASE NOTE THAT THERE MAY BE A CHARGE FOR MATERIAL SUPPLIED TO YOU. IT IS NOT ALWAYS POSSIBLE FOR THE LIBRARY TO ANTICIPATE THESE CHARGES. WILL YOU ACCEPT ANY CHARGES?

_____ YES, UP TO _____
AMOUNT

_____ NO

REQUESTER'S NAME _____

STATUS _____

DEPARTMENT _____

NOTICE
WARNING CONCERNING COPYRIGHT RESTRICTIONS

The copyright law of the United States (Title 17, United States Code) governs the making of photocopies or other reproductions of copyrighted material.
Under certain conditions specified in the law, libraries and archives are authorized to furnish a photocopy or other reproduction. One of these specified conditions is that the photocopy or reproduction is not to be "used for any purpose other than private study, scholarship, or research." If a user makes a request for, or later uses, a photocopy or reproduction for purposes in excess of "fair use," that user may be liable for copyright infringement.
This institution reserves the right to refuse to accept a copying order if in its judgment, fulfillment of the order would involve violation of copyright law.

TELEPHONE _____

LIBRARY USE

VERIFIED IN _____
LOCATION VERIFIED _____
DATE SENT _____   SENT BY _____

Note: Based on a form developed by Nancy Stump, Interlibrary Loan Department, Sangamon State University, Springfield, Illinois.

form includes the required Warning Notice concerning copyright restrictions. The library has also included on both forms a reminder that there may be an unanticipated charge for materials supplied. A separate section on both forms provides space for the library staff to complete all preliminary work on the request. Requests initiated through interview with the user or by telephone or memo should be transferred to such application forms for ease of handling.

Verifying Citations

Once the requester has identified the material needed, the next step is to check the accuracy of the information and supply any missing elements. Is the journal title spelled correctly? Is the article in the issue cited? Has the book been published or is the citation from an advance flyer? This process is called verification. Citation or entry verification confirms the existence of the work and the correctness of the bibliographic information describing it.

Books can be verified in standard catalogs such as *Medical Books and Serials in Print*, the *National Library of Medicine Current Catalog*, or, if the library has access to the National Library of Medicine (NLM) databases, through CATLINE. If the hospital library has access to bibliographic utilities such as OCLC or RLIN, these can be used for monograph verification.

Journal citations can be verified in printed indexes such as *Index Medicus* or *Hospital Literature Index*, or through access to online databases such as MEDLINE or Health Planning and Administration.

An important distinction exists between the verification of monographs and journal articles. With monographs, it is sufficient to confirm that the title exists and that the information given is correct. With journals, it is necessary to confirm not only that the title exists but also that the article requested exists in the volume and issue noted and on the pages cited.

When verifying a citation, the librarian should add necessary information that is often missed or abbreviated by the requester. The author's first name should be spelled out when known. The full title of a journal, and its place of publication if listed, should be noted. Spelling, especially of foreign titles, should be double-checked; a *Revista* may be several shelves distant from a *Rivista* at the lending library. The more accurate the information transmitted to the lending library, the faster the request is likely to be processed.

What should a librarian do if all sources available in the hospital library have been exhausted but the citation cannot be verified? The librarian can recheck the requester's source of reference or ask another library with more verification tools to check the citation over the telephone. If all attempts fail, then the sources tried should be noted on the request or attached on a separate list and sent to the lending library with the comment, "unable to verify." If the verification process reveals significant errors in the information supplied by the requester, it may be worthwhile to recheck the library's collection to be certain the item is not available in-house.

Deciding Where to Send the Request

In deciding where to send a request, the librarian should explore the interlibrary loan services offered through the RML program, state and multitype library networks, and local cooperatives. Connections with a variety of networks and cooperatives can be especially helpful if nonmedical materials are frequently needed. The RML network is a good choice for hard-to-locate health science materials since it provides a referral system. The RML network is discussed further in Chapter 19.

Whenever possible, libraries that own the requested material should be identified. Many local and some regional cooperative groups publish union lists of serials, and some maintain union catalogs. If such lists are not available, a quick telephone call to a likely source library will often confirm ownership. Lists of the serials holdings of many resource libraries in the RML network are available, as well as printed or microfiche book catalogs. SERLINE provides some location information; its usefulness will be greatly enhanced when it incorporates up-to-date holdings information for RML network resource libraries. This same information is also available on a subscription basis in microfiche, as *Health Science Serials*. OCLC and RLIN networks also provide location information. If a hospital library does not own the more comprehensive and expensive locator tools, the library may gain access to them through participation in a local cooperative.

Once locations of requested materials are determined, a librarian can choose one accessible through loan channels established under the library's interlibrary loan policy. Normally, the first choice would be a nearby member of a local cooperative group. The next choice would be the appropriate resource library in the RML network or a state or other non-medical network. If the material does not appear to be available through any established channels, the request may be sent to any library owning the material, subject to the provisions of the ALA National Interlibrary Loan Code. If, however, the only listed location is the National Library of Medicine, the request must be routed through the RML network.

If a librarian cannot locate the material, the request should be routed through the RML network or another network which has established procedures for processing such requests. These requests are usually not filled as quickly as those sent directly to libraries that are known to own the material, because the referral process itself takes time.

Transmitting the Request

Most libraries accept the ALA interlibrary loan form as the standard request form, though some networks and cooperatives use special forms. The four-part ALA form is available in quantity from several library supply houses, including Bro-Dart, Gaylord, and Demco. It is a good idea to have the form imprinted with the hospital library's name and address and any other important identifiers, such as a consortium name or a network ID number.

Figures 9-4 and 9-5 are examples of correctly completed forms for a book request and a journal article request. Request forms should always be typed, and only one item should be requested on each form. If it has not been possible to verify the request, the source of reference should be identified on the form. If neither verification nor source of reference is available, the comment "unable to verify" should be noted on the form along with a list of the sources tried. If the full title of a journal cannot be determined, then it is preferable to give the abbreviated form of the title rather than to make a guess. The maximum acceptable charge for microfilm or hard copy (that is, photocopy) should be indicated, and compliance with the copyright law or CONTU Guidelines noted.

After the form is typed, the staff member responsible for interlibrary loans should proofread and sign the form. If the citation proved to be a problem, then it is appropriate to append any additional information that might be helpful to the lending library.

Parts A, B, and C (white, yellow and pink) of the ALA request form should be mailed to the lending library, along with the requesting library's mailing label. Part D should be retained for the library's records. The in-house application form can be stapled to the back of Part D, in case more work is needed on the request in the future.

Some requesting and lending libraries use TWX or online systems to transmit requests. These requests require the same information, but in an altered format. Though few hospital libraries have TWX terminals of their own, they may be able to use one elsewhere in the hospital. Most major resource libraries have TWX terminals, and transmission via TWX is considerably faster than mail. A copy of the TWX message should be retained for the borrowing library's records with the in-

Figure 9-4

Completed Interlibrary Loan Request Form: Book

Date of request: 3/9/83 Not needed after: 5/1/83 Requester's order no.

Call No.

Borrowing library name and address

REQUEST

For use of M. Samuals Status Staff Dept. Cardiac Rehab.

Book author: OR: periodical title, vol. and date

Antonovskis, Aaron

Book title, edition, place, year, series: OR: periodical article author, title, pages.

☐ This edition only. Health, Stress, and Coping: new perspectives on mental and physical well-being. Jossey-Bass, San Francisco 1979.

Verified in: OR: item cited in Books in Print, 1982-83. V. 1 p. 135.

ISBN, or ISSN, or LC card, or OCLC, or other number if known. LC 79-83566 —

If non-circulating, & cost does not exceed $________, please supply

☐ Microfilm ☐ Hard copy

Lending library name and address

Request complies with

☐ *108(g)(2) Guidelines (CCG)*

☐ *other provisions of copyright law (CCL)*

AUTHORIZED BY: __________

(FULL NAME)

Title __________

Request for ☐ LOAN or ☐ PHOTOCOPY

According to the A.L.A. Interlibrary Loan Code

REPORTS: Checked by

SENT BY: ☐ Library rate ☐ ________

Charges $______ Insured for $______

Date sent ________

DUE ________

RESTRICTIONS: ☐ For use in library only

☐ Copying not permitted ☐ ________

NOT SENT BECAUSE: ☐ In use

☐ Not Owned

☐ Non Circulating

☐ Request of ________

Estimated Cost of: ☐ Microfilm ______

☐ Hard copy ______

BORROWING LIBRARY RECORD:

Date received ________

Date returned ________

By ☐ Library rate ☐ ________

Postage enclosed $______ Insured for $______

RENEWALS: ☐ No renewals

Requested on ________

Renewed to ________

(or period of renewal)

Note: the receiving library assumes responsibility for notification of non-receipt.

house application form attached. Major online systems such as OCLC have developed interlibrary loan subsystems of their own, with special formats and procedures for transmission. The National Library of Medicine is also testing an interlibrary loan subsystem, DOCLINE, which should eventually become available to institutions with online access.

Some lending libraries accept telephoned requests. The requesting library should be prepared to supply all the standard information by telephone, and to follow up the telephone request with a completed ALA form.

Following Up the Request

The library to which the request is sent will usually respond either by filling the request or by returning it unfilled. Under certain circumstances, a library may refer the request to another source, or ask for more information in order to fill the request.

If the request can be filled, it will either be sent on loan and a return date specified, or a copy will be sent that need not be returned. When loan material is received, a copy of the request form indicating restrictions such as due date and limitations on use will normally be attached. This form should be matched to the copy retained by the requesting library, and the date of receipt noted on the form. The requester should be notified that the material is available, or the material should be delivered to the requester through in-house mail. The requester should be alerted to any restrictions on use; some lending libraries ask that their material be used only within the receiving library or, if material is fragile, that no photocopying be done. Due dates should be carefully noted, and the material returned by the user in time to mail back to the lending library by the date due. To help users remember any restrictions on use and due dates and to call attention to the library's service, some libraries provide a reminder message that also serves as a bookmark (see Figure 9-6). The librarian should inspect all loan material as it is returned by the user to be sure that the correct items have been received back and that the material has not been damaged.

Sometimes a lending library will return a request asking for additional information. There may be a problem with the citation, the material may not be immediately

Figure 9-5
Completed Interlibrary Loan Request Form: Journal Article

Date of request: 5/7/83 Not needed after: 6/2/83 Requester's order no.

Call No.

Borrowing library name and address

REQUEST

For use of J. Hanson Status Staff Dept. Admin.

Book author: OR: periodical title, vol. and date
Southern Hospitals, v. 46(5), Sept-Oct. 1978

Book title, edition, place, year, series: OR: periodical article author, title, pages.
☐ This edition only. Wolfe, A.V. Improving department productivity. p. 14-15.

Verified in: OR: item cited in Hospital Literature Index, v. 35, 1979, p. 677.
ISBN, or ISSN, or LC card, or OCLC, or other number if known ______
If non-circulating, & cost does not exceed $ 5.00 ______, please supply
☐ Microfilm ☐ Hard copy

Request complies with
☐ *108(g)(2) Guidelines (CCG)*
☐ *other provisions of copyright law (CCL)*

AUTHORIZED BY: Joan Howard (FULL NAME)
Title Librarian

Request for ☐ LOAN or ☐ PHOTOCOPY
According to the A.L.A. Interlibrary Loan Code

REPORTS: Checked by
SENT BY: ☐ Library rate ☐ ______
Charges $ ______ Insured for $ ______
Date sent ______
DUE ______

RESTRICTIONS: ☐ For use in library only
☐ Copying not permitted ☐ ______

NOT SENT BECAUSE: ☐ In use
☐ Not Owned
☐ Non Circulating
☐ Request of ______

Estimated Cost of: ☐ Microfilm ______
☐ Hard copy ______

BORROWING LIBRARY RECORD:
Date received ______
Date returned ______
By ☐ Library rate ☐ ______
Postage enclosed $ ______ Insured for $ ______

RENEWALS: ☐ No renewals
Requested on ______
Renewed to ______
(or period of renewal)

Note: the receiving library assumes responsibility for notification of non-receipt.

available, or the library may request confirmation before mailing an expensive photocopy. In such cases the librarian should either supply the necessary information or cancel the request.

If a lending library cannot fill a request and does not participate in a referral network (or if the request does not meet requirements for a referral), the request will be returned to the initiating library. The reason for the return should be noted on the request form. If the reason listed is "not owned," or "missing" or "non-circulating," the only alternative is to begin the request process again with another library. If the reason listed is "on loan," the librarian may choose to resubmit the request at a later date. Many requests submitted through the RML or other networks are referred to other libraries if they cannot be filled by the receiving library and if they meet that network's criteria for referrable requests. In that case, the requesting library is notified that referral has been made to a particular library.

The requesting library should receive either the material requested or a report on action taken within a reasonable time. The librarian should keep an account of this "turn-around time," since it is a useful tool in deciding where to send a future request. If no report has been received within three weeks, the librarian should follow up the request with a phone call, a TWX message, or an ALA request form. Follow-up TWX transmissions and ALA forms should be exact duplicates of the original, with the addition of "Status Report Requested (date)" prominently in the first line. A request should not simply be resubmitted on the theory that the first one went astray; the result may be two sets of material and two bills.

The requesting library must notify the lending library of nonreceipt of loan material or receipt in damaged condition. According to the ALA National Interlibrary Loan Code, the responsibility for borrowed material rests with the requesting library from the time that the material leaves the lending library until it is received back in good condition. In practice, however, losses in transit to the requesting library are often covered by the lending library's insurance. Prompt notification is essential.

Returning Material

Materials should be sturdily packaged for return; commercial paper bag mailers are usually not sufficient. Care should be taken to return material to its rightful owner; if the material was received through a referral, this will not be the library to which the request was initially addressed. The ownership stamp should be double-checked and the address on the mailing label verified. Material should be returned fourth class mail (library rate) or via UPS or another delivery service, and should always be insured.

If a renewal is requested, the lending library should be contacted before the due date. Some libraries accept tele-

phone renewals. Others require a copy of the original TWX message or ALA request form requesting renewal. If the lending library grants a renewal, the appropriate records should be annotated and the user notified. If the library does not grant a renewal, then the requesting library must ensure prompt return of the material.

PROCEDURES FOR LENDING PRINT MATERIALS

Even the smallest hospital library can potentially lend material and is more likely to do so if the library is a part of a local cooperative group. Even if the lending volume is not high initially, such libraries should establish procedures for responding to interlibrary loan requests so that the requests can be handled promptly. Procedures for lending audiovisuals are covered in Chapter 10.

Screening a Request

When a hospital library receives a request, it should first screen the request for eligibility. Does the request conform to the library's lending policy? Has the necessary copyright compliance been indicated? If the request is eligible, then the card catalog or serials list should be checked to verify ownership. Next a decision should be made whether the material can be loaned or copied under the library's loan policy. Finally, the material must be located and a determination made whether it can be supplied prior to any "not needed after" date.

Figure 9-6
Information Bookmark for Users

WEST CENTRAL HOSPITAL LIBRARY

This material has been made available to you through interlibrary loan from another library.

_____ You may keep the material.

_____ Please return the material to West Central Library on

_____
(date)

Contact the West Central Hospital Library before the due date if you will need a renewal.

Note: Based on a form developed by Nancy Stump, Interlibrary Loan Department, Sangamon State University, Springfield, Illinois.

Filling a Request

As the first step in filling a request for an original document, the appropriate circulation records must be completed and the due date stamped in the book. On the appropriate sections of the ALA form, the date sent, date due, and any restrictions should be noted. The A copy of the form should be retained by the lending library, the C copy enclosed with the material, and the B copy sent separately to the requesting library (some libraries eliminate this latter step). Finally, the material should be prepared for mailing and insured.

If a photocopy is requested, the lending library first should check to be certain that copyright compliance has been indicated. Then the article should be copied, a notice of copyright added, and the "Reports" section of the ALA form completed. Copies are normally mailed first class to the requesting library, with the B and C copies of the ALA form enclosed.

Some libraries enclose a bookmark with loan material or attach it to a photocopy as an additional reminder of the lending library's policy (see Figure 9-7).

If a lending library accepts telephone requests, use of a form similar to the in-house application form may be necessary, and follow-up ALA forms should be requested. TWX requests should be handled in the same manner as ALA request forms.

Handling a Request That Cannot Be Filled

If the library cannot fill a request, the "Not Sent Because" section of the ALA form should be completed. The A copy is retained by the lending library and the other copies returned to the requesting library. If the request cannot be filled because of a citation problem, that problem should be noted on the form. Requests should not be referred to other libraries unless there is a specific agreement to do so. Instead, if another location is known, that information can be noted in the "Not Sent Because" space on the ALA form, under "Request of." If the request was received via TWX, the appropriate information should be transmitted to the requesting library in the same manner, and a reference made to the initiating library's request number.

RECORDS MANAGEMENT

The purpose of maintaining effective interlibrary loan records is to ensure compliance with institutional and legal requirements for records retention and to provide useful data for evaluating services and collection development. Records management policies and procedures should be carefully designed so that they require no unnecessary time or storage space.

Maintaining Borrowing Records

Four files are important for good borrowing records management:

• *Copyright compliance.* The CONTU Guidelines state that records of photocopy transactions should be retained for three full years after the end of the calendar year during which the transactions occurred. Requests filled with photocopies should be filed in alphabetical order by journal title, in one-year increments. Such records should include information on compliance decisions. For example, if permission to copy was received from the publisher, or if a royalty fee was paid, that information should be noted in the file. Judgments about the applicability of Section 107 or Section 108(g)(2) should be recorded. This file will also be useful for collection development since it indicates which titles have been in frequent demand.

• *Requests pending.* These are materials requested for which no answer has yet been received. This file may be kept by requester's name, by title, or by date the request was initiated. Most libraries find that filing by title and

Figure 9-7
Information Bookmark for Lending Library

WEST CENTRAL HOSPITAL LIBRARY

This material is being supplied to you through interlibrary loan from the West Central Hospital Library.

_____ You may keep the material.

_____ The material is due back in the West Central Hospital Library no later than

_____
(date)

Restrictions:

If a renewal is needed, please contact the West Central Hospital Library before the due date.

When returning material, please insure it and mail to:

West Central Hospital Library
901 James Street
Goodtown, Anystate 00000

Note: Based on a form developed by Nancy Stump, Interlibrary Loan Department, Sangamon State University, Springfield, Illinois.

maintaining a separate listing by requester's name is the most effective method.

• *Requests circulating.* Records of materials received on loan should be filed by due date, with the earliest due date at the front of the file. This will act as a "tickler file," reminding the librarian that materials are soon due. If the file is large, index cards separating due dates might be helpful.

• *Requests completed.* Closed requests for material returned to the lending library, or for which copyright compliance information was not required can be filed either by title or by requester's name. Most libraries find that filing by title is preferable, both for handling inquiries from lenders and for collection development purposes.

Maintaining Lending Records

The Copyright Act of 1976 does not require that records be retained by lending institutions, but institutional policies may have a bearing on the nature of lending records and the length of record retention. For example, if the hospital is charging for interlibrary loan service, fiscal policy may require that records be retained for several years.

Three files are basic to a lending operation:

• *Requests circulating.* These are materials currently on loan to other libraries. This file should be kept in the order of the dates due, with the earliest date due at the front of the file to serve as a "tickler." If its volume of lending is high, a library may wish to maintain a separate file by titles, so that records can easily be located when material is returned. A record of the loan kept with the circulation charge cards will serve this function.

• *Requests completed.* A file of closed requests contains forms on loan material that has been returned or for which copies have been made and sent. Such a file is usually maintained separately, by title.

• *Requests returned unfilled.* Requests that could not be filled are usually filed by title. This file is useful when answering inquiries by the requesting library.

If a library is involved in billing for its loan services, then additional files for pending and paid bills will probably be necessary. These files should be set up in consultation with the hospital business office.

Keeping Additional Statistical Records

If the volume of interlibrary loans is high or a variety of sources, such as the hospital administration, a consortium, a state network, and the RML network, all require statistical reporting, then a library might wish to develop summary forms. An advantage of working with summary forms is that it is then not necessary to sort and count request forms several times each month.

One useful format is illustrated in Figure 9-8. As each request is handled, the next successive number is crossed off, so that the last number crossed off is also the number of total transactions. The same procedure can be used to keep an account of categories other than those shown in Figure 9-8, as for example, the number of transactions carried out with specific libraries.

EVALUATION OF INTERLIBRARY LOAN SERVICE

The primary purpose of evaluating interlibrary loan service should be to determine whether the service benefits the library's users. Measuring the quantity of interlibrary loan service is easy; translating numbers into measures of effective service is more difficult. It may appear, for example, that a high rate of borrowing measures "good" interlibrary loan service; further examination may reveal instead that collection development is inadequate and that the library has failed to purchase material that it ought to own.

In evaluating the effectiveness of interlibrary loan services, it is essential to develop performance criteria against which the service can be measured. These criteria will vary depending on such factors as the library's level of development, its staff needs, and its location; and the criteria are likely to change as library and staff needs change. Some examples of measurable criteria for interlibrary loans are:

• X percent of all interlibrary loan requests initiated have been filled.
• X percent of all filled requests have been provided at a charge of less than $\$X$ per loan.
• X percent of all requests received from other libraries have been filled.
• X percent of all requests initiated by hospital staff members have been processed within one day of receipt.
• X percent of requests initiated have had citations verified.
• X percent of users have reported satisfaction with the service, turn-around time, and format.

Once objective measures of success in meeting criteria are developed by the staff and are measured by an analysis of requests and comments by users, then effective service can be evaluated by determining why each criterion was or was not met, and if there is anything that can be done to improve the service. If the number of requests filled for the library does not meet the established criterion, for example, perhaps it is because the library lacks the necessary tools for verification, or staff training is inadequate. On the other hand, it may be because the library's basic collection is so comprehensive that only material that is very difficult to locate is requested on loan.

Evaluation of the effectiveness of interlibrary loan service can be included in reports to the administration and also can be useful in budgeting for library services. Evaluation helps the library staff decide where to focus its

Figure 9-8
Interlibrary Loan Summary Transaction Record

WEST CENTRAL HOSPITAL LIBRARY

Interlibrary Loan Borrowing   _____ **Month**

Requests Initiated					Requests Filled				
MONOGRAPHS									
1	10	19	28	37	1	10	19	28	37
2	11	20	29	38	2	11	20	29	38
3	12	21	30	39	3	12	21	30	39
4	13	22	31	40	4	13	22	31	40
5	14	23	32	41	5	14	23	32	41
6	15	24	33	42	6	15	24	33	42
7	16	25	34	43	7	16	25	34	43
8	17	26	35	44	8	17	26	35	44
9	19	27	36	45	9	18	27	36	45
JOURNALS									
1	10	19	28	37	1	10	19	28	37
2	11	20	29	38	2	11	20	29	38
3	12	21	30	39	3	12	21	30	39
4	13	22	31	40	4	13	22	31	40
5	14	23	32	41	5	14	23	32	41
6	15	24	33	42	6	15	24	33	42
7	16	25	34	43	7	16	25	34	43
8	17	26	35	44	8	17	26	35	44
9	18	27	36	45	9	18	27	36	45
AUDIOVISUALS									
1	10	19	28	37	1	10	19	28	37
2	11	20	29	38	2	11	20	29	38
3	12	21	30	39	3	12	21	30	39
4	13	22	31	40	4	13	22	31	40
5	14	23	32	41	5	14	23	32	41
6	15	24	33	42	6	15	24	33	42
7	16	25	34	43	7	16	25	34	43
8	17	26	35	44	8	17	26	35	44
9	18	27	36	45	9	18	27	36	45

Note: Based on a form developed by Nancy Stump, Interlibrary Loan Department, Sangamon State University, Springfield, Illinois.

energies and how to compensate for external problems over which it has no control. Evaluation may also make evident how more control can be exerted. For example, if a hospital does not belong to a local cooperative and refers most of its interlibrary loans to libraries in another city, the material is probably delayed in getting to the user. An examination of this and other data may build up a strong case for joining the local cooperative; changes in service as a result of joining the cooperative can be documented.

EFFECTIVE INTERLIBRARY LOAN SERVICE

Since interlibrary loan is intended to provide access to materials not available in-house, it is vital to the library's overall goals and to the sense of service conveyed to the library's users. The provision of interlibrary loan service depends on effective interaction with other libraries. The basic tenets of this interaction can be summarized as:

- Follow the rules
- Expand contacts with other libraries
- Provide good service as a lender
- Educate users

If the users of a hospital's interlibrary loan service understand its limitations and know what information they need to provide; if the library staff "follows the rules" when initiating requests; if the librarian has a network of contacts for resource sharing and a thorough understanding of local, state, regional and national network channels; and if the library provides fast efficient service when called upon to do so, then interlibrary loan service will be an effective extension of the library's resources.

REFERENCES

1. American Library Association. Reference and Adult Services Division. National Interlibrary Loan Code Revision Subcommittee. National interlibrary loan code, 1980. RQ 1980 Fall;20:29-31.

2. Joint Commission on Accreditation of Hospitals. Accreditation manual for hospitals. 1983 ed. Chicago: Joint Commission on Accreditation of Hospitals, 1982:147-149.

3. Drake MA. User fees: a practical perspective. Littleton, CO: Libraries Unlimited, 1981.

4. Medical Library Association. The copyright law and the health sciences librarian. Chicago: Medical Library Association, 1978.

5. Miller JK. Applying the new copyright law: a guide for educators and librarians. Chicago: American Library Association, 1979. 1979.

READINGS

American Library Association. Librarian's copyright kit: what you must know now. Chicago: American Library Association, 1978.

American Library Association. Reference and Adult Services Division. National Interlibrary Loan Code Revision Subcommittee. Model interlibrary loan code for regional, state, local or other specific groups of libraries. RQ 1980 Fall;20:26-28.

Sanford L. Interlibrary loan and copyright. Chicago: Medical Library Association, 1981. (MLA courses for continuing education; CE 111).

Audiovisual Services

Frances Bischoff
Coordinator of Media Services
Wishard Memorial Hospital
Indianapolis, Indiana

CHAPTER 10

Audiovisual Services

Frances Bischoff
Coordinator of Media Services
Wishard Memorial Hospital
Indianapolis, Indiana

Appendixes

Figures

Health professionals have been using audiovisuals for many years. Since 1970 the use of audiovisuals has increased in many hospitals. Equipment has also become more sophisticated. In addition to slide and film projectors, many hospitals now own video playback units, closed circuit television stations, production facilities, and large numbers of audiovisual programs. The demand for audiovisuals to support educational activities in medicine, nursing, staff training, and patient education continues to grow. Many hospitals see a need for a systematic approach to providing audiovisual services. Such an approach can help control costs and can also ensure access to these services.

Librarians are well-equipped to play an active role in organizing audiovisual services. The skills and techniques used by librarians to locate, select, organize, and circulate books and periodicals can be applied to audiovisual resources. Also, providing audiovisuals is compatible with the library's goal of making educational and informational resources available to medical and hospital staff.

HOSPITAL AUDIOVISUAL SERVICES: A CONTINUUM

Many types and levels of audiovisual services are possible within the hospital. Figure 10-1 presents these services as a four-part continuum, from the most basic services at Level I to the most complex at Level IV. Full-scale audiovisual services can include all the items in the figure. However, such comprehensive service is not always possible or even desirable. Each hospital should determine the types of services that meet its individual needs.

Just as no one blueprint exists for the types of audiovisual services needed in a hospital, there is no single organizational model for the delivery of these services. Depending on the hospital, audiovisual services may be provided wholly or in part by the library, the education department, or a separate audiovisual or communications department. In many cases, responsibility for providing services is divided among several hospital departments.

The extent to which the hospital library becomes involved with audiovisual services may depend on many factors. These factors include the library's resources, the services currently available from other departments, the effectiveness of those services, and the willingness of other departments to work with the library. The hospital administration's understanding of the benefits of coordinated audiovisual services is also important.

Certain audiovisual services, particularly those listed in Levels I and II on the continuum, are most logically handled by the library. Services such as controlled circulation, cataloging and classification, selection, and organized reference are often lacking when the education department or a separate audiovisual department is responsible for audiovisuals. By starting with these services, the librarian can minimize "turf" problems with other departments already involved with audiovisuals. A good strategy for dealing with these departments is to include them in the planning stages and to stress the benefits of centralized and supplementary audiovisual services. Keeping the administration informed of both goals and progress is also important.

This chapter will focus on audiovisual services that hospital librarians can provide. Basic information about audiovisuals, such as the types of equipment available or procedures for labeling slides, can be located in the resources listed at the end of the chapter. For the purposes of this discussion, audiovisual services will be divided into three categories: software services, hardware or equipment services, and production services. Within each category, the various levels of service in the continuum will be covered. A discussion of copyright laws, management issues, and professional associations and journals in the audiovisual field is also included.

SOFTWARE SERVICES

In the context of this chapter, the term "software" refers to all types of audiovisual programs, including films, filmstrips, slides, and videotapes. The use of software generally falls into two categories: use by an instructor, lecturer, or presenter and use by individuals in the library itself. Examples of the first category include grand rounds and lectures, in-service sessions for employees or affiliated students, showings at departmental meetings, and public relations presentations. The second category includes all uses of software in the library, whether by medical staff, nursing or hospital staff, or affiliated students. In most cases, audiovisual materials that are part of an instructional activity get the heaviest use.

Software programs and the equipment needed to use them are expensive. Thus before embarking on any plan of software services, the librarian should look at the way software is currently used in the hospital and assess the potential for future use. Patterns of software use tend to change as users grow more sophisticated in audiovisual techniques. Instructors often begin by combining an audiovisual program with a lecture. Later they may identify specific programs and assign them to students as required viewing.

Identifying Users of Software Programs

The use of software programs in the hospital is not limited to students or those with formal instructional responsibilities. All staff connected with medical, nursing, and allied health educational programs are potential users of software programs. Administrative staff, department heads, supervisors, in-service trainers, patient education personnel, community and public relations personnel, and volunteers may also wish to use audiovisual materials.

Figure 10-1
Continuum of Audiovisual Services

Level I: Organization of resources already in hospital

SOFTWARE SERVICES

Collection:
Small circulating collection, usually consolidation of materials already in hospital
Reference services:
Producers' catalogs
Referral of questions to local media sources

Software for onetime use:
Loans from libraries, companies, associations, or agencies

HARDWARE SERVICES
Equipment pool:
Consolidation of equipment in hospital

Circulation and reservation system
Viewing area:
Small area in library

PRODUCTION SERVICES
None

Level II: Limited budget and staff (Level I plus)

SOFTWARE SERVICES

Collection:
Limited collection development
Cataloging/classification
Reference:
Producers' catalogs
AV reference tools
Media searches—manual or computer

Software for onetime use:
Loans from libraries, companies, associations, or agencies
Rentals

HARDWARE SERVICES
Equipment pool:
Purchase of needed hardware
Circulation and reservation system

Viewing area:
Permanent area with carrels and dedicated equipment
Accessories:
Carts for mobile equipment use
Equipment accessories

PRODUCTION SERVICES
None

Level III: Budget and staffing support (Level I, II, plus)

SOFTWARE SERVICES

Collection:
Active collection building to meet user's ongoing needs
Cataloging/classification
Printed catalog
Reference Service:
Producers' catalogs
AV reference tools
Media searches—manual or computer
Media utilization

Software for onetime use:
Loans from libraries, companies, associations, or agencies
Rentals

HARDWARE SERVICES
Equipment Pool:
Full range of AV equipment
Circulation and reservation system
Special purpose equipment

Viewing area:
Permanent carrel areas
Classrooms for AV use
Accessories:
Carts for equipment
Equipment accessories
Educational accessories

PRODUCTION SERVICES
None

Level IV: Full-scale audiovisual services (Level I, II, III plus)

SOFTWARE SERVICES
Same as Level III

HARDWARE SERVICES
Same as Level III plus equipment needed for production

PRODUCTION SERVICES
Production services can be provided on three levels: Small-scale, Medium-scale or Large-scale

Small-scale Production
Copying non-copyrighted audio-tapes
Making or assisting users to make
transparencies
posters
filp charts
Laminating
Dry mounting
Simple graphics

Medium-scale Production
Making audio recordings
Copying noncopyrighted video-tapes

Simple slide-tape shows
Simple video programs
(no editing)
Expansion of graphic area

Large-scale Production
Productions requiring instructional design
Slide-tape shows
Video production
Multi-image Slide-tape programs
Programmed instruction modules
Broadcasting and producing for patient television station

Offering a Continuum of Software Services

As Figure 10-1 demonstrates, several levels of software services are possible. Each of these levels will be discussed below.

Level I

Level I represents the organization of resources already available in the hospital and the provision of basic reference services. This level of service can be achieved with a very small budget. The software collection consists mostly of programs purchased by various hospital departments. Planning and tact are critical in any attempt to centralize these materials in the library. The librarian must convince personnel that they will benefit from programs being centrally stored, maintained, cataloged, and circulated. Administrative support is almost always essential for the consolidation of existing resources into a centralized collection. If a few departments resist, it is usually best to proceed without them. In many cases they will cooperate once the advantages of a centralized collection are demonstrated.

Software programs can be circulated in a manner similar to other library materials. They may or may not be classified, depending on the size of the collection. A collection of fewer than 20 titles with little potential for growth can be organized by title and subject. However, formal cataloging and classification should be considered for even small collections with growth potential.

The librarian can also collect the catalogs of local libraries, media centers, companies, and agencies that lend software programs without charge. An audiovisual reference service can be provided using producers' catalogs and a file of media resource personnel in the local area.

Level II

Software services can be expanded to Level II in libraries that have a limited budget for purchase and rental. Level II services usually require more of the librarian's time. The librarian can identify, purchase, and catalog software that will be used frequently. Appropriate materials can be identified using producers' catalogs, printed reference tools, or databases. A more extensive service of loans and rentals can also be offered.

Level III

With a larger budget and more staff, software services can be expanded to Level III. The librarian can develop the audiovisual collection based on user needs, and a printed catalog can be produced. Reference services can include not only answering questions but also assisting with the selection and use of appropriate media.

Level IV

At Level IV, production services are added to the library's audiovisual services. Software not available commercially is produced locally. Production services will be discussed later in this chapter.

Managing the Software Collection

Suggestions for managing the software collection are given below. Each librarian must choose the procedures that are best suited to his or her individual environment.

Circulation

Software can be circulated in a manner similar to books and journals. Cards can either be interfiled in the circulation file or kept in a separate file. If cards are interfiled, use of another color is advisable. Since the typical audiovisual loan period is very short, a separate file is often simplest.

Each piece of software should have its own circulation card, including title and format.

For some types of software, card pockets can be easily attached. It is sometimes difficult, however, to find a place for a pocket on smaller items. An alternative for a small collection is to place circulation cards for each piece in a separate file. When a software program is charged out, the card can be pulled and placed in the charge-out file. A third method is to require the user to fill out a blank transaction card for each loan, although many users find this inconvenient. If the software collection is very small and the material is unclassified, circulation cards can be filed by title. When the collection is classified, cards can be filed by number or by title. In larger collections, the circulation file can be divided by format.

If the library frequently circulates three or four audiovisual items to one person at a time, a circulation method in which all items are recorded on one card and filed under the user's name can be convenient. The major disadvantage of this system is that items are not filed individually. However, because loan periods are short and the number of loans is generally small, identifying who has individual items is usually not a problem. Using this circulation method, one card can be used as both a circulation card and a reservation form (see Figure 10-2).

Software items are usually checked out for use in specific activities. Thus short loan periods of either half a day or one day are not only feasible but desirable. By encouraging users to pick up the program shortly before they need it and to return it promptly, the librarian can stretch the availability of a small collection. Because loan periods are variable, the audiovisual circulation file should be checked once a day. Users with overdue materials should be contacted immediately.

The librarian should also develop written policies about who may use audiovisual materials, for what purposes, and whether materials may be taken off hospital premises. Such policies are necessary even in small collections. Problems are most likely to arise with the use of materials by people not directly affiliated with the hospital, such as friends or relatives of staff members. The use of materials by hospital personnel for outside functions can also cause problems. A sample policy statement covering use of audiovisuals is given below.

West Central Hospital's audiovisual programs and equipment may be used in the hospital or may be taken off the hospital premises by medical and hospital staff for activities provided or sponsored by the hospital.

Reservation and Reserve Systems

A reservation system is suggested to ensure that audiovisual programs are available when needed. Users should be encouraged to request items as far in advance as possible. This alerts the library staff to periods of heavy demand for particular items.

For a small collection, reservations can be kept on a calendar along with reservations for the hardware needed. The length of time materials will be needed should be noted as well. For a large collection, a book with a page for each date is suggested (see Figure 10-3). With either the calendar system or the logbook, repeating requests can be recorded. For example, a department may wish to reserve a particular film for the first Monday of every month. In addition to the calendar or logbook, a reservation form may also be used (see Figure 10-2). Some librarians attach the reservation form to the software item to prevent its being borrowed by a walk-in user just before its scheduled use.

Housing and Shelving

Since audiovisual programs come in many shapes, they do not always fit conveniently on the shelf nor are they always packaged conveniently for circulation. In addition, many programs have several parts. Decisions about housing audiovisual programs should be made in light of both shelving and circulating considerations.

Audiovisual materials may be shelved in several ways. They may be interfiled with books; filed separately by class number, title, or accession number; or filed separately by format and class number, title, or accession number.

Figure 10-2
Reservation Form/Circulation Record

AUDIOVISUAL REQUEST FORM

Name _____   PICK-UP DATE/TIME _____

Dept. _____   RETURN DATE/TIME _____

Phone _____   Person Taking Request _____

Number of Viewers _____   Today's Date _____

EQUIPMENT/ACCESSORIES	Unit #	PROGRAMS	Format/Call #
1. _____		1. _____	
2. _____		2. _____	
3. _____		3. _____	
4. _____		4. _____	
5. _____		5. _____	
6. _____		6. _____	

Location:

☐ In Hospital _____   ☐ AV Classroom _____

☐ Out of Hospital _____   ☐ Pass on File

Signature _____   Date _____

Interfiling audiovisuals with books requires that both be classified using the same system. One advantage of interfiling is that all material on one subject can be shelved together, thus allowing subject browsing. Interfiling also minimizes the differences between books and audiovisuals and can increase the use of audiovisuals. Arguments against interfiling include the fact that full classification for a small audiovisual collection is not always needed. Also, subject browsing can be done at the card catalog. The major disadvantage of interfiling is that the physical shape of audiovisuals requires that many formats be repackaged to stand neatly on the shelf in between books. Boxes for repackaging of filmstrips, slides, and slide-tapes are commercially available, although extra time and expense is involved in their use. Videotapes can generally stand by themselves, but 16mm films must either be stored in square film boxes or housed separately on wire racks. Also, users generally know whether they want a book or an audiovisual and often prefer that they be shelved separately. The disadvantages of interfiling usually outweigh the advantages. Thus interfiling is not generally recommended.

Software programs may also be classified and shelved separately. This arrangement brings together all the audiovisual programs on a specific subject and is convenient for users who know in advance whether they want print or nonprint formats.

A third option is to shelve by format. Special containers are available for many formats. Thus all audiotapes, filmstrips, and 16mm films can be neatly stored together in very little space. Within format categories, programs can be filed by class number, title, or accession number. The disadvantage of this system is that users most often are looking for a program on a particular subject rather than in a particular format. Thus primary access to programs is through the card catalog or a find-

Figure 10-3
Reservation Log Book

	16mm Projector & Reel	Cart	New Breath of Life	June 15, 1980			
7:30-8:00							
8:00-8:30							
8:30-9:00							
9:00-9:30	↑ 9 AM	↑ 9 AM	↑ 9 AM				
9:30-10:00							
10:00-10:30	Bill	Bill	Bill				
10:30-11:00	Martin	Martin	Martin				
11:00-11:30							
11:30-12:00							
12:00-12:30	↓ noon	↓ noon	↓ noon				
12:30-1:00							
1:00-1:30							
1:30-2:00							
2:00-2:30							
2:30-3:00							
3:00-3:30							
3:30-4:00							
4:00-4:30							
4:30-5:00							
5:00-5:30							
5:30-6:00							
6:00-6:30							
6:30-7:00							
7:00-7:30							
7:30-8:00							
8:00-8:30							
8:30-9:00							
9:00-9:30							
9:30-10:00							
10:00-10:30							
10:30-11:00							

ing list, since browsing requires looking in several areas for one subject.

If audiovisual programs are shelved separately, the librarian should consider subject cataloging so that cards can be interfiled in the card catalog. This provides subject access without regard to format.

The method of shelving will greatly influence the kind of packaging chosen for audiovisuals. If all parts of a program cannot be kept together in one package, this should be noted on each item and also on any records of the program.

All decisions on shelving and packaging audiovisuals should be made in light of the way materials are used, as well as the available space, budget, and personnel. For more information on these topics, consult the references at the end of the chapter.

Cataloging and Classification

The type of cataloging and classification chosen for audiovisuals depends on many factors. These factors include (1) size of the collection, (2) anticipated growth, (3) shelving arrangements, (4) available staff, (5) type of access required, and (6) the system currently used for cataloging print materials.

If the audiovisual collection will never grow beyond a very small number of titles, listing by title and subject may provide a measure of control. However, it will not allow card catalog access to the programs. With a collection that has any possibility of expanding, subject access, descriptive cataloging, and classification should be considered.

For a small collection (fewer than 100 titles), the librarian has a number of cataloging options. He or she must first decide what type of access is needed through the card catalog, how much descriptive information is needed, how items will be arranged on the shelf, and whether materials will be classified. These questions should be answered in relation to the library's patterns of use, growth potential, cooperative arrangements, and possibilities for automation. Broad subject access is probably necessary in all but the smallest collections. Suitable general terms for most concepts are found in the National Library of Medicine's (NLM) *Medical Subject Headings* (MeSH). Headings that correspond to local usage can be added as cross-references or used if no appropriate MeSH terms exist. Access by title and by other information, such as sponsoring body, is almost essential for locating materials quickly and easily.

Full descriptive cataloging, even in small collections, has many advantages. More information is available to the user, and the librarian becomes familiar with materials during the cataloging process. Extra information is easily included during initial cataloging. Also, using a standard format may make future participation in networking easier. Descriptions should include title, format, sponsoring agency, length, copyright date, audience level, and a brief summary of the program.

Even for small collections, it is useful to include audiovisuals in the main card catalog, by title, added entries, and subject. If possible a separate audiovisual catalog or drawer should also be available. If a separate catalog is not desirable or feasible, a subject heading such as "audiovisual aids" can be used for all audiovisuals.

For medium-sized collections (100-200 titles) and particularly for large collections (more than 250 titles), it is best to catalog audiovisuals in much the same way as books. OCLC and other bibliographic utilities include audiovisuals and can facilitate the use of the same cataloging system for both print and nonprint materials.

All cataloging systems and procedures for audiovisuals should be designed to avoid the need for future conversion or recataloging. Complete and standard cataloging provides users with better access to audiovisuals. It can also facilitate the library's use of automated circulation systems, databases, and library networks. The second edition of the *Anglo-American Cataloguing Rules* (AACR2) will help the librarian standardize cataloging of both print and nonprint materials. Further information on audiovisual cataloging is found in Chapter 5 and in the resources listed at the end of this chapter.

Processing

After cataloging and classification are completed, audiovisual programs must be processed. Processing involves stamping an ownership mark on each part of the program. An accession number, classification number, or other identification mark must also be stamped on each item. Some librarians label each slide so that missing slides can be easily returned to the proper program. Each librarian must weigh the time involved in detailed labelling against its benefits.

Printed Catalogs

Because the audiovisual collection often is relatively small, at least in comparison to the book collection, a printed catalog is often feasible. The major advantage of such a catalog is that it can be distributed to users and kept in their offices or at work stations. This may result in greater use of the audiovisual collection.

Printed catalogs also have disadvantages. They are time-consuming to produce and can become out-of-date quickly. Even when supplements are issued regularly, users tend to refer only to the main catalog, thus missing newer items. Because of the frequent need to update the catalog of a growing collection, some hospital librarians use a word processor for this purpose. Others arrange to automate catalog production with the help of the hospital's data processing department.

Maintenance

When a piece of software is returned to the library, it should be checked for damage. Damage is often visible in cassette tapes but may be harder to detect in 16mm film. Asking the user questions such as "Did everything go all right?" or "Any trouble?" can alert the librarian to hidden damage. If a user reports that a film skipped or fluttered, the librarian should check the film. If damage is irreparable, this should be noted on the item or on the catalog record.

Users should be instructed not to attempt any repairs themselves but to report all difficulties to the library. Library staff can learn to make simple repairs, such as splicing film. For sources containing detailed instructions on software repair, see the Readings section at the end of the chapter.

Because the software collection is usually smaller than the book collection, inventory and weeding can be done more frequently. It may also be possible to do both at the same time. The librarian should check each record against the corresponding software program, not only to verify that it is still on the shelf, but also to make sure that no part of the program is missing. All labelling on each item should also be checked.

The purpose of weeding is to determine if the audiovisual program still belongs in the collection. Some factors to consider are (1) how the subject fits into the total collection, (2) whether the format is useful and appropriate, (3) the condition of the program, (4) its age, (5) the accuracy and currency of its contents, (6) how often it is used, and (7) what users think of it. If an item is old or worn, the librarian should try to locate another program on the same subject that will fill users' needs. Because many educational activities may be keyed to the use of a particular audiovisual, it is best to consult with users before discarding any item. The librarian may also wish to involve users in a periodic review of the collection.

Developing the Software Collection

The approach to building a collection of audiovisual programs differs from that used in building a print collection, simply because of the differences between the two types of materials. Audiovisuals often center on a single concept and rarely contain comprehensive treatments of large subject areas, as textbooks do. Software programs are usually expensive, and they can become outdated quickly. Most audiovisual formats are relatively fragile. Also, audiovisuals are usually intended to be closely tied to educational activities.

Two basic approaches to developing the audiovisual collection exist. The first is a user-need approach, in which programs are added to the collection in response to a user's specific request. The librarian plays an active role in clarifying what the user needs and in helping to select the most appropriate program. Because each audiovisual is selected for a specific teaching, learning, or promotional situation, usage is almost guaranteed. The user-need approach is very cost-effective and usually results in frequent use of most titles. It requires a good deal of interaction between the librarian and users. It usually produces a small, though heavily used, collection. This

approach is generally recommended for libraries with a limited audiovisual budget.

The second approach to collection building is the core collection approach. In this approach, the librarian makes a list of titles that would be useful to a large number of users. Hospital personnel are often involved in the selection process, usually by previewing programs, providing critiques of titles, or suggesting how titles might be used if they were available. The most important difference between these two approaches to collection development is that in the core collection method, the initial request for a program does not grow out of a staff member's specific need. This difference often results in programs being used less frequently. To foster usage, the librarian may need to talk to instructors about using a particular program or publicize the program directly to the intended audience. The advantage of a core collection is that programs on basic subjects are immediately available if students or staff members need them.

Either approach, of course, can be supplemented by a rental and loan service. Several weeks' advance notice is usually required for rentals or loans.

Each librarian should determine which acquisition approach is most appropriate for the hospital library. A combination of the two approaches may be desirable. For example, a librarian may begin by purchasing only those programs specifically requested by users. A core collection might be built later based on the librarian's knowledge of users' needs. Other librarians may respond primarily to specific user requests but may also purchase one or more audiovisual subscriptions, such as the Network for Continuing Medical Education (NCME).

Identifying Software on Specific Subjects

In a typical hospital, audiovisual programs on a wide variety of subjects may be needed. These subjects include medicine, nursing, management and supervision, safety, patient education, and social services. Because hundreds of companies produce software programs, locating a program on a specific subject is often very difficult.

No source currently lists all audiovisual programs produced in the United States. To locate audiovisual programs by subject, librarians can use one or more of the sources and methods discussed below.

In-house File of Producers' and Distributors' Catalogs

Building a comprehensive collection of producers' and distributors' catalogs takes time but has many advantages. It involves only a small expenditure of money. Also, it can quickly increase the librarian's knowledge of audiovisuals in the health care field.

The librarian should first identify as many audiovisual companies as possible in all fields that might be interest to hospital personnel. Lists of companies that produce management and supervisory programs are often difficult to locate. A partial list of these companies appears in Appendix A. The *AV Source Directory* lists many audiovisual companies, as do other references listed at the end of the chapter. Catalogs should be requested from all companies. This process can be streamlined by using a form letter. Since the object is to get on as many mailing lists as possible, a catalog request should be sent every time a new company is identified. When the catalog arrives, it can be discarded if it contains no appropriate materials.

The next step is to set up a filing system. The librarian may wish to use a file folder for each producer. Although folders can simply be arranged alphabetically by company name, some form of subject access is usually needed. An in-house subject file is very useful for this purpose. First, the librarian should develop a list of subjects headings. Such a list might include MeSH terms, the names of departments and services in the hospital, and current topics in the health care field. This list of subjects will vary depending on the individual needs of the hospital.

The next step is to make a file card for each subject. As each catalog arrives, the librarian should scan it and write the company name on all appropriate subject cards. Although this process requires a concentrated effort for a month or two, it quickly provides comprehensive subject access to a wide variety of companies. In addition, the librarian using this system can quite quickly become an expert in the field of hospital audiovisual programs.

Once the catalog collection is established, maintaining it is fairly simple. The librarian should send for catalogs of new companies, index catalogs as they arrive, and replace old catalogs with new editions. These tasks may also be carried out by a volunteer or an assistant. However, the librarian should look through each catalog to learn of new programs and developments in the audiovisual field.

Printed Reference Works

A number of reference sources list audiovisual programs by subject. These sources can be used as a substitute for a catalog collection, although such use has several drawbacks. Even with an extensive collection of audiovisual reference books, subject coverage is usually not as comprehensive as that provided by a catalog collection. Complete information on initial evaluation, ordering, and previewing of programs is not always listed in reference sources. Also, a reference collection is more expensive than a catalog collection.

An audiovisual reference book collection, however, is an excellent supplement to an in-house catalog collection. The information listed in the annotations in reference books is often more objective than information in catalogs. For a listing of audiovisual reference sources, see Appendix B.

Online Access to Audiovisual Material

More than 15 online databases currently include information about audiovisual materials. See Figure 10-4 for a listing of databases with citations to audiovisuals.

Two databases consist entirely of audiovisual materials. They are AVLINE, the NLM's audiovisual database, and NICEM from the National Information Center for Educational Media.

AVLINE, which became operational in 1975, is geared toward the health professional. It contains more than 11,000 citations to all types of audiovisuals in the health sciences. AVLINE is the only audiovisual database that is reviewed for educational and technical quality. Searches for specific audiences can also be conducted using AVLINE.

NICEM is a more general audiovisual database. It contains more than 310,000 citations from the fields of health and safety, psychology, social science, and management and supervision. All audiovisual formats are included in one database. Names and addresses are given for producers and distributors. Purchase and rental prices are not included. NICEM is an excellent source for materials on topics related to the health sciences, such as hospital safety.

The OCLC database contains more than 216,000 title and author citations for audiovisuals, as well as summaries of certain programs. Names of producers and distributors are included, although producers' addresses and prices are not always given. Subject access is not available. Library holdings are displayed, thus OCLC can also be used for information on interlibrary loans.

Many hospital libraries may not have access to databases. These libraries should consider the possibility of contracting for these services from a local library.

Acquiring Software

After selecting an audiovisual program on a specific subject, the librarian must choose the most appropriate method of acquiring the program. Several options are possible, including purchase, preview for possible purchase, rental, or loan. The decision should be made based on the library's policy for audiovisual acquisition, the proposed use of the program, and the relative cost of each acquisition method.

The library's acquisition policy should be flexible enough to allow the librarian to acquire materials in a variety of ways. An example of such a policy follows.

The library will attempt to acquire audiovisual programs on specific subjects for users. Working with the user, the library will locate an acceptable program and determine the best alternative for acquisition. The purchase, preview, rental, or loan of audiovisual programs will be based on the user's need, the availability of the program, and budgetary constraints. The library will also assess hospital audiovisual needs and purchase programs according to need, usage, and available funding.

Purchasing

The purchase of audiovisual materials is complicated by the wide variety of company policies and procedures. Conditions for payment, shipping, and return may vary widely. Access to the company's catalog is almost a necessity.

Internal library records, in addition to a purchase order, should include arrival date, department or person requesting the material, and date the order was placed. Figure 10-5 is an example of an all-purpose software order log.

Preview for Purchase

In most cases, it is best to preview audiovisual programs before they are purchased to avoid expensive mistakes. Some companies allow free previews or charge a fee that can be deducted from the purchase price. Others charge a flat fee. If a previewing fee is too high, the librarian should try to locate a library or agency that owns the program and is willing to lend it free of charge. The OCLC database is an excellent source for this type of information.

Programs obtained for previewing should be used for that purpose only. Companies are understandably concerned about the abuse of previewing privileges.

Involving users in the previewing process is essential. This subject is discussed in more detail elsewhere in this chapter.

Rentals

A well-organized and well-publicized rental program can be an important part of the library's audiovisual services. For libraries unable to build an in-house collection of audiovisuals, a rental service can serve many of the same needs. In addition, many audiovisual programs are used only a few times a year, instructors frequently change the focus of their teaching, and programs can become dated. Thus renting audiovisuals can sometimes be more cost-effective than purchasing them. Small hospital libraries might consider purchasing only a few essential audiovisual programs and renting any others that are needed.

A large number of audiovisual programs are available for rental. Many commercial companies rent their programs. Audiovisual departments at universities are often excellent sources for rentals and will usually supply their rental catalogs free of charge. The Hospital Educators Resource Catalogue (HERC) Free Film Reference is another source for loans and rentals.

Renting audiovisual programs can be complex. The librarian must deal with a variety of company policies and procedures. Materials must arrive on time and be returned promptly. Also, rentals often must be prepaid

Figure 10-4
Databases Containing Citations to Audiovisual Materials

I. Databases Containing Citations to Audiovisual Materials

Database	Search Service	Subject
AGRICOLA	BRS, DIALOG, SDC	Nutrition
AVLINE	NLM	All health sciences
AVMARC	BLAISE	All subjects
BIOETHISCLINE	NLM	Medical ethics
CATLINE	NLM	All health sciences
CHILD ABUSE & NEGLECT	DIALOG	Abused child
DRUG INFO	BRS	Drug/alcohol use or abuse
ECER	BRS, DIALOG	Exceptional child
ERIC	BRS, DIALOG, SDC	Education
FAMILY RESOURCES	BRS	Family life
IRIS	DIALOG	Water
LIBCON	SDC	All subjects
NARIC	BRS	Rehabilitation
NCJRS	DIALOG	Criminal justice
NICEM	DIALOG	All subjects
NICSEM/NIMIS	BRS	Handicapped child
NIMH	BRS	Mental health
OCOC	OCLC	All subjects
RLIN	RLIN	All subjects
SPIF	BRS	Education

ii. Databases Containing Citations to Audiovisual Catalogs or Directories

Databases	Search Service
AGRICOLA	BRS, *LRS, SDC
BOOKS INFO	BRS
CATLINE	NLM
ECER	BRS, *LRS
ERIC	BRS, *LRS, SDC
GPOM	BRS, *LRS
LIBCON	SDC
MEDOC	BRS
NARIC	BRS
NICSEM/NIMIS	BRS, *LRS
NTIS	BRS, *LRS, SDC

*Now DIALOG

© Ann Van Camp, 1981

Note: Reproduced with permission from Ann Van Camp, "Health Science Audiovisuals in Online Databases," *Database* 3(3): 17-27, September 1980. Revised A. Van Camp, 1981.

or a purchase order supplied in advance of shipment. The librarian must maintain complete records and monitor each transaction carefully. The software order log shown in Figure 10-5 is useful for this purpose.

Users should notify the librarian at least three weeks before a program is needed. If the librarian feels that a program may not arrive on time, the user should be notified immediately. In most cases, orders should be placed by telephone. If programs consistently arrive late, the rental service's credibility will be damaged and usage is likely to decline. In order to ensure the prompt arrival of programs, the librarian should be alert for potential problems and call the supplier immediately if a program doesn't arrive on the scheduled date.

Rental programs must also be returned on schedule. The librarian should note the return date, insure the material, and keep a copy of the insurance slip. This slip can be attached to the purchase order or to any other form used to record information on rentals. It can save the library hundreds of dollars if materials are lost.

Borrowing and Lending

Many libraries, agencies, and companies lend audiovisual programs. The key to a successful borrowing program is to know which sources lend materials and to acquire their lists or catalogs. If catalogs are not available, the librarian can make notations on the subject strengths of each collection.

Libraries and media centers are good places to start when looking for sources of audiovisual loans. Many other agencies and institutions also have audiovisual collections with either one-way or reciprocal borrowing arrangements. Drug companies are a standard source of audiovisual loans for hospitals. Local chapters of associations such as the American Heart Association often lend audiovisual materials. Other sources are local medical and nursing associations, state and local boards of health, public libraries, colleges and universities, businesses and industries in the community, and centers such as the National Medical Audio-Visual Center.

The mechanics of the loan will depend on the policy of the lending library, agency, or company. However, certain considerations apply regardless of the lender's policy. When acquiring audiovisuals on loan, the librarian should consider the following:

- Verification of correct title
- Borrowing costs, if any
- Name and address of company or institution
- Company or institution's rules for use
- Record-keeping system to monitor borrowing, arrival dates, and fees

The librarian should also try to ensure the proper and efficient use of borrowed materials. This includes:

Figure 10-5
Software Order Log

Date Ordered	Title	Name of Order Source & Address	Expected Arrival Date	Date Received ⎯⎯⎯ Date Due Back	Ordered For: Name, Dept., Ext.	Check One				Rental Time	Date Returned to Order Source
						Pur-chase	Pre-view	I.L.L.	Other		

- Preventing damage to borrowed materials (Teach users correct operation of equipment.)
- Following copyright restrictions (Do not permit users to copy borrowed materials.)
- Establishing a record-keeping system to contact patrons requesting materials

The following are important considerations when returning borrowed audiovisuals:

- Correct packaging of materials for mailing
- Insurance for all items sent by mail (Retain insurance claims.)
- Record-keeping system to prevent late returns and penalty costs

Although borrowing audiovisuals is somewhat similar to borrowing books, there are some important differences. Union lists of audiovisuals are rare. The number of programs that can be borrowed inexpensively is rather limited, especially compared to the amount of print material available for a small fee. Some institutions will lend books but not audiovisuals. Also, libraries are only one of a number of potential borrowing sources for audiovisuals. Many of these sources do not use traditional interlibrary loan rules and forms.

When borrowing from other institutions or agencies, it is important to remember that the lender must arrange the loan to fit its own planned use of the material. Often a short-term loan is the most feasible, especially if the material can be returned by messenger. When working with institutions and agencies that do not have formal policies, procedures for each loan can often be worked out individually.

Libraries, even those with small audiovisual collections, should consider lending materials as well as borrowing them. The process of lending audiovisuals is somewhat different from that of lending books and journals.

Audiovisual programs are often reserved in advance and periods of heavy student use can usually be predicted. Thus the librarian can often identify slack periods when short-term loans are possible. Each library should determine its lending policy, including length of loans, method of pickup and delivery, insurance forms or record-keeping required, and responsibility for damage. If two institutions lend materials to each other frequently, they can formulate a borrowing and lending agreement. Standardization of borrowing and lending arrangements is often undertaken by hospital library consortia.

Many institutions are reluctant to lend audiovisuals because of the possibility of damage. Damage does occur, but not as frequently as might be expected. Routine inspections and agreement on packaging and methods of return can reduce the possibility of damage. The policy on responsibility for damage should be clear before material is loaned.

Libraries with larger or more developed collections can often help the development of libraries with smaller collections by being generous with loans. Collections of all sizes can be greatly extended when loans are easily available. For this reason, and also because of the high cost of audiovisuals, sharing through consortia is becoming more common. Although obstacles to lending audiovisuals do exist, all parties benefit when these difficulties are resolved.

Providing Software Reference Services

The term "software reference" is used to refer to the services that the hospital library must provide in order to answer the questions of software users. On the simplest level, questions about software usually concern purchasing information, such as prices and names and addresses of companies. Most questions of this type can be answered by consulting producers' catalogs in the library's collection or the reference works listed in Appendix B. The librarian should also get to know the personnel in local audiovisual centers and departments and consult them regarding questions that cannot be answered from the library's own reference collection

The librarian must also be prepared to answer users' questions regarding media utilization and to teach hospital staff to use audiovisual materials effectively. The successful use of media depends on many factors, some of which the user may not have considered. The librarian should encourage the user to think about not only the content of the program but also its length, production style, and level of difficulty. The choice of format is important as well, and should be compatible with the concept being taught, the size of the group, and the physical setting. The librarian may help by suggesting, for example, that slides rather than transparencies be used for a group of 200 people; that videotapes or films might be best for teaching procedures that involve complicated actions; or that three audiovisual programs in a one-hour teaching session may be too many. See Figure 10-6 for suggestions on selecting formats.

In addition to answering factual questions about software and instructing staff in media utilization, the librarian should also assist users in locating programs that meet specific needs. This process involves the four steps discussed below.

Initial Interview with User

The librarian's purpose in the first interview with the user is to determine the following: (1) the subject of the software program; (2) the type and size of the audience it is intended for; and (3) where and how often the program will be used. This type of information can be gathered by asking questions similar to those asked by audiovisual producers when they are trying to determine what kind of program to make. Such questions might include the following:

- What concepts are you trying to teach? What are your objectives?

Figure 10-6
Guidelines for Use of Audiovisuals

Software Format	When and How to Use	Audience Size and Room Arrangement	Equipment and Approximate Cost	Lead Time & Expense to Acquire	
				Producing Locally	Acquiring from Vendor
16 mm film	Use when color and motion are needed, or an emotional response to a particular subject is desired; use as an introduction to concepts.	1 to 100+ people Darkened room Screen	16mm projector $800-$1,500	Approx. $1,000 per minute; time consuming and costly.	Time: A few days to a month or more. Cost: $75-$500+
8 mm film	Excellent for patient education in smaller groups; equipment is easy to operate.	1 to 20 people Darkened room Screen	8 mm projector $500+	Cost varies; not quite as expensive as 16mm but still very costly.	Time: Same as above Cost: $75-$250
Videotape	Use when color and motion are needed; ideal for individual or small group use; multiple monitors or ceiling mounted monitors should be used for larger groups.	1 to 15 people With standard monitors, room does not need to be darkened.	Video playback Equipment $1,500-$2,000	Cost varies; less expensive and easier to produce than film.	Time: same as above Cost: $75-$300+
Slide-Tape	Excellent for patient education; versatile format; one of the easier formats to produce locally.	1 to 100+ people Darkened room Screen	Slide projector and tape recorder $400-$600; or dual projection type slide projector $500+	Cost varies; takes few weeks to several months depending on situation.	Time: Same as above Cost: $50-$200+
Slides	Excellent for live presentations when speaker wants to narrate; speaker controls the pace of the presentation.	Same as Slide-Tape arrangement	Standard slide projector $300+	Takes a few days to a week	Time: Same as above Cost: $50-$200+
Filmstrip-Tape	Use is similar to Slide-Tape presentation; generally a commercially produced format.	1 to 50+ people Darkened room Screen	Filmstrip projector $100-$400; new dual projection filmstrip projectors can be used with large groups.	Generally not locally produced	Time: Same as above Cost: $50-$150
Audiotape	This is used when only an audio message is needed.	Size varies; no special room arrangements necessary	Tape recorder or player $50-$200	Simple and inexpensive	Time: Same as above Cost: $5-$20
Overhead Transparencies	Excellent teaching format when presenter wants to be involved; some preparation time is involved, but visuals can be retained and reused.	5 to 75 people Semidark room	Overhead Projector $300+	Quick and easy; photocopying machine or special transparency-making equipment can be used.	Generally not a commercially available format

Software Format	When and How to Use	Audience Size and Room Arrangement	Equipment and Approximate Cost	Lead Time & Expense to Acquire	
				Producing Locally	Acquiring from Vendor
Opaque Projections	Requires no preparation time; printed material is simply inserted into projector; faster to use than transparencies, but sometimes visuals are a little unclear.	Medium size groups 10 to 40+; semidark room depending on the visual	Opaque projector $500	No preparation time; no cost involved	NA
Flip Chart	Ideal for informal brainstorming sessions; can be used when material needs to be retained.	Small groups 1 to 10+; flip chart toward front of room	Flip chart and pads $50-$100	Negligible cost; usually created on the scene	NA
Chalkboard	One of the oldest and most often used teaching devices; material can be placed on chalkboard in advance.	Small to medium size groups; chalkboard toward front of room.	Chalkboard $50-$200	Negligible cost; usually created on the scene	NA
Model	Models can be used in place of actual objects when object cannot be demonstrated: for example—the heart.	Depends on model	Equipment usually not needed: cost varies.	Usually very expensive	Depends on model
Actual Object	Often the actual object is more effective than an audiovisual; use of actual objects depends on situation.	Depends on object being demonstrated	Equipment usually not needed; cost varies	Situation varies	Depends on object

- Who are you teaching? Who is your client group? (Nurses? Physicians? Social workers?)
- Where will you be teaching? (In a classroom? In a unit?)
- How often will you be teaching this material? (Every day? Once a week?)
- How many people will you be teaching? (1? 15? 75?)
- When will you be teaching this material? (Next week? Next semester? Tomorrow?)

During this first interview, the librarian may also provide or suggest other services that may be useful in developing the user's educational project. For example, the librarian might suggest books or articles that contain information on the user's topic. In addition, the librarian might offer to do a literature search on the topic.

The Media Search

After gathering as much information as possible during the initial interview, the librarian must conduct a media search. A media search, like a literature search, is a systematic procedure used to locate material on a particular subject. The librarian should use sources that are likely to provide information on programs dealing with the user's topic. Usually, the first step is to consult the library's own collection of producer catalogs, previously assembled and indexed by general subject. Programs on hospital safety, for example, could quickly be retrieved if that topic were included in the original subject list. However, a particular topic may not appear on the subject list, or additional programs on the topic may be needed. In these cases, the librarian should consult the appropriate printed reference works listed in Appendix B. A search of AVLINE, NICEM, or other relevant databases may also be necessary.

Ideally, several suitable titles should be located. For each title, the librarian should locate as much information about the program as possible. This information should include the following: (1) producer's name and address; (2) format; (3) color or black-and-white; (4) program length; (5) production date; (6) summary of contents, preferably not by the producer; and (7) level of difficulty. A review of the program is also useful. The librarian should try to determine which institutions own the program and what the conditions are for its rental or loan. In certain cases the librarian may suggest that the program be previewed and evaluated for possible purchase.

The information gathered during the media search must be organized before it is presented to the user. The method of organization described below takes a minimum of time, and certain tasks can be carried out by an assistant or a volunteer.

• Photocopy the pages from producer's catalogs or reference works that list the programs selected. Circle the appropriate items on each.
• Photocopy any catalog pages that detail conditions of use, or note these conditions next to the item entry. This information is usually found in the front of the catalog.
• Add additional information from other sources to the photocopied pages. Jot down any comments about the company or the program. For example, the user may need a program on crisis intervention to show 50 people in an auditorium. If the librarian locates a videotape on this topic, the following comment would be appropriate: "Videotape—would need multiple monitors to show to 50 people." Other notes can explain how the program can be previewed, rented, borrowed, or purchased.

Second Interview

Once the media search has been completed and its findings organized, the librarian should arrange a second interview with the user. During this interview, the librarian should present the information gathered during the media search and also guide the user in deciding on a course of action. The librarian is the media expert and should not hesitate to make recommendations. However, it is important that the librarian be sensitive to the user's reactions and perceptions, since it is the user who must be satisfied with the final selection.

During this discussion a program should be selected and the most appropriate method of acquisition chosen. The librarian should take the lead in recommending that the material be purchased, rented, or borrowed, based on several factors. These factors include the number of times the program is likely to be used, either by the user or others in the hospital; the conditions under which the program may be rented or borrowed; and the relative cost of each method of acquisition.

Obtaining the Material

After the librarian and user have decided on the appropriate method of acquisition, the librarian should make arrangements for obtaining the program. In most cases, material that has been recommended for purchase should be previewed. The librarian should select a date that is convenient for the user to preview the material and should work closely with the purchasing department and the mail room to make sure that the material arrives on time. For some programs the user may wish to involve others in the evaluation, such as members of the department using the material, other instructors, or members of the group that will view the material. The librarian should provide evaluation forms to be filled out following the preview (see Figure 10-7). The librarian should then meet with those most likely to use the program in order to get their recommendations about whether to purchase the program or not.

HARDWARE SERVICES

Because audiovisual software requires hardware for use, librarians providing software services should consider providing hardware services as well. Every library needs a minimum amount of hardware to use in the library with audiovisual programs. Hospital librarians should also consider providing equipment for software use outside the library for a number of reasons.

A centralized equipment pool is cost-effective for a hospital. It eliminates the need for each department to own its own equipment, and thereby reduces unnecessary duplication of costly hardware. An equipment center also maximizes use of the hospital's equipment, spreading that use evenly over all pieces and ensuring the availability of equipment. It also simplifies the acquisition of supplies like projector bulbs and allows for routine maintenance and coordination of repairs.

Given the rationale of a centralized equipment pool, the library is often the ideal department to provide one. Library systems and techniques for circulation can easily include the controlled distribution of equipment. The library is usually open during convenient hours, and staff is available to assist with any problems. In addition, users appreciate having both software programs and hardware in one location.

Because software and hardware services are interrelated and dependent on each other for their success, the library should be involved with hardware services in order to control, plan, and provide for optimum software services. If the provision of hardware services is not possible, active cooperation and coordination with the department providing that services is essential.

Offering a Continuum of Hardware Services

A hospital library can provide four levels of audiovisual services to clients. Figure 10-1 describes each of the four levels for software and hardware. Librarians should analyze the unique character of their own hospital and its needs before planning the level of hardware services that will most appropriately meet its needs.

Level I

Level I services focus on centralizing existing audiovisual equipment and setting up a distribution system

Figure 10-7
Audiovisual Preview and Examination Form

DATE _____ NAME _____ DEPARTMENT _____

Title of Program _____

Format of Program

16mm film _____   Other _____

8mm film _____

sound _____

silent _____

cartridge _____

Filmstrip

record _____

cassette _____

Videocassette _____

Slide-tape _____

						Rating Scale	
1. CONTENT							
Meaningful to audience	(1)	(2)	(3)	(4)	(5)		
Well organized	(1)	(2)	(3)	(4)	(5)	5	Excellent
Accurate	(1)	(2)	(3)	(4)	(5)		
2. PRODUCTION QUALITY						4	Very Good
Sound	(1)	(2)	(3)	(4)	(5)		
Visual	(1)	(2)	(3)	(4)	(5)		
						3	Good
3. EDUCATIONAL DESIGN							
Appropriate vocabulary	(1)	(2)	(3)	(4)	(5)		
Interesting presentation	(1)	(2)	(3)	(4)	(5)	2	Fair
Length of program	(1)	(2)	(3)	(4)	(5)		
4. Opinion of the program as a whole	(1)	(2)	(3)	(4)	(5)	1	Poor

5. Do you think this program will get enough use to warrant its purchase?

Yes _____   No _____   Rental _____

6. Please state in two or three sentences what the program is about and describe its probable audience.

ADDITIONAL COMMENTS:

that provides access to the hospital's audiovisual equipment for all departments. At this level, the librarian may also consider answering reference questions related to audiovisual hardware, such as questions about specific models and prices.

Level II

Level II involves assessing the hospital's needs for audiovisual equipment and expanding the equipment pool accordingly. Because new purchases are required, Level II depends on some funding. However, a centralized service usually makes the hospital's equipment needs very obvious, so justification of need is relatively easy. At this stage cf development, as in Level I, a limited equipment pool is often "stretched" by reserving materials and moving equipment from the viewing area to the circulation pool as needed.

Level III

Level III hardware services include a full range of audiovisual equipment and necessary accessories for its use. This equipment should be available in sufficient quantities for all departments to have access, preferably for short-term loans. Facilities include a viewing area and one or more rooms for small group use.

Level IV

Level IV hardware services include equipment needed for production. The library may provide equipment and work space to produce small-scale instructional materials, such as transparencies, posters, dry mounts, and laminations. In a few cases, the library department may also provide production equipment for videotaping, producing slide-tapes, or broadcasting for the hospital's closed circuit television station.

Assessing Equipment Needs

Librarians can determine equipment needs in several ways. If the library has a small collection of audiovisual software programs, librarians can discern from the circulation and usage patterns what types of equipment are needed, by whom they are needed, and how often they are to be used. By talking with users librarians can become aware of problems with current access systems and discover where service gaps exist. The sample survey provided in Figure 10-8 may help to determine current and potential usage patterns by recording equipment needs. Such a survey also evidences teaching activity and identifies potential users of expanded services.

The documentation of user needs can form the basis for discussions between the librarian and the hospital's administration or other hospital departments on the best way to provide for equipment needs. For example, most administrators can readily see the financial advantages of a centralized equipment pool as opposed to decentralized acquisition of audiovisual equipment by individual departments. A survey of existing equipment, more detailed than the survey on needs assessment, may confirm the decision to centralize. Acquiring equipment to meet these documented needs may then be accomplished by voluntary donation of equipment from other departments, centralization of existing equipment directed by the administration, or by purchase.

Setting Up an Equipment Circulation System

If the library is responsible for the audiovisual equipment pool, the librarian should set up a circulation system that can provide all departments with access to equipment for short loan periods. The equipment circulation file can be maintained separately, or equipment can be incorporated into the existing system for circulating software. The librarian should assign a number to each piece of audiovisual equipment. Each numbered piece of equipment can then have its own charge card, on which the user signs his or her name, departmental phone number, and length of borrowing time. When the equipment is not circulating, cards can be kept in an "in" file behind the file of circulating material. Cards in the circulating file may be arranged by type of equipment or by user's name. The latter system allows cards for all items borrowed at the same time to be clipped together.

In an alternative circulating system, the user request form serves as a reservation form and a circulation card. It is used for both hardware and software equipment. See Figure 10-3 for a sample form.

Policies governing the circulation and use of software can be written so that one policy governs both software and hardware. The policy should include the loan period; who will pick up and return the equipment; who may use the equipment; for what purposes the equipment should be used; and where the equipment will be used.

Organizing a Hardware Reservation System

A hardware reservation system ensures accessibility of the equipment and increases the availability of a limited number of items. Reservations for both software and hardware can be noted on a calendar for a small operation or on special forms as services expand. Figures 10-2 and 10-3 illustrate sample forms for recording reservations. When the librarian provides equipment to all departments on a "first-come" reservation system, even the smallest department can have audiovisual equipment available for its use most of the time. A well-organized reservation system also maximizes the use of equipment so that one piece of equipment may be used several times each day, by different departments, in different locations.

Acquiring Equipment

Centralizing equipment increases the visibility of materials and encourages an increase in their use. As this occurs, librarians may need to purchase additional equipment to meet the needs of the growing service.

Figure 10-8
Audiovisual Equipment Needs Survey

Please help us assess the hospital's needs for audiovisual equipment by completing the questionnaire below.

Name _____

Department _____

Extension _____

I. Indicate the audiovisual equipment that you currently need or would use if available.

Equipment	Program and Use	Frequency	Current Source of Equipment
16 mm film projector	_____	_____	_____
8 mm film projector	_____	_____	_____
Slide projector	_____	_____	_____
Slide-tape projector	_____	_____	_____
Dual projection slide-tape	_____	_____	_____
Filmstrip projector	_____	_____	_____
_____ cassette			
_____ record			
_____ dual projection			
Audiotape player	_____	_____	_____
Videotape playback equipment	_____	_____	_____
Overhead projector	_____	_____	_____
Opaque projector	_____	_____	_____
X-ray view box	_____	_____	_____
Portable chalkboard	_____	_____	_____
Portable easel and flip charts	_____	_____	_____
Electric pointer	_____	_____	_____
Other (please specify)	_____	_____	_____

II. Add any special needs or requests for audiovisual equipment that have not been covered above.

Please return the questionnaire to the library no later than _____.

Thank you for your help in establishing an audiovisual equipment pool.

Selection and Purchase

There are many sources for gathering purchasing information about audiovisual equipment: other librarians who are knowledgeable about audiovisual equipment; audiovisual professionals in schools, universities, business or industry; and reference books such as the *Audio-Visual Equipment Directory.*

Equipment selection involves a process of matching the users' needs with the capability of the equipment. When this is determined, the librarian can identify the appropriate models from the *Audio-Visual Equipment Directory.* Seeing a demonstration of the machine in action at another audiovisual center or a dealer's showroom is very useful. Some factors that should be considered when selecting equipment are listed below:

- How much money is available?
- How long is the equipment expected to be used? (Two years? Five years?)
- How often will the equipment be used? (Every day? Once a week?)
- Who will be using the equipment?
- What size groups are generally at each viewing session?
- Should the equipment be mobile? Where will the equipment be used?
- What other equipment is already available in the hospital?
- What features or capabilities does each specific model provide in relation to cost and in relation to other models already available?
- How easy is the equipment to use?
- Is local repair service available?
- Is a repair budget available?

After the librarian selects the brands and models desired, he or she should have the selection confirmed by the hospital's purchasing department. Audiovisual equipment may be considered capital equipment and may be subject to specific regulations, such as the necessity for bids. In such a case, the librarian should be active in the choice of a vendor. A local vendor's service and repair capabilities are often more valuable than a small savings in initial price.

Processing

Librarians may find it expedient to use the following procedures when processing newly purchased audiovisual equipment:

- Check ordering records against equipment received.
- Inspect equipment to determine if it is in working order, if there are defects, and if all accessories have been received.
- Assign a number to the new piece of equipment for circulation records.
- Engrave equipment with a departmental and hospital

ownership mark. If hospital equipment requires a serial number, comply.
- Record the following information on an equipment inventory card:
  - Date purchased
  - Price
  - Vendor name, address, phone number
  - Model number
  - Serial number
  - Item number
  - Manufacturer
- Report equipment specifications to the hospital insurance department.

Figure 10-9 provides a sample inventory card.

Maintaining the Equipment

Maintaining the equipment pool in good working condition must be a high priority for the librarian since the use of the software collection depends on functional equipment. Effective maintenance includes the routine inspection and repair of equipment and periodic inventory and weeding of hardware.

Routine Inspections

The library staff should inspect all equipment as it is returned to the library. It is a good idea to ask users if

Figure 10-9
Inventory Card

ITEM _____
MANUFACTURER _____
VENDOR _____
_____
_____
TELEPHONE _____

MODEL NO. _____
SERIAL NO. _____
COST _____
PURCHASE DATE _____
P.O. NO. _____
REPRESENTATIVE _____

LOCATION _____
ACCESSORIES _____

PARTS AND WARRANTY _____

they encountered any problems with the equipment. Consistent routine checking may identify problems at an early stage and help keep repair costs and user dissatisfaction down.

Routine Repair

Library staff should also perform preventive maintenance checks and routine repairs, such as changing bulbs, cleaning film tracks and lenses, and freeing jammed film or tape. Brown and Lewis offer suggestions on routine repair of audiovisual equipment.

Outside Repair

If the library needs assistance beyond routine maintenance, repair agreements can often be worked out with other departments in the hospital, such as Medical Engineering, Maintenance, or Engineering.

If such arrangements are not feasible, service contracts may be obtained from local audiovisual dealers or equipment may be sent out on a one-time basis, as needed. If good relationships have been established with local dealers, they are often willing to diagnose problems over the telephone. If an item is sent out for repair, the history of its repair should be documented on an inventory card.

Inventories and Weeding of Hardware

An inventory of all the audiovisual equipment should be taken periodically, perhaps once a year when preparing the budget requests. To take an inventory, a librarian should match the equipment inventory card with each piece, checking serial numbers, accessories, and ownership labels.

The equipment cards should also indicate any repairs done in-house as well as repairs done outside. This repair history helps to determine which pieces of equipment should be weeded from the collection because of age or condition.

Providing Equipment Delivery and Projectionist Services

Some audiovisual departments, usually those not affiliated with libraries, deliver equipment to classrooms and provide technicians to operate equipment. Such services are convenient for users but are generally only available when a staff member is employed for this purpose. Although the library staff may include an audiovisual technician, it is better if the library develops workable alternatives to delivery and projectionist services. Users rapidly adjust to a policy that requires them to pick up and return their own equipment when they realize that the volume of equipment used makes delivery very difficult. Users will also understand that staffing limitations necessitate either the operation of their own equipment or use of staff from their own departments to provide operators. An active program of instruction for hospital staff in equipment operation will ensure that most users have the skills to operate their own equipment.

Providing Instruction in Use of Equipment

Repair costs can also be kept down if the library staff routinely instructs users on the correct operation of audiovisual equipment. Before staff members can teach patrons about the equipment, however, they must feel comfortable operating it themselves. Then they should be encouraged to demonstrate the operation of equipment when equipment is being checked out by patrons unfamiliar with its use. In addition to "on-the-spot" instruction, librarians may also hold informal classes in equipment operation, scheduled at the user's convenience. Taping instructions to the equipment is another means of ensuring correct operation.

Providing Hardware Reference Services

Hardware reference service involves answering questions and providing information about audiovisual equipment and its use. Typical questions the library staff encounters concern price information, specifications on equipment models, and recommendations for equipment that will be by a particular group size or in a specific setting.

If the library staff is providing audiovisual hardware services at more advanced levels, the staff may be recognized as audiovisual experts, and users may turn to the library for their audiovisual information. In essence, audiovisual information then becomes just another type of information provided by the library.

Librarians who develop a positive rapport with the staff of nearby audiovisual centers, production facilities, and dealerships can build a base of contacts for answering future reference questions and provide a continual source for audiovisual information.

Maintaining Viewing Area in the Library

Audiovisual equipment is often checked out for use in classrooms, on the floor and in clinics. Frequently, however, patrons may prefer to use the equipment and programs in the library. If the hospital is a teaching hospital or has an active patient education program, students and patients may be required to read or view assigned materials. Other users may be requesting information on their own. In either case, some type of viewing area is essential. Ideally, several viewing options should be available, including a general area with individual carrels, one or more small rooms for three to four users, and a classroom that allows instructors full use of audiovisual equipment.

If a carrel area or an audiovisual classroom is not possible, due to lack of space or insufficient equipment, the librarian should use the reservation system to adjust the amount of available space and equipment between check-out use and in-library use. If this arrangement becomes difficult to maintain because of increased use of programs and equipment, the extent of the increase should be documented. Such documentation would support requests for more equipment and more space.

PRODUCTION SERVICES

If library-based audiovisual services continue to expand, and other hospital departments are not currently responsible for production services, the library might consider providing in-house production services with varying levels of complexity. In a small number of hospitals, libraries and audiovisual departments have been merged—frequently under the overall direction of the library. This merger reflects the view that unified management of educational resources, whether print or nonprint, is cost-effective and provides coordinated, efficient service. When audiovisuals are produced in-house, they become an educational resource and provide one more service in an overall educational resources operation.

Some practical advantages of coordinating in-house productions and purchased programs under single management are listed below:

• When a thorough search of commercially available material produces an unsuitable selection of software for a specific need, in-house production may answer the need. In-house productions are usually more expensive than purchased programs, however, and are usually produced only when suitable material is not available elsewhere.
• Some of the audiovisual equipment needed by the production staff is similar to the equipment needed by library-based audiovisual services.
• All the support components of hardware and software are available from one department, thus allowing for maximum coordination, maximum convenience for users, and minimum expenses.
• Since the library is already set up to handle the distribution of materials, it can fit audiovisual equipment and the locally produced programs into its existing systems for access, circulation, and use. Freeing the production staff from the responsibility of circulating equipment and organizing access to programs allows more time for primary interests.

With all the advantages that a complete educational resources program provides, a librarian in a hospital without existing production services may wish to consider developing these services. In situations where it is not feasible or desirable to combine library audiovisual services and production services, librarians should encourage coordination and cooperation between the two departments.

Unlike audiovisual equipment services that can be incorporated into the daily routine of the library staff, however, production services involve specialized training and specialized equipment. The advantages of involving the library in production services should be weighted against the time and effort required to manage the production of programs.

Two types of production services can be provided in hospitals. The more traditional service involves pro-

ducing a variety of educational aids, including slides, transparencies, slide-tapes, videotapes, and occasionally, films. The second is less frequently seen but provides a wide variety of inexpensive teaching aids. It is the do-it-yourself graphics lab.

Traditional Production Services

Traditional services can be provided by a librarian, an audiovisual technician, or a production specialist. The types of services include copying noncopyrighted audiotapes, audio-recording grand rounds, and making transparencies, slide-tapes, and scripted videotapes. Level IV of Figure 10-1 describes the varying degrees of library involvement in production services. For medium and large-scale production, additional, specialized staff is necessary, thus augmenting the existing well-established library-based audiovisual program.

Do-It-Yourself Graphics Lab

The second type of production service provides small-scale graphics, such as transparencies, posters, flip charts, and others. The library furnishes the equipment for small-scale productions, but the users make the materials for themselves. This procedure expands the number of aids that can be produced. Given appropriate equipment, most graphic aids are relatively simple to make. Users can provide for their own graphics needs quickly and inexpensively.

Figure 10-10 describes one type of do-it-yourself graphics lab. The librarian can arrange the lab so that each major activity or category of equipment has a separate station. Each station should contain complete instructions for operation to lessen the number of times users need to contact the library staff after the initial instruction.

Librarians may find much of the equipment needed for a simple lab available in the hospital. By tactfully stressing the advantages of a do-it-yourself lab and centralized access to materials, the librarian can often obtain support for setting up a lab with the existing equipment. A library's established patterns of service, such as long hours, available staff, and involvement with other educational resources make the library an appropriate choice for the location of the lab.

COPYRIGHT RESTRICTIONS

Libraries involved with audiovisual services need to be informed about copyright laws as they pertain to audiovisuals. Two basic guidelines should be kept in mind. Lending of audiovisuals is legal, unless prior restrictive arrangements have been made. Copying audiovisuals is illegal, unless specific permission has been received.

Most libraries having audiovisuals are probably involved in lending these materials. Interlibrary loans of

Figure 10-10
Do-It-Yourself Graphics Production Lab

FORMATS
  Transparencies
  Posters
  Flip Charts
  Flyers
  Signs
  Dry mounts
  Laminations

EQUIPMENT
  Transparency maker
    (or photocopy machine capable of making transparencies)
  Letter systems
    Kroy or similar lettering system
    Transfer letters
    Stencils
    Leteron or similar lettering system
  Laminator
  Large paper cutter
  Dry-mounting press

SUPPLIES
  Supplies required for presses and lettering systems
  Poster board
  Paper in various colors
  Scissors, rulers, felt-tip markers of various colors
  (See *Figure 10-11* for additional supplies)

STATIONS
  Lettering
  Laminating
  Cutting
  Transparencies
  General Work

audiovisual materials is legal, unless the library signs a contract waiving these rights. Some companies require the buyer to sign an agreement before purchase, stating that the program will not be loaned out to other institutions.

Copying audiovisual materials without permission is illegal, unless companies give permission for archival purposes. Librarians should check with each individual company before copying materials, since each company has its own rules and procedures. All requests for permission to copy should be made in writing. Librarians should also request a written permission from the company. If copying needs are known before purchase, and the librarian has already received permission to copy materials from the company, a statement indicating

permission to copy for archival purposes can be included on the purchase order form.

Sometimes an audiovisual program is unavailable in a preferred format. With company approval, the library can modify the program in-house, providing the library has the appropriate equipment. Audiovisual companies allow this practice, if permission is requested. Librarians who request this in the form of letter or purchase order should document all permissions received. They should also adhere to any conditions in the permission agreement. If one format has been designated an archival copy, for example, it should not be used for other purposes. Librarians should always ask if they are in doubt about company practices. The use of illegal copies of programs, rather than the rental or purchase of the program, is directly related to the high cost of audiovisuals.

MANAGEMENT ISSUES

The same management issues facing librarians in libraries that provide only print materials, face librarians who provide audiovisual services. These management issues include budgeting, staffing, planning space and facilities, and designing promotional activities.

Budget

The budgetary support required by audiovisual services varies with the types and levels of service provided. When librarians plan the audiovisual budget, the following categories should be considered: hardware purchase, software purchase, software rental or preview, hardware repair, audiovisual supplies, and special categories for production supplies and contractual production services. A list of commonly used audiovisual supplies appears in Figure 10-11. Additional information on budget requirements can be found in Chapter 13.

Staff Positions

In most libraries the existing staff provides audiovisual services. Many programs never require specialized staff positions. Frequently, however, when audiovisual services are organized efficiently, they expand rapidly, enabling the librarian to justify additional staff positions on the basis of new programs, volume of services, and user needs. The following list of staff positions includes those that can be created to meet expanded needs:

• *Audiovisual coordinator or audiovisual librarian.* With either title, this position's responsibilities include assessing audiovisual needs, planning and providing services, making budget recommendations, cataloging and processing audiovisuals, and working with hospital staff to use media effectively.
• *Audiovisual technician.* A technician's responsibilities include operating the equipment checkout system, maintaining and repairing the equipment, recommending

Figure 10-11
Commonly Used Audiovisual Supplies

GENERAL AUDIOVISUAL SUPPLIES

Extension cords
Slide trays
Slide boxes
Remote control advances
Various adapters and connectors
Film repair and splicing kits
Soldering iron
Various sizes of cables
Projection bulbs
Film take-up reels
Gaffers tape
Repair tools
Bulk eraser
Portable screens
Portable easels

PRODUCTION SUPPLIES

Audiotape
Videotape
35 mm film

GRAPHICS SUPPLIES

Poster board
Colored construction paper
Rubber cement
Dry mount tissue
Laminating film
News print paper
Various sizes of lettering pens
India ink
Various sizes and colors of felt-tip markers
Transparency acetate
Transparency mounting frames
Clip art
Dry transfer letters
Letter stencil sets
Ruler
T-square
Paint brushes of various sizes
Rubber art erasers
Chalk and erasers
Heavy duty stapler
Masking tape
Adhesive tape
Opaque watercolor paint
Tacking iron

equipment for purchase, providing projectionist services as needed, and developing a file of equipment catalogs.

• *Audiovisual assistant or associate.* As a support staff position, responsibilities may include assisting with cataloging and media searching, handling software orders, loans, previews and rentals, and basic media reference duties. The level at which this position operates depends on the amount and type of service provided, the number of other staff positions, and the experience of the individual.

• *Audiovisual clerk.* Typical clerical duties include filing producers' catalogs, determining precataloging information, staffing the users' service desk, checking equipment in and out, making basic repairs, and typing.

• *Production specialist.* If medium-scale or large-scale production activities are planned, one or more production specialists are usually needed. Usual preparation involves a master's degree in Instructional Systems Technology or Communications, and relevant production experience. Responsibilities can include producing slide-tapes or videotapes, operating a patient television station, and supervising the do-it-yourself graphics lab.

• *Medical photographer or illustrator.* Often outside the production department, this position can be part of production responsibilities. A professional medical photographer, with relevant training and experience, is necessary for this position.

These positions are indicative of the variety of responsibilities involved in providing full-scale audiovisual service. Only the largest audiovisual service operation would have a separate full-time person for each position.

Space and Facilities

The space and facilities required for hospital library audiovisual services also varies with the level of service provided. Ideally, audiovisual services should be one of many services the library provides for the entire hospital. The space and facilities needed for the operation of the services should be centralized in the library. Often, this is not possible, and facilities are organized outside the library. In such a case, librarians need to coordinate procedures and establish cooperation between the two separate units. General considerations involved in planning space for library services are discussed in Chapter 16. For more complete information on the design of audiovisual facilities, consult the references at the end of this chapter.

Promotional Techniques

All library activities benefit from promotion. Audiovisual services, especially when first introduced, should be advertised. Librarians can inform hospital staff about the new services through flyers, brochures, posters, demonstrations, newsletters, and one-to-one selling. Because audiovisual services are highly visible, they are promotional items in themselves, continually advertising library service. More information on promotion techniques appears in Chapter 17.

PROFESSIONAL ASSOCIATIONS AND JOURNALS

Librarians who are interested in professional organizations that address the issues of audiovisual services in a health care setting should consider joining the Medical Library Association (MLA) and its regional chapters, the Health Sciences Communications Association (HESCA), the Health Education Media Association (HEMA), the American Society for Healthcare Education and Training (ASHET), or the American Society for Training and Development (ASTD).

All of these associations have journals that are also excellent sources of information on audiovisual services. A list of these and other journals appears in Appendix C.

The need for some type of audiovisual service exists in almost every department of the hospital. The librarian is in an excellent position to organize and develop services that fill these very real and often unmet needs for educational resources.

READINGS

CATALOGING AND CLASSIFICATION

American Library Association. Anglo-American cataloguing rules. 2d ed. Chicago: American Library Association, 1978.

Brantz MH. Classification and audiovisuals. Bull Med Libr Assoc 1977 Apr;65:261-264.

Olson NB. Cataloging of audiovisual materials: A manual based on AACR2. Mankato, MN: Minnesota Scholarly Press, 1981.

Tillin AM, Quinly WJ. Standards for cataloging non-print materials. 4th ed. Washington, DC: Association for Educational Communication and Technology, 1976.

COPYRIGHT

Are you guilty of copyright rip off? Training HRD. 1979 Apr;16: 39-42.

Association for Educational Communications and Technology. Copyright and educational media: a guide to fair use and permissions procedures. Washington, DC: The Association for Educational Communications and Technology, 1977.

Golob, Melinda V. Not by books alone: Library copying of non-print, copyrighted material. Law Library Journal. 1977 May;70:153-170.

Russell TK. Television videotaping and copyright law: a selective bibliography. Audiovisual Instruction 1979 Apr;24:52-53.

GENERAL

Educational media yearbook. Littleton, CO: Libraries Unlimited, 1973-. Annual.

Elsesser L. Patient education. Chicago: Medical Library Association, 1982 MLA courses for continuing education: CE-636.

Harris CL. Hospital-based patient education programs and the role of the hospital librarian. Bull Med Libr Assoc 1976 Apr;66:210-217.

Kronick DA. Nonprint media as information resources: software and hardware. Bull Med Libr Assoc 1974 Jan;62:19-23.

McIlvaine PM, Brantz MH. Audiovisual materials: a survey of bibliographic controls in distributors' catalogs. Bull Med Libr Assoc 1977 Jan;65:17-21.

Meiboom E. A film program in a teaching hospital. Bull Med Libr Assoc 1973 Oct;61:416-421.

Midwest Health Science Library Network. The librarian as a service professional: a promotional kit. Chicago: Midwest Health Science Library Network, 1980.

Robinow BH. Audiovisuals and non-print learning resources in a health sciences library. 1979 Mar;6:14-19.

Sparks SM, Mitchell GE. The National Medical Audiovisual Center. J Nurs Educ 1979 Sept;18:47-55.

Tonkery D, McIlvane MF. Bibliographic control of non-print educational material. Biomedical Communications 1978 July;5:28-30.

HARDWARE SERVICES

Brown JW, Lewis RB. Audio-visual instruction: technology, media and methods. 5th ed. New York: McGraw Hill, 1976.

Ebock SC, Cochern GW. Operating audiovisual equipment. 2d ed. San Francisco: Chandler, 1968.

National Audio-Visual Association. Audio-visual equipment directory. Fairfax, VA: National Audio-Visual Association, 1953-. Annual.

Reinhart RC. How to select your audiovisual equipment. Public Relations Journal 1979 May;35:27-29.

Rosenberg KC, Doskey JS. Media Equipment: a guide and dictionary. Littleton, CO: Libraries Unlimited, 1976.

Schroeder D, Lane G. Audiovisual equipment and materials: a basic repair and maintenance manual. Metuchen, NJ: Scarecrow Press, 1979.

Smith J. Choosing and using the new breed of film projectors. Training HRD. 1979 Feb;16:39-43.

Smith J. Why and how to choose video receivers and monitors. Training HRD. 1979 Jan;16:53-58.

MANAGEMENT ISSUES

Bock DJ, LaJeunesse LR. The learning resources center: a planning primer for librarians in transition. New York: Bowker, 1977. (LJ Special Report Series: no. 3).

Brooks ML. Primer for media resources librarians. Atlanta: National Medical Audiovisual Center, 1976.

Denman JP. Environmental and physical considerations in planning multimedia libraries. Amer Pharm Educ, 1973, Dec;37:755-759.

Hampton CL, Hurwitz GH, Shaffer MC. Management of a learning resource center: a seven-year study. J Med Educ 1979 Feb;54:90-95.

Hunter GH. Establishing a learning resource center in a medical library. Atlanta: National Medical Audiovisual Center, 1974.

Moreland EF, Craig JF. Developing a learning resource center: a guide to organizing a learning resource center in health science educational institutions. Atlanta: National Medical Audiovisual Center, 1974.

Wimmer K. Media management in a hospital library. Biocommun 1981 May;9:20-22.

ONLINE ACCESS

Bridgman CF, Suter E. Searching AVLINE for curriculum-related audiovisual instructional materials. J Med Educ 1979 Mar;54:236-237.

Slusser MC. NICEM, the non-print database. Database 1980 Sept;3: 63-67.

Sparks SM, Kudrick LW. AVLINE: An audiovisual information retrieval system. J Nurs Educ 1979 Sept;18:47-55.

Van Camp A. Health science audiovisuals in online databases. Part 2. Database 1982 Aug;5:23-29.

PRINTED CATALOGS

Bogen B. A computer-generated catalog of audiovisuals. Bull Med Libr Assoc 1976 Apr;64:224-227.

Moulton BL, Wood WI. A computer-produced catalog for non-print materials. Spec Libr 1975 Aug;66:357-362.

PRODUCTION SERVICES

Bensinger C. The video guide. 2d ed. Santa Barbara, CA: VideoInfo Publications, 1979.

Harwood D. Everything you always wanted to know about portable video tape recording. 3d ed. Syosset, NY: VTR Publishing Company, 1978.

McCavitt W. Basic television production techniques. Video Systems. 1979 Feb;5:18-20.

Minor E, Frye HR. Techniques for producing visual instructional media. 2d ed. New York: McGraw-Hill, 1977.

Orgren, Carl F. Production of slide/tape programs. Unabashed Librarian 1975 Summer;16:25-28.

Quick J, Wolff H. Small-studio video/tape production. 2d ed. Reading, MA: Addison-Wesley, 1976.

SOFTWARE BORROWING

Crowley CM. Interlibrary loan of audiovisual materials in the health sciences: how a system operates in New Jersey. Bull Med Libr Assn 1976 Oct;64:367-371.

SOFTWARE REFERENCE

American Hospital Association. Media handbook: a guide to selecting, producing and using media for patient education programs. Chicago: American Hospital Association, 1978.

Cabeceiras J. The multimedia library: materials selection and use. New York: Academic Press, 1978.

APPENDIX A
Sources: Management Training Audiovisuals

American Management Associations
AMACOM Division
135 West 50th Street
New York, New York 10020

American Media, Inc.
5907 Meredith Drive
Des Moines, Iowa 50324

Barr Films
P.O. Box 5667
Pasadena, California 91107

BNA Communications, Inc.
9401 Decoverly Hall Road
Rockville, Maryland 20850

Bureau of Business Practice
24 Rope Ferry Road
Waterford, Connecticut 06386

Cally Curtis Company
1111 North Las Palmas Avenue
Hollywood, California 90038

Creative Media
820 Keo Way
Des Moines, Iowa 50309

CRM/McGraw Hill Films
110 Fifteenth Street
Del Mar, California 92014

Dartnell
4660 Ravenswood Avenue
Chicago, Illinois 60640

Education for Management, Inc.
85 Main Street
Watertown, Massachusetts 02172

MTI Teleprograms, Inc.
3710 Commercial Avenue
Northbrook, Illinois 60062

National Education Media, Inc.
21601 Devonshire Street
Chatsworth, California 91311

Pyramid Film
Box 1048
Santa Monica, California 90406

Ramic Productions
58 West 58th Street
New York, New York 10019

Resources for Education and Management, Inc.
544 Medlock Road
Decatur, Georgia 30030

ROA Films
914 Fourth
P.O. Box 661
Milwaukee, Wisconsin 53201

Roundtable Film and Video
113 North San Vicente Boulevard
Beverly Hills, California 90211

Salenger Educational Media
1635 12th Street
Santa Monica, California 90404

Thompson-Mitchell & Associates
3384 Peachtree Road N.E.
Atlanta, Georgia 30326

Time/Life Video
Time and Life Building
New York, New York 10020

Vantage Communications, Inc.
P. O. Box 546
Nyack, New York 10960

VIS-U-COM Productions, Inc.
Box 5472
Redwood City, California 94063

Xicom Video Arts
Sterling Forest
Tuxedu, New York 10987

APPENDIX B
Catalogs and Other Audiovisual Finding Aids

About aging: A catalog of films, 1977. Allyn MV, ed. 3d ed. Los Angeles: Ethel Percy Andrus Gerontology Center, University of Southern California, 1977.

Audiovisual market place: a multimedia guide. New York: Bowker Company, 1969-. Annual.

Audiovisual resources for diabetes education. 4th ed. Ann Arbor, MI: University of Michigan, 1982.

Benschoter RA. 8mm films in medicine and health sciences. 3d ed. Omaha, NE: Biomedical Communications Division, University of Nebraska Medical Center, 1977.

Catalog of audio-visual aids in hypertension. Bethesda, MD: High Blood Pressure Information Center, 1975.

Educational film locator of the consortium of university film centers. 2d ed. New York: Bowker, 1980.

Educational materials for obstetrics and gynecology. Chicago: American College of Obstetricians and Gynecologists, 1974.

Guide to audiovisual resources in the health care field. 1981 ed. Pittsburgh: Medical Media Publishers, 1981.

Health sciences audiovisual resource list: 1978-79. 2d ed. Farmington, CT: University of Connecticut Health Center Library, 1978.

Hospital educators resource catalogue. Lincoln, NB: Hospital Educators Resource Catalogue, 1976-. Annual.

Hospital/health care training media profiles. New York: Olympic Media Information, Vol. 1-, 1974-.

Index to audiovisual serials in the health sciences. Chicago: Medical Library Association, Vol. 1-, 1977-. Quarterly.

Index to health and safety education. Vol. I & II. 4th ed. Los Angeles: National Information Center for Educational Media (NICEM), 1980.

Management media directory. Detroit: Gale Research, 1982.

Media resources for gerontology. Sahara, JP, Comp. Ann Arbor, MI: Institute of Gerontology at the University of Michigan, 1977.

Medical audiovisuals: a comprehensive catalog. Baltimore: Welch Medical Library Audiovisual Division, Johns Hopkins University, 1977.

Medical catalog of selected audiovisual materials produced by the United States government. Washington, DC: National Audiovisual Center, 1980.

National Library of Medicine audiovisuals catalog. Bethesda, MD: National Library of Medicine, 1977-.

National medical audiovisual center catalog: films for the health sciences. 1981 ed. Bethesda, MD: National Library of Medicine, 1981. (NIH publication no. 81-506).

Roper FW, Boorkman JA. Introduction to reference sources in the health sciences. Chicago: Medical Library Association, 1980.

Selected audiovisuals on mental health. Rockville, MD: National Institute of Mental Health, National Clearinghouse of Mental Health Information, 1975.

Shanteau D, ed. Audiovisuals about birth and family life: 1970-1980. 10th ed. Minneapolis. International Childbirth Education Association, 1981.

Simmons G, Floyd K. Alcohol film bibliography: a sourcebook of titles and reviews. Fayetteville, AK: Rehabilitation Research and Training Center, University of Arkansas, 1976.

Spencer DA, Duke P. Source list for patient education materials. Milledgeville, GA: Health Sciences Communications Association, 1978.

The health sciences videolog. 1981 ed. New York: Video-forum, 1981.

Video source book. 4th ed. Detroit: Gale Research, 1983.

Videotape catalog: continuing medical education and medical training instruction. 7th ed. Fort Sam Houston, TX: Academy of Health Sciences, 1976.

APPENDIX C
Journals Related to Audiovisual Services

Audiovisual Communications

Audio-Visual Communications
United Business Publications
475 Park Avenue South
New York, New York 10016

Biomedical Communications

Biomedical Communications
United Business Publications
475 Park Avenue South
New York, New York 10016

Bulletin of the Medical Library Association

Bulletin of the Medical Library Association
Medical Library Association
919 North Michigan Avenue
Suite 3208
Chicago, Illinois 60611

Cross Reference on Human Resource Management

Cross Reference on Human Resource Management
American Society for Health Manpower Education and Training
840 North Lake Shore Drive
Chicago, Illinois 60611

EPIE Report

Educational Products Information Exchange
EPIE Institute
Box 620
Stony Brook, New York 11790

Instructional Innovator

Instructional Innovator
Association for Educational Communications and Technology
1126 Sixteenth Street, N.W.
Washington, D.C. 20036

Journal of Biocommunications

Journal of Biocommunications
Association of Medical Illustrators and The Health Sciences
    Communications Association
3215 Haddon Road
Durham, North Carolina 27705

Library Technology Report

Library Technology Report
American Library Association
50 E. Huron Street
Chicago, Illinois 60611

Training and Development Journal

Training and Development Journal
American Society for Training and Development
P.O. Box 5307
Madison, Wisconsin 53705

Training: The Magazine of Human Resources Development

Training: The Magazine of Human Resources Development
Lakewood Publications, Inc.
731 Hennepin Avenue
Minneapolis, Minnesota 55403

SECTION III:

*Managing
Library
Services*

The Hospital Librarian's Administrative Role

Gertrude Lamb, Ph.D.
Director, Health Science Libraries
Hartford Hospital
Hartford, Connecticut

The Hospital Librarian's Administrative Role

Gertrude Lamb, Ph.D.
Director, Health Science Libraries
Hartford Hospital
Hartford, Connecticut

The primary commitment of the hospital librarian is to meet the information needs of the hospital staff. Consequently, the librarian's most demanding role is service-oriented. The current emphasis on cost containment in health care delivery reasonably assumes that the hospital librarian will make wise use of limited resources. Therefore, another task of the hospital librarian is to allocate library resources to get the most for the money spent. This is the librarian's management role.

In addition to service provision and management, a third possible role should be considered: an administrative role. Current thinking about organizations classifies the administrator's major responsibility as the decision-making that determines an organization's future course of action and maintains it as a viable institution.

This chapter looks at these three possible roles of service provision, management, and administration. It assesses, in terms of organizational theory, their applicability to the hospital librarian.

HISTORICAL PERSPECTIVE

A review of the history of administration's emergence as a separate discipline gives some insight into these three distinct roles. Administration as a field of study developed from two fundamentally different points of view, one focusing on the work process and the other focusing on the executive process. The work-process approach functioned from the bottom up. It aimed to maximize profit by maximizing the productivity of employees. The executive-process approach functioned from the top down. Its goal was to create a profitable system through efficient organization. The technical expert, as the chief executive, organized and controlled the various elements of production, such as the plant, machines, raw materials, and workers in order to increase the profit margin.

The Work-Process Approach

The work-process focus has its roots in the turn of the century when Frederick W. Taylor and other problem solvers conducted intensive and systematic studies to find out how much workers could accomplish when given the proper tools and materials. Taylor was an engineer and production expert who applied scientific (as opposed to trial-and-error) methods to problems of factory production. Taylor's experiments ranged from carefully-timed trials of yard gangs using various sizes of shovels to move large tonnages of coal, to observations on the best cutting speeds and feeds for boring mills. He used time and motion studies, cost analyses, and incentive pay scales to motivate employees to achieve higher rates of production.

The Executive-Process Approach

The executive-process approach was developed by Henri Fayol, based on his experience in organizing profit-able industrial firms. Fayol himself had worked at a variety of jobs, from pit miner to chief executive. He observed the processes of production, experimented, and then drew up a set of operating principles to create the most efficient design of such processes. His principles are widely recognized today. They include the following axioms:

- Specialization must be a factor in structuring an organization.
- Responsibility must be accompanied by authority.
- Unity of direction is necessary, with one head and one plan for each activity.
- Unity of command must be established with each person reporting to only one boss.

The tools Fayol used to increase efficiency were planning, organizing, command, coordination, and control.

Scientific Management

To replace trial and error with what they and their followers considered to be a science, both Taylor and Fayol laid down rules and set standards. Managers were led to expect that if they followed these rules exactly, high profit productivity would result. The basis of scientific management was the assumption that identified organizational goals could be achieved by applying such prescriptions. Scientific management did not seek to establish rigorous analytic methodologies. The science assumed only that practical results could be achieved by the systematic study of problems and situations.

Future Planning

Administration as a discipline emerged when managers had sufficiently mastered scientific management to turn their attention to planning in terms of the whole complex of external conditions that determine an industry's form and survival. For example, administrators in the automobile industry are currently planning for the survival of their industry in the context of an external environment that includes predictions of gasoline shortages, consumer demand for a small but luxurious car, and fluctuating government regulations. Today's automotive administrator is responsible for deciding how the company can remain viable in such a changing environment.

HOSPITAL STRATEGIES FOR SURVIVAL

The responsibility of today's hospital administrator is to maintain the viability of the institution in the changing context of health care delivery. How can the hospital survive when faced with a shortage of nurses, government regulation of fees, escalating malpractice insurance costs, and pressures from Health Systems Agencies (HSAs) to reduce the number of beds?

As a part of long-range planning, today's hospital administrator is making decisions about health care services to be added, and services to be dropped; new staff positions to be created, and positions to be eliminated; construction to be rushed, and construction to be postponed. These decisions reflect the administrator's considered opinion of the shape the institution will assume in 5, 10, or 20 years. The chief administrator does not make such decisions in isolation but depends on advice given by the hospital's board of directors, its medical staff, and others on how the hospital should adapt to its environment. To make predictive decisions for the institution, the hospital administrator must anticipate the future far in advance of any actual crisis in order to make the least possible number of errors.

LIBRARY STRATEGIES FOR SURVIVAL

The hospital librarian, no less than the hospital administrator, stands at the end of a long tradition of scientific management and administrative theory. Yet it is as an on-the-line provider of information service that the hospital librarian first builds up a reputation.

A Systematic Approach

The preceding chapters 3-10 have dealt with the major services of a hospital library and how these services can be organized. In this, the first arena in which the librarian is accountable, the librarian follows in the footsteps of Frederick Taylor and develops the work process. Chapters 12-20 examine the techniques used by librarians to manage resources allocated to the library and to compete for resources with other hospital services in a climate of cost containment. Here the librarian enters a second arena of accountability, and in the tradition of Henri Fayol, focuses on the executive process. By synthesizing the work process and the executive process into one operation, the librarian becomes a "scientific manager," that is, a manager who achieves practical results by a systematic approach to problems and situations.

Predictive Decision Making

The first two roles of the hospital librarian—as a provider of services and as a scientific manager—have been established. Does the librarian have an administrative role as well? Our definition of an administrator was one who is concerned primarily with decisions that anticipate the changes the organization must make if it is to survive in its competitive environment. The librarian performs such a role when contributing to the decisions that keep the hospital evolving in the face of change.

Supplying Information

The major integrating force that draws the hospital librarian into partnership with other administrators is the administrative decision-making process. The administrator must act on sound information. The librarian is the gatekeeper of information and can provide studies on the habits and preferences of health consumers, the admitting practices of staff physicians, the response of consumers to promotion, the characteristics of competitors and their capabilities for providing health care, recent trends in health care delivery, and many other topics.

To provide the most relevant information, the librarian needs to have a broad understanding of a hospital's goals and of its decision-making practices. Without knowledge of the rationale behind hospital policies, the librarian cannot accurately appraise the hospital's long-range planning and provide the appropriate information. The hospital librarian acquires this understanding through exposure to the thinking of key hospital officials.

The librarian begins to learn about hospital goals and practices by reading material such as the hospital's charter, annual reports to incorporators, and reports of medical staff committees. If the librarian is responsible for maintaining hospital archives, then there is no problem in gaining access to policy reports. If the librarian does not exercise this archival function, then the librarian must make an effort to collect the significant documents.

The librarian should not only read reports but should also write reports, identifying the factors in the hospital that have an impact on library service and detailing ways to make the library more responsive to its public. If the librarian writes reports only once a year, when the budget is due or an annual report is required, both the development of the library and of the librarian will be hampered.

The best time to begin writing reports is when a librarian first takes a job. In the prehiring interviews, hospital representatives will usually express their expectations and hopes for the hospital library. The new librarian's first report might be a written summary of the goals for library service as understood from the prehiring interviews and an outline of how those needs and expectations might be met. Such a report will lead the administrator to conclude that the new librarian is a well-organized, articulate person capable of intelligent planning and, in short, worth talking to again.

The initial report might be followed up at the end of the first 100 days by a written reassessment of the goals in the light of the newly acquired working experience and suggested means of achieving them. Thereafter, short reports might identify specific problems and describe how solutions have been achieved. To maintain the hospital library's position and a fair share of finances, the librarian must compete against other departments within the hospital. Good reports are effective competitive tools.

Adapting to Change

In some ways the hospital library is a microcosm of the larger institution of which it is a part. The librarian must develop the same capabilities of decision making for the future of the library as the chief executive director exercises for the hospital as a whole. The librarian takes on an administrative role when consciously using a decision-making process to relate library activities to the predicted changes in the hospital's delivery of health care.

The hospital librarian needs to think about what kind of library will be needed in five years' time, not only in terms of an ideal of library activity and service, but also in terms of the changing hospital setting. The librarian must also be attuned to the hospital's external environment and be willing to respond to the community's expectations from health care institutions. Local communities are demanding cheaper health care at the same time that they are demanding better and more elaborate health services. Obviously, the burden of satisfying the demand for more with less will be passed on by the hospital administrator to the various departments. Like other health professionals, librarians must accept that however desirable it might be to provide everyone the ultimate in service, hospitals cannot afford the ultimate in service.

The librarian must accept the realities of the library's environment. Unless the library program has a high priority with the medical staff, the hospital administration may conclude that library service is a nonessential frill and, therefore, wasteful of the hospital's limited resources. To survive and even flourish in such an environment, the librarian must develop strategies for achieving general recognition of the importance of library service in the hospital setting. This may involve changing the medical staff's basic approach to patient-care information.

One of the most subtle, persuasive activities of the medical librarian is educating the medical staff in information retrieval techniques. Often the medical librarian's most effective teaching occurs, not in a formal setting, but in a one-to-one situation. Such teaching occurs, for example, when a physician comes to a librarian with a specific patient-care problem and the librarian helps find in the literature the experience of other physicians with the same problem. To create a climate of support for the library, librarians must deliver the results required by the consumer.

A physician probably will not only require specific information about a patient's symptoms, physical signs, and laboratory findings but also about the experience of other physicians in dealing with similar patterns. The primary record of this experience is contained in medical books and journals.

The gathering of books, journals, and other resources in one central place—the library—makes easily available to everyone information on any aspect of medicine in whatever depth required. Since published information is such a vital tool of the health care practitioner, it is reasonable to require that information should also be easily and immediately available in the work area. Clinical practice can be additionally supported by decentralizing information resources and supplying working tools for special groups on patient floors. In a growing number of hospitals, the librarian has transformed the inadequate, outdated collections on patient floors into up-to-date ref-erence centers with current titles selected by the medical specialists on that floor.

The library committee can serve for the librarian the same function that a board of directors serves for the chief administrator. A librarian can plan for a library ably without a library committee if the librarian knows the hospital staff well and can ask advice from the staff member best qualified to give it. The entire staff then serves as a committee without the formalities of a chairman, agendas, motions, or minutes. However, a library committee with representatives from the various groups served by the library—administrators, physicians, nurses, allied health professionals—can be a most important channel of communication between the hospital staff and the librarian.

Most library committees exist primarily to advise on library policy. They approve policy revisions as the need arises and interpret policies to the hospital staff. Committee members can also be an invaluable resource for interpreting the hospital's goals and objectives to the librarian. Good communication between the library staff and those who take care of patients improves the library's effectiveness in the provision of patient care. It also helps the librarian to synchronize the long-range plan for the library with the long-range goals for the hospital.

The hospital librarian can also use national standards for hospital library service to make the library more responsive to its environment. In 1978 the Joint Commission on Accreditation of Hospitals (JCAH) strengthened its standards for professional library services. (See Chapter 2 for further information on standards.) To facilitate use of the standards, the Medical Library Association (MLA) has prepared a guide to library services for JCAH surveyors (1).

Standards and guidelines are not blunt instruments that can be used to force hospitals to support their libraries. They are, however, helpful in raising the consciousness of decision makers as to what their peers consider to be appropriate, minimal service in a hospital. The hospital librarian should provide promptly the data relevant to libraries in the JCAH presurvey questionnaire submitted by the administration. For the survey itself, the librarian should assemble the documentation suggested in the MLA guidelines in a location convenient for the surveyors. Above all, the librarian should take an interest in library standards and contribute to their development. Standards are not intended to be static but to imply that hospital libraries can all move forward together.

THE GROWING ROLE OF THE LIBRARY ADMINISTRATOR

The hospital librarian soon finds that the job does not consist solely of a series of daily tasks for which medical librarians have been specifically trained. Instead, it requires the librarian to be information provider, manager, and administrator. The service role of meeting information needs is a familiar one. The role of manager, active in both the work process and the executive process, is often less expected by the librarian. Some librarians resent the obligation to manage, citing an already over-loaded work schedule. The librarian should also recognize that along with a need for service and management there is a need for long-range planning. The most accepted and well-defined administrative task is planning for the future. The hospital librarian, in accepting the responsibility of library administrator, must become skilled in predictive decision making. The administrative role of the librarian develops as the librarian learns to adapt the library to its changing environment.

REFERENCES

1. JCAH guide to professional library services for surveyors. MLA News 1980 Sept; (127):1-2.

READINGS

Chen C-C, ed. Quantitative measurement and dynamic library service. Phoenix, AZ: The Oryx Press, 1978.

Dillon RD. Zero-based budgeting for health care institutions. Germantown, MD: Aspen Systems, 1979.

Lancaster FW. The measurement and evaluation of library services. Washington, DC: Information Resources Press, 1977.

Wren GR. Modern health administration. Athens, GA: University of Georgia Press, 1974.

Planning and Evaluating Library Services

Nardina L. Nameth
Director of Library Services
Henry Ford Hospital
Detroit, Michigan

CHAPTER 12

Planning and
Evaluating
Library
Services

Nardina L. Nameth
Director of Library Services
Henry Ford Hospital
Detroit, Michigan

THE PLANNING PROCESS

TYPES OF PLANNING
    Program Planning
    Project Planning
    Long-Range Planning

EVALUATION
    Classes of Evaluation
    Types of Measurement Criteria
    Evaluation Strategies
    Quality Assurance

Figures

Planning is essential to the management of any complex activity, including running a library. Faced with pressures to provide services, librarians are sometimes tempted to neglect planning in favor of immediate action. Planning, however, ensures organized and effective activity. It takes time, but that time is recouped in more efficient operations after implementation.

Planning not only helps a librarian to organize the activity of the library, but it also provides the means by which a librarian can obtain approval to expand that activity. A detailed plan for a projected new service or for the expansion of an existing service shows the administration what is suggested; why it is suggested; how much it will cost; and what impact it will have. The same plans, once approved, can then direct the new activity.

Trial and error consumes time, causes confusion, and damages the credibility of the librarian. By developing plans that identify worthwhile activities, determining the steps needed to accomplish those activities, identifying necessary resources, and establishing policy and procedures, librarians can make the library operate more smoothly.

THE PLANNING PROCESS

The planning process can be divided into a series of separate activities that provide an organized and logical framework. The following activities provide a step-by-step approach to the planning process:

- *Determining goals.* What are the goals of the institution? Do the library's goals reflect institutional goals?
- *Assessing needs.* What are the needs for library and information services in the hospital?
- *Setting objectives.* What specific actions will meet these needs?
- *Determining priorities.* Which objectives are most important? How much of the library's resources will be spent on each objective?
- *Establishing policy.* What conditions or principles will guide the provision of services?
- *Developing procedures.* Who will do what and how?
- *Scheduling.* When will the tasks be done?

TYPES OF PLANNING

Although the activities involved in all types of planning remain essentially the same, three types are useful in hospital libraries: (1) program planning, (2) project planning, and (3) long-range planning.

Program Planning

Program planning involves library activities as a whole. During this type of planning, a librarian decides what services the library will provide, gives a philosophical basis for the library services, and describes how the services will be provided. At this time the librarian has a chance to list goals, determine how much time and

money are necessary to accomplish the goals, and establish the guidelines or rules that govern the activity. Program planning organizes library activity and demonstrates the logic of that activity.

Ideally, librarians should develop a program plan when first establishing library services in a hospital. After library services have been established, librarians can use the planning process to rethink the priorities of their programs and record the decisions for the hospital administration. Librarians undertake the development of formal planning documents, including goals, objectives, policies, and procedures at various times. They may develop these documents after assuming a new position, before adding a new program, or when studying, changing, or expanding an existing service. After planning documents have been prepared or revised, they should be submitted to the hospital administration for approval. When planning programs, librarians should follow the steps described below.

Determining Goals

Determining goals is the first step in the planning process. It involves identifying institutional goals and then formulating library goals to support the goals of the institution. Hospitals may have a variety of formal documents expressing their philosophy. Some hospitals are guided by a mission statement and then develop annual goals from that statement. Other institutions may not have formally labeled mission statements, but they publicize their philosophy in the hospital's motto. In most hospitals, the philosophical statements emphasize patient care first and then may include education and research. Figure 12-1 illustrates a sample hospital mission statement.

Goal statements are usually general statements that project what is to be accomplished. In this sense, library goals define the library program. Because goals should be broad enough to encompass an entire program and yet specific enough to identify the major components, some librarians develop one generalized library mission statement and then develop goal statements for specific library services. A general mission statement usually relates× to the goal or mission statement of the hospital. Figure 12-2 illustrates a typical mission statement for a hospital library.

Figure 12-1
Hospital Mission Statement

West Central Hospital shall maintain high standards of practice to provide quality, comprehensive, accessible health care services with emphasis upon ambulatory and selected tertiary care programs; to promote research in the health sciences; and to contribute to the education and training of students in medical and allied health fields.

Figure 12-2
Mission Statement of a Health Sciences Library

The library will support the work of all hospital employees involved in patient care, research, teaching, and administration by providing a dynamic information service. The library collects and organizes information for this purpose in the form of books, journals, and audiovisuals. The library is dedicated to finding answers to all requests for health care information and can identify and deliver published materials from the worldwide library community.

Specific goal statements describe each of the library's major services. Some librarians identify each of these major services as a program area, and then refer record keeping, reporting of statistics, and sometimes budgeting to these program areas. Whether or not specific areas are identified within the total library program, the identification of specific service goals will help define the components of library service. One possible set of program goals for library service is illustrated in Figure 12-3.

Assessing Needs

An accurate needs assessment is the foundation of any planning process. It provides planning data for librarians and solid evidence of the need for library services. The needs assessment should be carefully planned, based on what the librarian wants to know and how that information will be used. A librarian might need to know what information the hospital staff needs, what sources they already use, how often and how quickly they need material, and whether they would use particular services and sources if they were available.

Knowing how to phrase assessment questions is also important. In general, librarians should avoid library jargon and phrase questions in the user's terminology. Some users might respond that they have little need for interlibrary loan. If they had been asked about their needs to consult journals not available in the hospital, the responses might have been different. Librarians should also ask questions that relate to what the user really needs, rather than to what the library offers.

Although questions should be designed to reflect specific situations, some general questions pertain as well, such as:

- What types of information do you require in the performance of your job?
- Where do you get information at the present time?
- What are the three most frequent problems you encounter in getting infomation?
- Which information sources do you need? (How often? How quickly?)
- Which formats do you prefer? (Photocopies? Original

material? Bibliography? Summary? Highlighted article?)
- How often do you require a list of articles on a particular topic?
- How many times per month do you need journals that that the library does not have?
- How many times per month would you use a film or videotape if it were available on a subject of your choice?

In addition to determining what questions to ask, the librarian must also decide *who* to ask and what method of data collection to use. When assessing needs prior to planning programs and services, librarians should survey nonusers as well as users. Grouping potential respondents by type of user will allow the librarian to determine the most effective way to survey each one. The librarian may decide for example to interview all department heads, to hold a needs-assessment discussion at a medical staff meeting or a head nurse meeting, to send a questionnaire to the medical staff and the housestaff, and talk to a representative group of floor nurses.

Before deciding to send questionnaires or interview in person, a librarian should consider the nature of the questions. If the questions are self-explanatory, such as "How often do you use a 35 mm slide projector?," a questionnaire will suffice. However, if the range of possible answers goes beyond "yes" or "no" or a short checklist, a librarian may prefer a personal interview to

Figure 12-3
Program Goals of a Health Sciences Library

INFORMATIONAL AND EDUCATIONAL RESOURCES
The Health Sciences Library provides book, journal, and audiovisual collections to meet the informational and educational needs of the medical and nursing staff and all other departments and programs of the institution.

INFORMATION SERVICE
The Health Sciences Library provides information services, including answering factual questions, and compiling bibliographies in a timely manner and in a usable format.

DOCUMENT DELIVERY (Interlibrary Loan)
The Health Sciences Library will attempt to obtain any needed document through interlibrary loan or other appropriate means. Photocopying services are available in the library.

COOPERATIVE LIBRARY SERVICES
The Health Sciences Library maintains active, cooperative relationships with local, and where possible, nonlocal libraries. Such cooperation may include interlibrary loans, collection development, reference referrals, technical processes, and other project areas.

determine exactly what the interviewee needs. Interviews with key hospital staff—such as clinical chiefs, administrators, and department heads—give a librarian the opportunity to explain existing services as well as to test the need for new ones.

When the need for a particular service is disclosed in questionnaires or interviews, a librarian may wish to test that need by providing the service on a limited basis as a pilot project. This would show concretely how the service is used, and how effectively that service is meeting needs. For example, a librarian interested in demonstrating the need for MEDLINE might plan a pilot project that requires a funded searcher to be available at the hospital one day a week. Data on the results of such a project would show how the service meets identified needs.

Setting Objectives

Although definitions of planning terminology vary considerably, the term "goal" usually refers to a general statement that projects what is to be accomplished. An "objective" is a concrete statement of specific action. In some institutions that require measurable objectives, entire management systems such as Management by Objectives (MBO) are designed to define the actions that achieve goals and to judge performance according to the accomplishment of those actions. In most institutions, however, objectives represent statements of actions that do not always include levels of expected activity.

Since objectives represent specific actions, more than one objective is necessary to achieve a program goal. If a librarian wants to be specific, several objectives can be written. Although broad objectives are easier to write, they are less easy to measure and reveal less about the library's activities. Specific objectives take more thought, but they are also more useful in organizing activities and showing personnel outside the library what the library does. Figure 12-4 gives an example of a general program goal and the specific objectives chosen to achieve that goal. Objectives not only show the administration what the librarian plans to do, they also provide the librarian with a guide. When objectives need to be more specific than those in Figure 12-4, a second level of objectives can be added. Figure 12-5 shows possible operational objectives for an objective covering selection of new materials.

Many institutions require that each department set objectives for periods of time, usually six months to one year. Even if objectives are not required, the use of annual or semiannual objectives to direct activity is often considered a sign of good management. Objectives can be used to establish the overall activities of the library program and also accommodate yearly changes. For example, a librarian can use the same program objectives from year to year but modify operational objectives for each year's activity. Operational objectives can include a mix of objectives that reflect ongoing activities and special projects for a particular year.

Figure 12-4
Program Objectives of a Health Sciences Library

INFORMATIONAL AND EDUCATIONAL RESOURCES

Goal:
  The Health Sciences Library provides book, journal, and audiovisual collections to meet the informational and education needs of the medical and nursing staff and all other departments and programs of the institution.

Objectives:
1. Select, with the input of appropriate departments, 50 new books, 1-5 new audiovisual programs, and 1-2 new journals each year. Subject areas to be considered are internal medicine, nursing, dermatology, pathology, pediatrics, obstetrics and gynecology.
2. Identify, evaluate, and acquire the most recent editions of books currently in the collection.
3. Acquire selected material.
4. Evaluate and withdraw dated material.
5. Produce and distribute a list of new books four times a year.
6. Produce and distribute once a year a list of journals owned by title and subject.
7. Update the audiovisual catalog annually.
8. Provide a mechanism for staff to request specific titles in specific subject areas.
9. Design and maintain systems for the circulation of appropriate resources and the in-house use of non-circulating materials.

Figure 12-5
Operational Objectives of a Health Sciences Library

INFORMATIONAL AND EDUCATIONAL RESOURCES

Objective: Selection
  Select, with the input of appropriate departments, 50 new books, 1-5 new audiovisual programs, and 1-2 new journals each year. Subject areas to be considered are internal medicine, nursing, dermatology, pathology, pediatrics, obstetrics and gynecology.

Operational Objective:
1. Identify possible titles from users' requests, flyers, journals, and recent editions of standard lists (see selection policy).
2. When appropriate, seek the advice of subject specialists by routing bibliographic information and reviews, if available.
3. Design and implement a new form for departmental input into selection (August 1982).

Determining Priorities

Many hospital librarians experience a continuous shortage of time. Therefore, they should decide which library objectives are the most important and so should be accomplished first. By ranking objectives in order of priority and by referring to these rankings when scheduling, librarians can organize events apart from the day-to-day crunch of activities. Objectives can be listed in order of importance or grouped under specific categories of priority. The librarian can then assign realistic completion dates to operational objectives.

To be effective, objectives and priorities must not only be set but also adhered to. Librarians should incorporate objectives into scheduling, task assignments, and policies; post them in a visible place; or schedule a specific time during the week to review their status. Although the mechanics of the reviewing process are not important, regular review is vital. Setting objectives and then filing them away until next year defeats the purpose of the entire process.

Establishing Policies

Policies are the general guidelines or rules that govern the way an objective will be accomplished. By establishing these rules in advance, the librarian can anticipate operational problems, design solutions, obtain administrative approval, and publicize the ground rules to both library staff and users. If a library committee exists, its endorsement and support of library policy is invaluable. In many institutions, policies that affect the entire hospital must be reviewed by administration and filed in the hospital policy manual. Whether the library policies become part of hospital policy or remain only as departmental policy, they facilitate the smooth operation of library activity and provide a vehicle for obtaining the approval and support of the library committee and the administration. Writing policies is discussed further in Chapter 15.

Developing Procedures

Writing procedures is an essential part of planning. During this step, a librarian decides how each objective will be implemented. Once the procedures are used, librarians can modify them, if necessary. Even if the procedures will be implemented only by the person writing them, they are still valuable. Procedures require the logical analysis of a task, provide a written record of the standard practice, and can be used to estimate the amount of time necessary to complete a task. The writing of procedures is discussed in Chapter 15.

Scheduling

Part of planning involves determining how much time a task should take, and how much time a librarian should devote to the task per day or per week. For ongoing library programs, librarians should estimate how much time will be spent on each objective per week. Allotting specific amounts of time to tasks may signal the need for priorities or realistic cuts in programs. When planning a new service, librarians should schedule a specific amount of time for each objective in order to integrate the new service into the existing services.

Project Planning

The process used by librarians for program planning can also be used for planning individual projects. Some librarians avoid formal project planning, realizing that it is time-consuming. However, project planning involves systematizing and documenting decisions that must be made in any case. The dividends gained through increased efficiency and administrative awareness of library activity outweigh the few additional hours involved. For a list of documents often used in project planning, see Figure 12-6.

Long-Range Planning

A third type of planning, often the most neglected type, is long-range planning. This process anticipates institutional changes and analyzes how these changes may affect library services. Librarians often begin long-range planning with a question: "What will this institution require in the way of library services in the next five years?" A librarian makes this inquiry to determine what new programs will be required; how old programs will adapt to new information demands; and what personnel, equipment, space, and additional budget will be necessary to support these changes. The long-range planning process often results in a written five-year plan that the librarian presents to the administration and the library committee for approval and support.

Effects of Long-Range Planning

Long-range planning prepares the library for future contingencies. New residency programs, additional outpatient clinics, and new allied health training programs all have an impact on information needs. Budget increases take time to justify and also must be planned

Figure 12-6
Project Planning Documents

Library Goals

Needs Assessment

Project Plan (goals, objectives, estimated costs)

Project Proposal

Policies

Procedures

Project Completion Memo

Project Evaluation

for. Furthermore, the administration is more apt to support requests for collection development and new staffing if they are anticipated a year or two before the actual requested date.

Long-range planning is essential in today's dynamic library environment. The effects of automation alone have a dramatic impact. Librarians need to anticipate developments in electronic publishing, telecommunications, and information handling, and integrate these changes into regular library policies and procedures when useful. Increased networking among libraries continues to make a variety of new services available. Librarians should keep informed of these services and anticipate how they can affect their own institutions.

Finally, long-range planning ensures logical development of new operations and services. It anticipates problems before they occur, examines alternative operations and services as possible plans, and reduces impending crises.

Elements of Long-Range Planning

Long-range planning focuses on three major elements of the library: collection development, staffing, and new services.

As the hospital institution develops and changes, so does the library collection. Therefore, collection development becomes an important element of long-range planning. New librarians who are initiating a long-range plan should ask the administrator if a plan for the hospital exists. If a plan has not been established, the techniques discussed in the needs-assessment section of this chapter can be used to gather the necessary information. Additional information can be gained by asking representatives of medical education, the medical staff, health educators, nurses, and the administration about the five-year plans they are proposing in their area. How these plans may affect their need for library services can also be asked. After acquiring information, the librarian should evaluate the existing collection with the new programs in mind and make recommendations for additions.

When the approximate additions are identified, the librarian should project what impact they will have on the budget. For example, a librarian may evaluate the immunology section or related areas of the library collection after hearing about the hospital's plans to begin a new residency program in two years. The result of the evaluation may show that there are materials that should be added to support the program: specifically, six basic level books and three reference books. To estimate the cost for these new materials, the librarian would use the following formula:

$$\left(\begin{array}{c}\text{average cost} \\ \text{for books}\end{array} + \begin{array}{c}\text{inflation} \\ \text{factor}\end{array}\right) \times \begin{array}{c}\text{number} \\ \text{of books}\end{array} = \begin{array}{c}\text{increase in book budget} \\ \text{for new program}\end{array}$$

In our example,

$$\left(\begin{array}{c}\text{\$29 average} \\ \text{cost}\end{array} + \begin{array}{c}\text{30 percent inflation} \\ \text{factor (15 percent for} \\ \text{each year)}\end{array}\right) \times 9 = \begin{array}{c}\text{\$339.30 increase in} \\ \text{book budget}\end{array}$$

This amount is then added to the budget request, along with documentation for the increase. Since the program would not begin for two years, during the first year the librarian could work on budgeting, and during the second year could acquire all needed materials. Anyone who has participated in a crash acquisitions program can appreciate the advantages of long-range planning.

The second element of long-range planning is staffing. Librarians should justify requests for increased staff by projecting increases in workload. These increases can be projected in several ways. One standard way is to study growth trends in the past five years, using some standard indicator such as patient days, number of employees, or bed count. Trends toward cost containment in the eighties, however, may result in growth patterns different from those seen in the seventies. Therefore, projections based on growth in personnel or bed count may not be as useful today as they have been in the past. Whenever possible, librarians should discuss the problems of projecting growth with the administrator or the hospital planner, using an indicator similar to the one used to project growth for the hospital as a whole.

Another way to project increases in workloads is to calculate increases in the use of services due to marketing services to new user groups and the addition of new services. The increase is calculated by multiplying the estimated number of additional units of service for a procedure (100 new interlibrary loans) by the average time spent on each procedure. By adding the totals of all expected increases, librarians can estimate the number of additional staff needed.

By calculating the percentage by which services are expected to increase, librarians can also project the level of the workload. Suppose, for example, that documented use of library services has been increasing an average of 5 percent over the past five years. Based on the recent addition of MEDLINE, plans for increased marketing, and the addition of a family practice residency, the librarian might project an additional 5 percent growth each year, or a total of 10 percent annually. Based on a projected 10 percent growth rate, 48 extra hours will be required in five years. Such projections should be backed by documentation. The information should include current hospital figures, showing an expected increase in the number of primary users; past data, indicating the correlation between the introduction of an educational program and library use; and studies from the literature, documenting increases in use following implementation of a new service such as MEDLINE.

The third element in long-range planning is the five-year service plan, which starts with the needs assessment. When needs have been documented, the new services are planned by methods outlined earlier in the chapter. With a five-year lead time for planning, however, thorough needs assessments may be conducted and major budget requests or grant proposals initiated. As long-range service planning progresses, librarians should document each stage in the annual report and in the annual review and update of the library's five-year plan.

EVALUATION

Evaluation is essential to the entire planning process. A librarian cannot formally plan unless programs, services, and procedures are analyzed to determine their function, effectiveness, and need for improvement or change. The purpose of evaluation is threefold: (1) to determine the effectiveness of existing programs, (2) to determine specific changes that will improve existing programs, and (3) to justify continuing budget support. Evaluations of individual programs or services are more helpful in making improvements than evaluations of an entire program of services. Generalized statements about the worth of library programs do not provide specific data to support appropriate changes.

Classes of Evaluation

In order to understand the evaluation process, librarians should examine the four classes of evaluation suggested by Knightly: effort evaluation, process evaluation, effectiveness evaluation, and impact evaluation (1).

Effort Evaluation

Librarians can compare the resources used with the results achieved. In an interlibrary loan operation, for example, the following resources may be measured and then compared with the number of interlibrary loan transactions: staff time, salaries, supplies, and space utilized for borrowing materials.

Process Evaluation

Librarians can evaluate processes to determine whether the procedures used in the performance of a service are efficient and appropriate. For example, if a librarian has used two different procedures to determine which library owns a particular journal title, process evaluation can indicate which method is more efficient. The method of consulting a union list of serials for journal title information is certainly more efficient than calling every source in the area.

Effectiveness Evaluation

Evaluating program effectiveness determines whether a service accomplishes its objectives. An effectiveness evaluation of interlibrary loan service might, for example, assess whether users receive the material in time for

the information to be helpful. If the librarian's objective is to supply 80 percent of interlibrary loan requests in three weeks, the evaluation can indicate if the objective is being met.

Impact Evaluation

The most powerful form of evaluation is impact evaluation. It assesses the extent to which accomplished objectives actually meet the needs of the parent institution. This class of evaluation could be used to measure whether library service is improving patient care by making information available that would normally not have been accessible. It also determines whether programs are meaningful to the institution. Reliable, statistical data acquired from impact evaluation can be the most instrumental type of support for the hospital library. It can show that the library's information service has a positive effect on patient care.

Types of Measurement Criteria

In addition to identifying different classes of evaluation, Knightly describes seven types of measurement criteria. The criteria also represent seven different techniques of evaluation: user opinion, expert opinion, ideal standards, comparison with other organizations, quantifiable outputs, quantifiable processes, and cost or unit costs.

User Opinion

The opinion of the user is one of the most important measurement criteria from a service standpoint. Measurement of user opinion is usually taken after a new program is launched or when an existing program is reviewed. In either case, a librarian should be prepared for negative feedback, be willing to balance negative and positive responses, and make alterations in a program that gets poor reviews. Librarians can use the survey questionnaire, the suggestion box, or interviews with a cross section of library users for collecting their data. MEDLINE services, for example, are frequently evaluated by obtaining users' opinions of the service.

Expert Opinion

Assessment on the basis of expert opinion varies from a professional communication with colleagues in other libraries to a contract with a library consultant. Although experts can be used in evaluating total library operation, their recommendations may tend to be broad and general. Expert opinion is probably more helpful in evaluating a specific program, such as computerized information services, audiovisual services, or a clinical medical librarian program. Although evaluation by expert opinion is probably used less frequently than other types of evaluation, it provides the librarian, the library committee, and the hospital administration with an objective assessment of library service. For additional information on the use of consultants, read Chapter 18.

Ideal Standards

Although "perfect" standards for hospital libraries cannot be determined because of the variables within each institution, several commonly accepted types of standards do exist. The Joint Commission on Accreditation of Hospitals (JCAH) publishes standards for professional library services. At this writing, quantitative standards are also being developed by the Hospital Library Standards and Practices Committee of the Medical Library Association. Chapter 2 contains a list of available standards and guidelines and describes their characteristics.

The advantage of using standards as an assessment tool is that the criteria have already been developed, presumably from a broad base of experience. The major disadvantages are that standards for many library services and operations are not available, and most standards define minimum requirements in broad program areas only. Where standards such as those of the JCAH do exist, librarians can list separate components of the standards on one side of an evaluation sheet and the data from the library on the other.

Comparisons with Other Organizations

Since hospital libraries vary greatly in size and scope, librarians can usually identify several institutions with programs similar to their own. When comparing one library with another, librarians should assess only data that are not associated with a particular institutional situation. For example, comparing book budgets in institutions of similar size and scope might be helpful, but comparing titles in the collections would not be appropriate because collections are developed to serve the specific needs of institutions. Probably the most widely used application of assessment by comparison is the salary survey.

The process of comparing one organization with another often poses problems that are not immediately obvious. Significant dissimilarities in the institutions may not be recognized. Mistakes can be made in the information provided by other institutions, and unwillingness to share certain types of information can be encountered.

Quantifiable Outputs

Generally, measuring quantifiable outputs relates to a specific goal, such as processing a certain number of items in a set period of time. Assuming that there is a standard number of books that can be cataloged in one month, the output of books during a given time period or under special circumstances is measured against the standard. Usually, the standard is based on the experience in one library. If a library has cataloged twenty books per month for several years, for example, that number might be taken as the standard. If acquisitions grow and the librarian modifies procedures to increase the number of books cataloged per month, he or she should evaluate the new procedures by quantifiable output. A monthly chart showing goals and actual performance, plus last year's performance, would be a helpful guide.

Quantifiable Processes

Evaluating quantifiable processes is similar to evaluating quantifiable outputs except that the processes themselves are being analyzed in addition to the results they produce. This type of assessment is also goal-oriented. It measures the completion of a certain number of procedures in a given time. In this type of assessment, the tasks involved in the total process, however, are as important as the number of completed items. If a librarian evaluates an interlibrary loan by quantifiable process, for example, he or she would identify the individual steps involved in an interlibrary loan and measure the time spent on each, as well as the total time and average time per request. Librarians would find this type of evaluation particularly useful in determining staff requirements and staff performance.

Cost or Unit Costs

Assessment of a program on the basis of costs or unit costs is an excellent way to study the cost-effectiveness of a new program. Cost-benefit analysis frequently justifies a new program. Therefore, a follow-up evaluation on the basis of costs is often useful. Determining precise costs for services is a complex and a time-consuming activity. Often, however, librarians find that estimating costs works just as well. When making estimates, it is possible to include all relevant factors, including overhead. Such a thorough approach, though, is often not necessary, so many librarians limit their considerations to staff time, supplies, and resources. Elements included in estimating cost for an average manual search in *Index Medicus* might include the following: average time per search, average cost of *Index Medicus* per use (cost of subscription divided by number of searches), and cost of supplies. Such an approach is fairly superficial and does not make allowances for many variables, but often this level of estimating costs is a useful indicator.

Evaluation Strategies

To create an evaluation strategy, librarians should measure any of the four evaluation classes by using any one of the seven assessment criteria. The choice of class or criteria depends on the situation being evaluated and what information the librarian expects from the evaluation process.

The choice of evaluation class should be made first. Librarians should study the library service being evaluated and choose the evaluation class that would produce the type of information they desire. The following summary illustrates the best use of each class of evaluation.

- *Effort evaluation*—determines whether the resources

being used (money, space, manpower) are appropriate for the service
- *Process evaluation*—determines how efficient the procedures are
- *Effectiveness evaluation*—determines how well the service accomplishes its objectives
- *Impact evaluation*—determines how the service meets the user's actual needs

After selecting an evaluation class, librarians should choose a tool or type of measurement criterion. Each of the seven measurement criteria has unique characteristics that can be applied to some or all of the four evaluation types. Librarians can use the evaluation strategy worksheet in Figure 12-7 to organize evaluation decisions.

Quality Assurance

Quality assurance (QA) is another example of an evaluation process. It has become increasingly important in hospitals during the last decade. The JCAH stresses QA for clinical departments, although it is an institution-wide program in many hospitals.

QA programs identify and solve problems that relate to patient care. The JCAH QA process contains five steps (2).

1. Identification of problems
2. Objective assessment and determination of priorities for investigating and resolving problems
3. Implementation of plan to eliminate problems
4. Monitoring to ensure desired result
5. Documentation to substantiate effectiveness of plan

It is assumed that as problems are identified and resolved the quality of patient care will improve.

The JCAH also stresses interdisciplinary cooperation in the QA process. Librarians should take advantage of this emphasis by participating in multidepartmental studies to show the relationship of library service to patient care. For example, an assessment of how nurses obtain information to develop patient care plans would involve the library and its service.

QA studies should be based on the objectives of the library and the activities of the library staff that support those objectives. Librarians should involve the library staff in the process of selecting evaluation criteria and ask for agreement on the importance of the processes and services to be assessed. By involving staff, librarians are assured of cooperation and support when the results of the process are known. To conduct a QA audit in a one- or two-person library, librarians may also invite library users to participate.

Figure 12-7
Evaluation Strategy Worksheet

CLASSES OF EVALUATION	User Opinion	Expert Opinion	Ideal Standards	Comparison with Other Organizations	Quantifiable Outputs	Quantifiable Processes	Costs or Unit Costs
Effort Evaluation							
Process Evaluation							
Effectiveness Evaluation							
Impact Evaluation							

The evaluation techniques described earlier in the chapter can also be applied to a QA audit. A QA project related to patient care is easily recognizable as "impact evaluation," the most powerful form of evaluation available to hospital librarians. When selecting measurement criteria, user opinion seems to be one of the strongest criteria to use, since only the user can describe how available information changed patient care. Another criterion to be considered in the QA study is quantifiable outputs. Careful audits of patient care related to the user of library information may be an excellent method of evaluating the impact of library services on patient care.

Evaluation of the clinical librarian program, LATCH, and similar patient care information programs provide a unique opportunity to show the relationship between library service and patient care.

Although a librarian may do many evaluation studies regarding the efficiency and acceptability of library operations, the focus of hospital quality assurance is patient care (3). This focus on patient care, coupled with its accompanying contact with other departments, makes hospital QA one of the most valuable programs in which the library can participate.

REFERENCES

1. Knightly JJ. Overcoming the criterion problem in the evaluation of library performance. Spec Libr 1979 Apr; 70:173-178.

2. Joint Commission on Accreditation of Hospitals. Accreditation manual for hospitals. 1983 ed. Chicago: Joint Commission on Accreditation of Hospitals, 1982.

3. Self PC, Gebhart KA. A quality assurance process in health science libraries. Bull Med Libr Assoc 1980 July;68:288-292.

READINGS

Angrist S. Evaluation research: possibilities and limitations. JABS 1975 Jan 1;11:75-91.

Bell JA, Keusch, RB. Comprehensive planning for libraries. Long Range Plan 1976 Oct;9:48-56.

Kahalas H. Look at major planning methods: development, implementation, strengths and limitations. Long Range Plan 1978 Aug;11:84-90.

Matheson NW, West RT. NLM Medical Library Resource Improvement Grant Program: an evaluation. Bull Med Libr Assoc 1976 July; 64:309-319.

McClure CR, ed. Planning for library services: a guide to utilizing planning methods for library management. Journal of Library Administration 1981 Summer/Fall/Winter;2.

Roach AA, Addington WW. The effects of an information specialist on patient care and medical education. J Med Educ 1975 Feb;50:176-180.

Sellers DY. Basic planning and budgeting concepts for special libraries. Spec Libr 1973 Feb;64:70-75.

Suchman E. Evaluation research; principles and practice in public social service and social action programs. New York: Russell Sage, 1967.

Tagliacozzo R. Estimating the satisfaction of information users. Bull Med Libr Assoc 1977 Apr;65:243-249.

Webster D. Planning aids for the university library director. Washington, DC: Association of Research Libraries, 1971.

Budgeting for Library Services

Sally Harms
Director, Health Science Library
St. Luke's Methodist Hospital
Cedar Rapids, Iowa

Budgeting for Library Services

Sally Harms
Director, Health Science Library
St. Luke's Methodist Hospital
Cedar Rapids, Iowa

Figures

The hospital library is a vital professional service that must be supported with adequate resources in order to be effective. To secure sufficient funding the librarian must demonstrate both the importance of library services and the importance of adequate financial support. The budget is one tool that can be used to show the relationship between library support and library service.

This chapter discusses the purposes of budgeting, the librarian's role as a resource manager, the sources of hospital library funds, the process of budgeting, and budget review during the course of a financial year.

BUDGETING AS A MANAGEMENT TOOL

Various misconceptions about budgeting often cloud understanding of this important process. Budgeting is neither a mysterious manipulation of money nor an inflexible shield to ward off requests for increased service. The budget is a device to help identify and coordinate both the resources put into an organization and their impact upon the organization. The experienced manager uses the budget as a tool for planning and organizing services and for communicating effectively in an institutional environment.

Although budgeting usually is thought of in financial terms, the concept can also be applied to any allocation of resources, including people, time, and space, as well as money. Effective management of library service involves careful budgeting of all forms of resources.

Fiscal Tool

Budgeting in a hospital serves a number of different purposes. First, a budget is a fiscal tool used to meet legal requirements. It provides the information necessary to meet hospital audit requirements and is the basic documentation for the entire corporate structure. A hospital's balance sheets, financial statements, ledgers, and annual reports furnish the information necessary for long-range planning directed towards financial stability and responsible corporate management.

Complete and accurate records of day-by-day income and expenses and a plan (budget) that anticipates income, expenses, and personnel needs will help the hospital management to monitor and maintain adequate supplies of cash for the necessary transactions. Maintaining an optimum day-by-day cash flow is important, since unused money must be quickly and profitably invested. The fiscal department, under the direction of the controller or business manager, generally prepares and monitors this information for the hospital.

The middle manager becomes directly involved with budgeting when transactions within his or her department require the assistance of the financial staff, and again during the budget cycle of the institution's financial year. At budget time, the department head has an opportunity to influence the plans of the organization for the coming year. The department head achieves this impact through effective use of the departmental budget as a communications and administrative tool.

Communications Tool

The budget functions as a communications tool among management levels in three distinct ways. First, the budget is the traditional method for bringing information upward to the proper level for decision making. It is the formal means by which a department tells the administration what resources it will need to perform its assigned responsibilities. By linking costs of resources to products or services, the budget gives management the information necessary to make decisions about the levels of activity it should support.

Second, the budget communicates to all levels of personnel what decisions have been made about activities or services. It also indicates what financial limits or guidelines have been placed on those activities.

Finally, the budget document is a public relations opportunity to communicate to the administration the services of a department, its resource needs, and its efficiency in resource management. Many hospital librarians feel that the budget presentation is the best opportunity to draw attention to what the hospital buys with the money spent on its library.

Administrative Tool

The department manager probably will use the budget mainly as an administrative tool to plan, organize, and control departmental activities.

The middle manager can view the budget as a major means of having input into the long-range decision making of an organization. Through the budget the librarian indicates the directions the hospital library program should take and which activities should be emphasized and strengthened. The budget then must reflect the librarian's total service plan for the department, not just for a year, but as one year of a longer plan.

To use the budget for planning, a manager must develop and present alternatives and identify the funding levels, the services, and, if possible, the consequences attached to each alternative. Administrative decision makers are thus made aware that when they choose a level of funding, they also choose a level of service. Even if an expanded service is not the alternative chosen, the plan is at least introduced and will be familiar to the decision makers the next time it is presented.

A budget helps organize departmental activities by imposing limits on the resources available and assigning priorities for the allocation of those resources. A budget also requires the accumulation and review of statistical information about the library's activity. Finally, the budgetary process can lead the manager to develop practical, achievable plans for implementing creative ideas. A library manager can come up with exciting new ideas regarding information delivery and education with relative ease but usually finds formulating concrete plans to carry out these ideas much harder. By converting ideas into categories of people, units of time, resources, and ultimately dollars and cents, the manager can formulate a practical approach that will have a better chance of gaining administrative approval.

In addition to its uses in planning and organizing, the budget is an essential tool for controlling and directing. The manager's budgetary responsibility divides into two parts: deciding how to allocate resources (planning); and spending those resources (controlling). As a part of control, the librarian chooses which expenditures to make, both in terms of the goals desired and the total assets available. The librarian then proceeds to monitor expenses and to redirect activities as necessary to comply with budgetary limits and to achieve objectives.

In order to control expenditures, the librarian needs records of expenses to date. Every organization provides some sort of budgetary feedback in the form of budget updates or expense summaries. The librarian should understand these financial reports and be able to use the information in managing expenses. If reviewing these reports is not part of the librarian's responsibility, the librarian may ask to read them periodically for general information. In addition to using the records distributed by the hospital, the librarian should also keep some sort of record of the library's own expenses.

ROLE OF THE RESOURCE MANAGER

An effective resource manager is not necessarily one who saves money but one who provides value for money spent. This distinction is vital because the manager is responsible for providing services as well as managing a budget. These functions are interdependent, and neither should be sacrificed for the other.

As a resource manager, the librarian has several responsibilities. The librarian must recognize the organizational value of library skills and services and communicate this to the hospital's administration. Library services contribute to quality patient care by providing other professionals, who are in highly technical and rapidly changing fields, with access to knowledge that is crucial for maintaining acceptable levels of skill.

Another responsibility of the librarian is to demonstrate the real costs of library services, as well as some of the problems inherent in providing good library service. One advantage of charging for services, even if only pro forma, is that it brings about an increased awareness of and appreciation for those services. Cooperative efforts, shared service arrangements, and extra hours of duty by the librarian may be valid cost-saving efforts, but because they tend to disguise the true cost of service, their presence and value should be clearly identified.

In addition, the librarian must prepare and present budgets that balance service expectations with realistic expenditures. Quality services cannot be provided without adequate funds. Librarians perform professional, not clerical, functions and should expect to be supported professionally and to be paid salaries that are comparable to salaries paid other related health professionals in the hospital. If hospital support is inadequate, the librarian must make clear the value of information services, the need for those services, and their true price.

Finally, the librarian must provide value for resources expended. As a professional, the librarian is expected to purchase the best services for the money. For example, the librarian may find that purchasing a subscription to a journal is more cost-effective than borrowing the journal. It is the librarian's responsibility to recognize which is the better alternative and to demonstrate that to the administration.

FINANCIAL POSITION OF HOSPITALS

In order to understand and prepare effective budgets, the librarian must recognize the financial context in which the hospital library exists. Both the present state of the health care industry and the fiscal position of a particular institution have considerable impact on the variety and extent of services supported. Such factors also influence the receptivity of the organization toward new services, particularly when the proposed services have an indirect, rather than a direct, effect on patient care.

Industry and Institutional Pressures

The external pressures upon today's health care industry are tremendous. Both state and federal regulations are bringing more and more areas of health care expenditures under close scrutiny. Legislative interest in health care costs, the cry for cost containment throughout the health care industry, and the response of the American Hospital Association (AHA) through voluntary cost containment guidelines, all have had an impact on individual institutions. A variety of special interest groups, including doctors, third party payers, the Joint Commission on Accreditation of Hospitals (JCAH), licensing groups, consumers, labor unions, and local businesses have all generated external pressures that influence the options available to hospitals and health care institutions of all types.

Many institutional variants also affect budgetary decisions. These include the current financial position of the hospital, the community in which the hospital is located, and the financial structure of the hospital—whether it is public, private, profit, or nonprofit.

Other variables within a hospital include the:

- Amount of competition faced
- Uniqueness of services offered
- General fiscal attitude of the hospital's governing body and administration
- Type of clientele served

- Specific goals of the institution
- Hospital's teaching status
- Extent to which the hospital is currently in debt

A knowledge of the major financial forces affecting the hospital should aid the manager in analyzing which budgetary requests are likely to be successful. The timing of such requests, particularly those for program expansion, can be critical. For example, a proposal for an additional staff position when layoffs are being contemplated probably would not be successful. On the other hand, an atmosphere of cost reduction should not automatically preclude the development of programs, especially if the new program or extended service can show savings or a better use of resources.

Hospital Financial Systems

Every hospital designates a division, office, or position with specific responsibility for financial control. Many institutions vest this responsibility in a controller's office, but the business office, a section of data processing, accounting, or purchasing can also exercise this function. In a smaller institution fiscal control may be one of the administrator's direct responsibilities. Generally hospital fiscal services are handled by a chief financial officer who has the title of controller, or accountant. In larger institutions both of these positions will be filled, with the controller handling the major financial activities, such as investment policy decisions, and the accountant handling the day-to-day internal activities and transactions.

A financial division may be set up either as a line operation or a staff operation. If financial affairs are handled in conjunction with other services, such as within the business office or purchasing, responsibilities will usually be structured in a direct reporting arrangement, or line operation. If the financial division is designed to handle only financial services, the financial officer may report directly to the chief executive officer, making it a staff operation. Usually a specific committee of the hospital's governing body will be designated to deal with financial activities. This committee will review financial decisions and make recommendations to the executive committee of the board. This mechanism is usually used to approve general salary increases and annual institutional budgets.

The librarian must become acquainted with the person or persons in the institution responsible for providing support during the budgeting process and for day-to-day handling of all financial affairs. By developing good working relationships with the financial management personnel, the librarian not only can obtain considerable assistance with these activities, but also can substantially increase his or her budgetary sophistication. Librarians will also find that a rudimentary understanding of the complexities of health care finance is useful. References for further reading are provided at the end of the chapter.

SOURCES OF FUNDING FOR THE LIBRARY

The hospital derives its funds from a variety of sources. All hospitals generate revenue, whether from patients who receive services or from reimbursement paid by third parties. Public hospitals also receive a portion of their funding from taxes or government sources, and almost all institutions receive other funding from educational programs, schools, auxiliaries, and gifts. Finally, most hospitals receive grants from government and private agencies.

Every hospital library must have a stable and dependable source of funding. Identifying and securing sources of funding is one of the librarian's foremost responsibilities. Library operating resources can be grouped into five major categories: hospital allocation, gifts, revenues, funding equivalents, and project funds.

Allocations

Many hospital librarians feel that the most stable funding arrangement is a departmental budget allocated from hospital operating funds. Under this arrangement, the hospital includes the cost of operating the library as part of its formal budgeting process, and the librarian goes through the same budgeting process as the heads of all other departments.

Monetary Gifts

Monetary library gifts include donations from professional associations, individuals, and auxiliaries; endowments; memorial grants; and bequests. The planning process and accountability for funds received under these special arrangements vary.

When a portion of the library's funding comes from gifts, the librarian should stay alert for an opportunity to transfer the funding responsibility to the operating budget. This change can be triggered by a reduction in gift funding levels, greater difficulty in administering and keeping records for gift funding, increased conditions imposed by the granting agency, or an annual renewal process that does not provide budgetary security. One must not assume, however, that funding from the hospital's operating budget is always preferable to gift-funding. As long as a library's budgetary source is renewable, is responsive to needs, and is a stable part of the hospital financial structure, the source should not be of concern.

Revenues

For the most part, the library is a service department, rather than a revenue-producing department. Most libraries, however, generate some income, and a few libraries are involved in revenue-producing projects on a larger scale. Whether the library produces $5 or $50,000 a year in revenue, the income is usually deposited in the hospital's general fund. Some hospital libraries do have special gift fund accounts, however. The librarian should keep a careful account of the revenue produced and should be certain that revenue information appears in the appropriate financial reports.

Because a record of producing even a small amount of revenue is often useful, some of the more common revenue-producing practices will be reviewed. Some hospital libraries charge fines. Almost all charge for misplaced or damaged books, and a few add processing fees to the cost of the lost items. Photocopying charges can also be considered revenue.

The most common sources of significant library income are fees for services. Services that lend themselves to fees are computerized and manual searches, interlibrary loans, and alerting services. Fees for such services can be assessed at several levels:

• As a partial subsidy, with the library sharing the cost with the user
• At cost, with the library charging the user any fees the library was charged; this involves billing the user only after the library is billed
• As a flat fee which is an average cost for the service; this eliminates the necessity of determining immediately the exact cost for each service or of billing the user later
• As a flat fee, which is an average service cost plus an increment to cover factors such as staff time and materials; libraries rarely attempt to cover all indirect costs, such as heating and lighting, in the fee charged

Limited fee-for-service arrangements are also common, with the library charging only certain user groups, such as users not connected with the hospital, or charging after an initial service limit is reached. For example, community physicians might be charged $3 per loan after the first ten loans, or law firms or other outside groups might be given 30 minutes free reference time and be charged $20 per hour thereafter.

A special example of fee-for-service is the charge-back system, in which costs are billed back to users' departments. This system places more responsibility on other departments to obtain financial support for library services. Even though the monetary transfers may exist only on paper, they help make others aware of the value of the services provided by the library.

Other opportunities for income to a library include professional dues' assessments through the medical staff association; contracts with local professional associations or institutions that offer health-related programs; contracted services either for or on behalf of the public library; and membership fees. While some of these possibilities may be more or less appropriate, depending on local circumstances, they all should be recognized as potential sources of income for day-to-day operations.

Funding Equivalents

Libraries receive varying amounts of nonfinancial support. Such support can come in the form of services from other libraries, from volunteers, and from donations of library materials.

When managed properly, all three types of support can expand and improve services. Gifts of materials are discussed in Chapter 3, volunteers in Chapter 14, and cooperative services in Chapter 19. In budgeting, the use of such equivalents should be documented and reported regularly, both in monthly reports and in the budgetary process. Each type of service equivalent can be assigned a value, and the total yearly value of each category entered as a source of support. These nonmonetary subsidies should be documented, not only to indicate the true cost of library service but also to hedge against the disappearance of the subsidy. Gifts of time or materials that are relied upon as a part of basic service must be replaced if they are discontinued. Sample forms for reporting funding equivalents appear in Figures 13-1 and 13-2.

Project Funds

Just as a hospital may attract funding from outside groups for highly visible projects, so may the library obtain funding for special projects. In addition to the grant programs of the National Library of Medicine (NLM), local, state, or national foundations and agencies can often be persuaded to support a well-documented project that will produce tangible results. Health education projects currently are enjoying popularity because of their potential marketing implications. Some larger institutions have a development officer or grant writer who helps with project applications. Librarians in smaller institutions can often find help for preparing grant applications by contacting their regional medical library, or local public library or public school library system. Board members and members of civic organizations are also often helpful. A good source for literature on planning budgets for special projects is the Grantsmanship Center. References for further reading are given at the end of the chapter.

BUDGETS

Budgets can be classified according to type, system used, or technique employed. Among the most common types are the operating or expense budget, the personnel budget, and the capital expenditure budget. Different systems for budgeting include item, formula, and program. Among the specific techniques used for budgeting, three will be discussed in this chapter. They are add-on, zero-based, and cost-based. These distinctions between various types, systems, and techniques often become blurred, since an institution will tend to develop its own terminology and will often mix systems or modify a single concept to suit its own particular needs. Although terminology and definitions differ considerably from one institution to another, once the ideas behind a particular term are grasped, the basic concepts can be identified no matter what label is applied.

Figure 13-1
Funding Equivalents: Volunteer Staffing

Task	Contributed Hours		Position Level of Task	Hourly Rate & Benefits	F.T.E. (Based on 2080 hrs./yr.)	Equivalent Staff Value	
	Monthly	Yearly				Monthly	Yearly
Tally statistics	4	48	2	$6	.023	$ 24	$ 288
Photocopying	8	96	1	$4	.046	$ 32	$ 384
Binding preparation	4	48	3	$7	.023	$ 28	$ 336
Volunteer bookcart	40	480	1	$4	.231	$160	$1,920
Circulation desk	80	960	1	$4	.462	$320	$3,840
Inventory	—	50	1	$4	.024	—	$ 200
Inventory	—	30	3	$7	.014	—	$ 210
TOTALS	136	1,712		**TOTALS**	.823		$7,178

Figure 13:2
Funding Equivalents: Cooperative Services and Gifts

Service	Yearly Quantity	Purchase Price and Cost of In-House Equivalents	
		Unit Price	Total
Interlibrary Loan	160 loans	$5	$800
Reference Referral	67 questions (20 hours)	$20/hr.	$400

Gift	Source	Value
Subscription: *Journal of Family Practice*	Dr. Smith	$ 15
Subscription: 2nd copy of *Journal of Nursing Administration*	Mrs. Jones	$ 20
Shelving: 6' x 3' x 1' used wooden section for reference	John Doe	$250

Types of Budgets

An institution's budgets are usually divided according to the type of expense being considered, most commonly operating expenses, personnel, and capital equipment. A department or subdepartment head prepares a budget for each of these and forwards them through an administrative cycle, where common organizational guidelines are imposed, to the top administrative levels of the institution. The department manager's role in setting levels of future expenses and monitoring current expenses may differ for each of these budget types.

Operating Budget

The operating or expense budget typically includes amounts allotted for such items as office supplies, minor equipment, books, journals, audiovisuals, telephone, postage, continuing education, travel, and various contractual expenses. The departmental manager usually recommends the needed expense levels for departmental operation and is then responsible for keeping expenses within the final, approved amount. The number and kind of authorizations needed to spend budgeted money from operating funds depend on the institution. Each manager is responsible for learning what the approval channels are for various kinds of expenses within the operating budget.

Personnel Budget

The personnel budget includes all expenses associated with the staff of a department, including salaries; individual and institution-wide changes in compensation; and fixed costs for employee expenses such as retirement, insurance, vacation, sick time, and federal and state taxes. Personnel expenses also include overtime pay and extra compensation granted to employees working second and third shifts. Because these expenses vary depending on hours worked, managers commonly budget staff in terms of full-time equivalents (FTEs), at a specified job description or salary range.

3 clerks, each 20 hrs/wk = 1.5 FTE
1 librarian, 40 hrs/wk = 1.0 FTE
                        2.5 FTE

The departmental manager usually has little control over the dollar amount budgeted for existing staff, although he or she may be responsible for initiating proposals for changes in salary ranges. In some institutions, the departmental manager may be asked to compute estimates for personnel expenses for the next year, figuring in institutional increases, anticipated prorated merit increases, anticipated overtime and shift differential required, and fixed amounts for benefits and taxes. These calculations are always made at some level in the institution; a librarian who does not directly participate in computing them should consider asking to see the breakdowns.

The departmental manager may also to some extent monitor personnel expenses during the year. Although usually little can be done directly to reduce fixed personnel expenses, adjustments can sometimes be made in overtime scheduling or in the scheduling of part-time staff. If the manager concludes that actual personnel expenses will exceed the budgeted amount, then the manager should discuss the situation with his or her supervisor, since the action taken will vary with the circumstances.

Personnel budgeting, so far, has been discussed in terms of existing staff. A departmental manager is also responsible for determining and documenting when additional positions are required, and for submitting the request for additional positions through established channels. Chapter 14 discusses requests for additional staff positions in more detail. Because personnel decisions involve long-lasting commitments for the hospital, these decisions are made at the administrative level, based on information provided by the requesting department. In general, administrators react more favorably to requests for operating money than to requests for staff.

Capital Equipment Budget

The capital equipment budget typically includes all items that will cost more than a specified amount and that will last more than a specified number of years. For example, capital equipment may be defined as anything that costs more than $500 and that will last more than three years. These limits vary among institutions, so departmental managers must determine the definition used in their institutions. Typically, capital equipment includes office and library furniture, machines such as typewriters and computer terminals, and some audiovisual equipment. Managers are usually asked to submit their documented capital equipment requests well in advance of actual need so that the capital equipment expenses for the institution can be systematically planned. Many state planning agencies require submission of three years of anticipated capital budgets from hospitals.

Systems for Budgeting

A budgeting system can be loosely defined as the framework that the hospital chooses to use for presenting budgetary information. Almost always one system is used for all departments throughout a hospital. A librarian beginning a new job should learn as much as possible about the system used in the hospital before the time for budget preparation arrives.

Typical budgeting systems include:

• *Lump sum.* A specified dollar amount is budgeted for each major category of expenditure, or in some cases, for each department (Figure 13-3).
• *Line item or object of expenditure.* Each item or category that is expected to be purchased is identified along with its anticipated cost (Figure 13-3).

Figure 13-3
Lump Sum and Line Item Budgets

Simple Lump Sum		Expanded Lump Sum or Simple Line		Expanded Line		
Personnel related	$10,000	Salaries	$9,100	**Supplies**		
Library materials	5,000	Social Security	800	4 reams paper	$	25
Contractual services	3,000	Books	2,000	Glue		8
TOTAL EXPENSES	$18,000	Clerical supplies	200	Covers		52
		Journals	3,000	Staples		26
		Audiovisuals	500	Pencils		13
Revenue offset	-5,000	Minor equipment	200	Tissues		16
DEPARTMENT BUDGET	$13,000	Phone	300		$	140
		Maintenance and parts	200			
		Film and equipment rental	500	**Dues**		
				Medical Library		
		Travel and continuing		Association	$	50
		education	500			
		Special services	2,000	**Books**		
		Revenue offset	-5,000	Nursing	$	640
			$14,300	Neurology		200
				Cardiology		150
				Radiology		200
				General		400
				Management		150
						$1,740

• *Unit performance or formula.* The number of anticipated units of service or materials is multiplied by the unit cost of such services or materials (Figure 13-4).

• *Program or matrix.* Many variations of this concept exist, including Program Planning and Budgeting System (PPBS) and zero-based budgeting. Program budgets identify subprograms within a department and then within those programs further define various levels of service. For each level of service, the resources required to achieve the stated objectives are specified. In the budget review the organization considers these programs on a level-by-level, service-by-service basis. This allows specific services, rather than entire departments, to be identified for support (Figure 13-5).

• *Grant budgets.* Proposals or budgets prepared specifically for grant opportunities fall outside of the normal organizational scope. Grant budgets should reflect the particular preferences of the granting agencies and must adhere rigidly to the agency's requirements. Such budgets often include amounts for contributed items, in order to demonstrate what an institution will be contributing as well as what is expected from the granting agency.

Figure 13-4
Formula Budgeting

Medline [Special Services]			Cost
17 searches per mo. x 12 mo.			
$7.50 avg. cost		=	$1,530
Film Rentals			
10 per mo. x 12 mo. $25.00 avg. cost		=	$3,000
Books			
150 nursing books	$25.00 avg. cost	=	3,750
200 medical books	$52.00 avg. cost	=	10,400
150 general books	$17.00 avg. cost	=	2,550
30 reference books	$100.00 avg. cost	=	3,000
			$19,700

Figure 13-5
Program Budget

Expense	Circulation	Book and Journal Collection	Reference	AV	Processing	Management
Salaries	5,000	12,000	3,000	8,000	5,000	8,000
Supplies	50	50	500	250	500	50
Books	0	16,100	100	100	0	100
Phone	100	100	500	200	0	200
Equipment	0	50	0	300	150	0
Dues	0	0	0	0	0	500
Journals	0	13,000	500	500	0	0
Audiovisual	0	0	0	14,000	0	0
Special services	0	0	1,280	0	0	0
Film/Equip. rental	0	0	0	2,500	0	0
Travel/Cont. ed.	0	250	250	250	0	250
Other	100	100	100	100	100	100
Subtotal	5,250	41,650	6,230	26,200	5,750	9,200
Revenue offset	2,720	0	1,280	0	0	0
Total	2,530	41,650	4,950	26,200	5,750	9,200

No. of circulations / No. of hours open / Annual inventory / % Collection review/yr — No. of subscriptions / No. of new books / No. of uses — No. of ref. searches / No. reader assists — No. of new programs / Delivery services / Production of slides and transparencies — No. materials processed / No. repaired, discarded — Staffing / Evaluations / Reporting / Procedures / Goals / Public relations

Examples of terms to help relate program objectives and activities to budget.

The budgeting system each institution chooses will reflect its own philosophy and management style. As institutions vary widely, so do budgeting systems. Ways in which budgeting systems differ include:

- Aspects of performance highlighted
- Control or flexibility
- Emphasis on function or program
- Amount of creativity allowed
- Level at which decisions can be made
- Length of budget process and time required
- Involvement by departmental manager
- Time required to prepare budget

The syllabus for the Medical Library Association's continuing education course on budgeting, listed at the end of the chapter, contains a good discussion of the advantages and disadvantages of various budgeting systems.

Techniques for Budgeting

Budget figures can be determined by using one of a number of different techniques. Each institution usually indicates the technique it requires or prefers. In reality none of these techniques exists in isolation. A good manager uses the method appropriate for each account and situation.

Add-on Method

The most common budget technique is the add-on method. Using this technique, the department manager reviews last year's expenditures, determines specific changes in needs and priorities, and then adds or subtracts a percentage or flat dollar amount from the previous year's base level to provide a budget figure for the coming year.

Add-on

This year	=	$1,000
Inflation at 10%	=	100
		$1,100
Growth at 10%	=	110
Next year	=	$1,210

Zero-based

Reference services this year	=	$1,000
Next year, cut to basic reference collection only	=	800
Next year, same level, services	=	1,100
Next year, searching on new database	=	1,500

Zero-based, with Decision Packages

A second common technique, which has been popular in recent years, is zero-based budgeting. Theoretically, each category begins at a level of zero, and the budget preparer individually tabulates all expenses to come up with an overall amount for the coming year. Decision packages are components of zero-based systems. Such packages include a brief description of a service, what is provided, why, and how much it will cost. A budget using this technique usually presents three packages for each service: (1) one that would be funded at about 80 percent of the current budget or less, (2) one at the same level plus inflation, and (3) one showing how additional money would be used. The librarian then ranks all packages for all services and allocates the money until it is depleted.

Decision packages help to summarize each activity and its cost. In theory, this budgeting process should encourage the library to be flexible in the selection of services offered. In reality, zero-based budgeting tends to protect existing services at the expense of innovative or creative projects. However, use of the decision package method can help gain psychological and financial support for change, since often the only way to start something new is to eliminate something old.

Cost-based

Cost-based budgeting, often used in combination with add-on or zero-based budgeting, involves determining the cost of a particular unit of service and then deciding how many units of service will be provided. For example, if providing one page of interlibrary loan material costs

Figure 13-6
Generalized Budgeting Process

Process	Actions	Done By
Information gathering	Identify institutional objectives Identify goals/needs for coming year	Department
Preparation	Determine levels of activity desirable for next year Evaluate feasibility: preliminary determination Calculate costs of activity Evaluate feasibility Obtain informal administrative review of plans Prepare request Prepare justification	
Review and preliminary approval	Review all requests Adjust to conform to institution-wide guidelines Prepare hospital-wide budget	Administration
Approval	Review hospital-wide budget Approve a level of spending for coming year	Board
Adjustment	Reassess plans to spend amended allocation Report consequences	Department

seven cents and 1,000 pages of interlibrary loan material will be required during the coming year, then $70 needs to be budgeted for this particular activity.

THE BUDGETING PROCESS

The process of preparing the actual budget will differ from one institution to another. A summary of a typical process is given in Figure 13-6. Because details of the process vary so widely, this section of the chapter will focus on planning and on the resources available to muster support for library activities.

Pre-budget Planning

The librarian should always work on the budget in the context of planning for services. The librarian should review institutional and departmental goals and note any changes in the library's focus. Budgeting is the art of making intelligent guesses about the costs required to meet program needs during a fixed period of time. For this reason, the planning component of the budget is critical. Chapter 12 discusses planning in detail. Some questions that might be used to guide budget preparation are:

- What have recent assessments of needs shown?
- What resources are necessary to meet recent needs?
- What new services or programs is the library planning?
- Are there new programs within the institution that have created new user groups?
- Is the library expanding services to previously unserved groups?
- Is the library expanding into new subject areas?
- What special circumstances will affect next year's operation?

Information for Budgeting

Before beginning budget preparations, the librarian should make an effort to collect all the information needed. Reports, market predictions, and institution and association guidelines will all help the librarian to determine the amounts to be allotted under specific entries and to justify those amounts.

Reports and Statistics

The librarian will find a variety of institutional and departmental summaries useful in preparing a budget. First among these is the institution's statement of goals for the coming year, as well as the library's own statement of departmental goals.

The budget preparer will also wish to consider all formal information given to the administration during the year, including reports on services, proposed programs, levels of interest, results of needs assessments, and accreditation results. Review of these documents will ensure that all communications with the administration are consistent with one another.

Statistics on library services for the current year to date and for the two previous years will help document trends or changes in services. The previous year's budget, internal expense records kept by the library, and financial reports distributed by the administration will be useful in tracking individual expenses, errors, and fluctuations.

Published Price Data and Predictions

Current reports from publications such as *Library Journal* and *Publishers Weekly* that analyze and predict book, journal, and audiovisual prices give credibility to estimates presented in the library budget. In February or March each year *Publishers Weekly* prints a report on the book publishing industry. Their report includes the average cost of medical hardback books, of medical trade paperbacks, and of all books for the last few years. A comparable report for periodicals appears in a summer issue of *Library Journal,* which also carries similar information on audiovisual materials. Occasionally articles in other journals can be found that document price increases. Citations of some recent articles with price information appear in the reading list at the end of the chapter; however, librarians will need to update the list for the coming year. Although data from the literature may be several months old, the librarian will find it useful for identifying inflation factors, which may be much higher than increases for normal clerical supplies, forms, or other types of hospital printed materials.

Institution and Association Guidelines

Most institutions provide managers with timetables for budget preparation, as well as specific instructions, forms, and inflation factor guidelines. Professional library standards, such as those issued by the JCAH, may prove useful in obtaining budget support. The librarian may be able to justify requests for new services, staff, or materials by referring to professional guidelines. In any case, the librarian should review such standards to make certain that the library service meets the criteria.

Miscellaneous Information

Other sources that might be utilized to prepare the budget or to influence its acceptance include special projects, special gifts, income estimates, request records, local or regional library survey information, and informal information. State library organizations, vendors, and core collection lists are additional sources for data. Local surveys among other libraries and data from comparable institutions are also effective in communicating the needs and normal costs of a library.

Other Departments' Requests

The librarian may find it useful to know what other departments are requesting or expecting, particularly in related accounts such as continuing education, travel, and telephone expenses. Developing good relations with other department heads and with financial management personnel can prove especially valuable at budget time.

Library Budget Categories

The budget categories, or accounts, depend upon the system used by the institution. Once established they usually require a long, formal process in order to be modified. If the librarian feels that the existing accounts do not allow library expenses to be recorded in useful ways, then he or she should discuss the problem with the hospital finance officer well in advance of budget time. If the library is new and no accounts exist for library materials, the librarian may be able to specify separate book, journal, binding, and audiovisual accounts. Sometimes, however, hospitals will not require such precise distinctions among these types of expenses, and the department manager must work within more general categories. More specific records can then be maintained within the library.

Some common accounts include:

- Books
- Audiovisual materials
- Dues
- Subscriptions
- Supplies
- Telephone expenses
- Postage
- Printing
- Rental
- Equipment repair
- Reimbursement
- Minor equipment
- Contractual services, such as binding, online contracts, cataloging, and maintenance contracts

Frequently categories can be combined into a single account. The librarian must clearly understand what is included by convention as well as by definition.

Sometimes library expenses are not kept separately but are included with the expenses of another department. In that case, the librarian may wish to learn which accounts are used and to keep a parallel internal record of the library's expenses, even though the hospital does not require it.

Estimating Current Expenses

The first step in estimating budget levels for the coming year is to analyze spending for the current year. Budgets for the year ahead are usually prepared around the middle of the current fiscal year, so the full current year's data is not available. The librarian must use the spending levels of the year to date (YTD) to determine whether the amount budgeted for the year will meet the department's needs. If spending is likely to be spread evenly throughout the year, the year's estimated expenses can be calculated by dividing the expenses to date by the number of

months to date and multiplying by 12:

$$\frac{\text{YTD expenses}}{\text{Number of months to date}} \times 12 = \begin{array}{l}\text{estimated current} \\ \text{year's expenses}\end{array}$$

If spending is not steady throughout the year, as would be the case in the account for journals, a more accurate estimate can be obtained by adding estimated costs of anticipated items to YTD expenses.

Journals, YTD	$3,200
Estimated increases	50
Estimated new subscriptions	100
Estimated current year's expenses for journals	$3,350

If the estimate of the year's expenses is more than the amount budgeted, the librarian must make a further analysis to determine why. Is the spending pattern for this item irregular? Was last year's figure too low or were expenses unusually high? Is this year's spending pattern the same as or different from patterns in previous years? By understanding the present situation in each account the librarian can better predict what will occur in the future.

Estimating Expenses for Next Year by Accounts

The best approach to use in setting the levels needed for the next year varies with different accounts, as well as with the system and techniques used. The following discussion of the major library accounts is based on a modified line-item expense budget.

Books

Figuring next year's budget using the add-on method is fairly straightforward. Each institution preselects the add-on percentage, or the librarian recommends one based on the predicted increase in book prices. Nevertheless, the librarian may wish to look at last year's expenses and predict next year's expenses in more detail. The librarian may use such calculations to determine needed budgetary levels, to show the inadequacy of current levels, or to show what can be done at given levels of funding. Useful figures for calculating budgets include:

- Average cost per book (Figure 13-7)
- Number of books purchased (Figure 13-8)
- Number of purchases by category or subject specialty
- Estimates of costs for purchasing new editions of titles already owned

The average cost per book can be determined from published sources or by estimating from departmental purchasing records (Figure 13-7). In some instances the librarian may find it useful to calculate the number of

Figure 13-7
Average Cost Per Book

To figure the average cost per book for the previous year, use:

$$\frac{\text{Amount spent}}{\text{Number of books}} \qquad \frac{\$\,2,700}{100} = \$27$$

To figure the average cost per book for the year-to-date, use:

$$\frac{\text{Amount spent YTD}}{\text{Books purchased YTD}} \qquad \frac{\$\,2,900}{100} = \$29$$

To estimate the average cost per book for next year, use:

(Average cost YTD x Inflation factor) + Average cost YTD

($29 x 10%) + $29 = $31.90

books purchased and the percentage of the total budget this represents: as a total and by category (Figures 13-8 and 13-9).

The librarian may wish to have an estimate of the percentage of the book budget required solely to maintain the current collection; that is, to buy new editions of titles already owned. That figure will allow the librarian to differentiate between maintenance and growth requirements and to calculate the amount remaining for purchase of new titles. This can be a powerful illustration to others of the costs required to maintain a library. To provide an accurate prediction, the librarian should base the estimate on the percentage of the budget spent on later editions over a period of years.

Some possible justifications to support title requests include:

- High numbers of interlibrary loan requests and costs in certain subject areas
- Low percentages of total collection published within the last five years, this figure is part of the documentation required for the JCAH survey
- Under-representation of hospital program areas in the library collection
- New student affiliation programs
- The number of new titles requested each year, perhaps listed by subject specialty
- Results of a structured departmental review of the collection (recommended by JCAH) or other needs assessments
- Specialty areas assigned as part of a cooperative acquisition program

Journals

The budget formula for journals can be estimated as follows:

| Cost of last year's subscriptions | — | cost of titles canceled | + | cost of titles added | × | inflation factor | = | Estimated cost of next year's subscriptions |

Estimating accurately the amount that journal prices will increase is very important because only salaries represent a larger share of most library budgets than do journal subscriptions. As mentioned earlier, some hospitals

Figure 13-8
Purchasing Potential

To estimate the number of books to be purchased during the current year, figure:

$$\frac{\text{This year's budget}}{\text{YTD average cost}} \qquad \frac{\$\,5,800}{29} = 200 \text{ books}$$

To estimate the number of books to be purchased next year, figure:

$$\frac{\text{Requested budget}}{\text{Estimated avg. cost next year}} \qquad \frac{\$\,6,280}{31.90} = 200 \text{ books}$$

To calculate the cost of acquiring a given number of titles, figure:

Needed titles x Estimated avg. cost next year
200 x $31.90 = $6,280.00

Figure 13-9
Comparison: Cost-Quantity-Use

Area	Budgeted Dollars for 1980	Number of Books Purchased in 1980	Average Cost per Book	Number of Uses
Medical	$ 5,000	100	$ 50	390
Nursing	4,000	200	20	650
Management	1,000	40	25	40
Support services	2,000	100	20	200
Reference	1,000	14	71	70
	$ 13,000	454	$ 29	1,350

Area	Percentage of Total Book Budget	Percentage of Total Number Acquired	Percentage of Total Use
Medical	38%	22%	29%
Nursing	31%	44%	48%
Management	8%	9%	3%
Support services	15%	22%	15%
Reference	8%	3%	5%

determine a set inflation factor to be used uniformly throughout the hospital unless a higher rate can be justified because of special circumstances. Although the librarian may wish to accept the standard rate in other accounts, he or she should be certain that this rate is not lower than the predicted estimates for journal inflation. The librarian should provide specific documentation from the literature to support a request for a higher rate. Sources for predictive data have already been referred to. Articles listed at the end of the chapter document journal inflation rates in past years.

Justifications for journal budgets can be divided into two categories: support for continuing existing subscriptions and advocacy for new ones. Usage statistics are the most compelling argument for current subscriptions. When the librarian anticipates difficulty in obtaining approval to renew an existing list, then he or she may want to keep detailed records of the following types of journal use:

- Circulation, bound and unbound
- Room use (easiest to record as journals are being shelved)
- Photocopy use
- Reference use by staff

In other situations, circulation statistics coupled with subjective observations for the other categories may be sufficient to obtain approval. The librarian can calculate the cost per use for each title, either using data from the previous full year or estimating for the current year (Figure 13-10).

Comparing the cost of the subscription with alternative ways of supplying the material allows the librarian to show the costs of interlibrary loan and at the same time point out other considerations, such as the value of timely accessibility. For such a comparison the librarian can use either the actual cost or an average or estimate of true interlibrary loan costs. Justification of new titles should include the requester, the projected user groups and levels of use, any interlibrary loan statistics, the cost per use of supplying that particular title through interlibrary loan or cooperative arrangements, and the impact of copyright limitations.

Supplies

After identifying the type and quantity of library supplies used during a year, the librarian can accurately figure a supply budget using the add-on method. Most hospitals recommend a percentage increase for office supplies. This same figure is normally adequate for library supplies.

The list of supplies needed can be used from year to year and can serve as an aid for timely ordering of supplies as well as for budgeting. Typical headings for a supply list appear below:

Type of supply	Usage rate	Yearly quantity	Cost
ILL forms	50/month	650	——
Date due slips	100/month	1200	——
Typewriter ribbons	2/month	24	——

If use increases or if experience shows that the estimate is inaccurate, the list of supplies should reflect that change. Otherwise the list loses its effectiveness as a planning tool.

Continuing Education and Travel

When preparing a travel budget, the librarian should be thoroughly familiar with the institution's policies and guidelines on travel as well as the practice of other departments. The librarian should discuss travel and educational needs as they relate to the library's program objectives with the administration prior to budget time, so that the budget request will be seen in an operational context.

The travel and education budget should be based on specific meetings or conferences and on an estimate of actual expenses. Typical expenses allowed are travel (airfare or mileage), transportation to and from airports, parking, lodging, meals, and registration fees. Most institutions have specific rules governing reimbursable expenses. Justification for travel expenses should include the titles and dates of the meeting, who will attend, the need for attendance, and the program of the meeting or description of the course.

Personnel

The financial office will usually compute the specific amounts for salaries and related personnel expenses. The major responsibility of the departmental manager is to make sure that the administration understands staffing requirements for the library. The information required to justify both new and existing positions varies from institution to institution. Justifying new positions is discussed further in Chapter 14.

New Services

Most librarians find budgeting for new services difficult because no historical data is available. Success in this situation depends on carefully considering the project and trying to anticipate all possible costs, including staff time and actual cash. Project planning layouts and decision packages can be useful. The librarian should discuss thoroughly proposals for new services with the administration, and perhaps the budget committee or budget officers, before the budget is presented so that they will be anticipating the new proposal.

Preparing the Final Budget

When the budget is ready to be submitted, the librarian should take a thorough look at the recommendations as a whole. Do they seem reasonable? Can each item in the budget be explained and justified? Is anything missing? At this point some managers routinely add 5 percent for "miscellaneous," spreading it throughout the budget. Although a hedge against a routine cut should not be necessary, managers should be aware that the practice does exist.

MONITORING THE BUDGET

As important as the planning aspect of the budgeting process, but less complex, are the control and review of financial activities. If the benefits and not just the efforts of budgeting are to appear, these activities must take place throughout the year. Financial reports generated by the hospital indicating the status of each department's budget are usually regularly available for analysis. The department manager must make adjustments whenever

Figure 13-10
Journal Usage Costs

To figure the cost per use last year, calculate:

$$\frac{\text{Cost of Subscription} + \text{Cost of Binding and Processing}}{\text{Number of Uses}}$$

To figure the cost of borrowing from other libraries last year,

first calculate the cost of labor for last year's interlibrary loans:

$$\left(\frac{\frac{\text{Avg. ILL Processing Time (minutes)}}{\times \text{ No. of Borrows}}}{60}\right) \times \begin{array}{l}\text{Hourly rate}\\\text{for librarian}\end{array}$$

then caluclate the total cost of borrowing:

$$\frac{\text{Cost of Labor} + \text{Total Yearly Fees for ILL}}{\text{No. of Borrows}}$$

To figure the estimated cost per use for the current year, calculate:

$$\frac{\text{Cost of Subscription} + \text{Cost of Binding and Processing}}{\left(\frac{\text{Number of Uses YTD}}{\text{Number of Months YTD}} \times 12\right)}$$

Figure 13-11
Monthly Financial Report: Sample

Health Science Library Monthly Financial Report   February 28, 1982

| | February 1982 | | | February 1981 | |
Description	Monthly Budget 1982	Monthly Actual 1982	Percent OV/UN- Budget	Actual 1981	Percent OV/UN- 1981
Unclassified Salaries	$3,229	$3,431	6.2	$1,855	84.9
Social Security Taxes	188	191	1.5	118	61.8
TOTAL EMPLOYEE BENEFITS	3,417	3,622	6.0	1,973	83.6
Instruments			0.0		0.0
Processing Supplies	38		100.0-		0.0
Clerical Supplies	148	57	61.4	346	83.5-
Printed Materials	2,489	3,495	40.4	3,119	12.0
Linen and Uniforms	1	2	100.0	1	100.0
Maintenance & Parts	12	10	16.6-		0.0
Minor Equipment	100	231	131.0		0.0
Sundry Other	12		100.0-	178	100.0-
TOTAL SUPPLIES	2,800	3,795	35.5	3,644	4.1
Purchased Maintenance	8		100.0-		0.0
Telephone & Telegraph	6	4	33.3-	2	100.0
Dues & Tuition	19		100.0-		0.0
Postage & Freight	4	15	275.0	28	46.4-
Equipment Rental	20	18	10.0-		0.0
Other Purchased Services			0.0-		0.0-
TOTAL PURCHASED SERVICES	57	37	35.1-	30	23.3
Travel Expense	15		100.0-		0.0-
Continuous Education	46	80	73.9		0.0-
Miscellaneous Expense	2		100.0-		0.0-
Revenue—Offset	250-	269-	7.6		0.0-
TOTAL MISCELLANEOUS	187-	189-	1.1	0	0.0-
DEPARTMENT TOTAL	$6,087	$7,265	19.3	$5,647	28.6

expenses exceed the budget. Awareness of opportunities, potential problems, and planning for the next budget cycle must begin almost as soon as the current budget is implemented.

Analysis

The department manager should review financial reports plus internal departmental records to assess spending patterns and to spot problem areas. Many managers construct monthly budgets allocating spending throughout the year in order to create meaningful benchmarks and to spot problems quickly. For spending that occurs at a regular rate throughout the year, monthly budgets can be determined by using one-twelfth of the annual figure. For irregular expenses such as calendar year subscription renewals, yearly budgets must be divided by allocating specific, varying amounts to each month.

However the monthly spending estimate is established, it should be compared with actual expenses. If actual expenses are less than the amount budgeted, a positive variance exists. If expenses exceed the monthly budget, a negative variance exists. By recording variances each month, the manager can quickly spot areas of potential trouble at the year's end. A typical monthly worksheet for monitoring expenses appears in Figure 13-11.

By using a monthly worksheet, the department manager can spot when a possibility for exceeding the budget exists. Negative variances should be watched closely. Any unusual variance, positive or negative, which is either large or continues over several months should be explainable, though not necessarily justifiable. Are costs per item higher than anticipated? Is the need for services exceeding the estimate? Have there been unanticipated changes in program or goals?

Because the library's budget is usually small, the library may be allowed a 5 or 10 percent variance, whereas the hospital as a whole can tolerate only a 1 percent variance (10 percent of $10,000 = $1,000; 1 percent of $1,000,000 = $10,000). Since each institution has its own policies, each librarian must identify and conform to local requirements.

Adjustments

As soon as a problem is detected or anticipated, the department manager must report it to the administration, along with a clear explanation and a suggested solution or response. No department head should ever report a budgetary problem without having facts clearly in mind and a plan for action ready to present. Both the explanation for the problem and the solution that is finally agreed upon should be documented.

When expenses must be reduced, a quick and simple solution is to cut all accounts by a fixed percentage. Yet the impact of limited funds can be lessened if each ac-count is carefully analyzed and cuts are related to services and needs. The librarian should assess the cost of each service, the value of that service to the institution, and the impact of restricting or eliminating it, as well as the possibility of locating alternate funding for it. Possible funding sources have been mentioned earlier. Charge-back systems, or allocating costs of services to those departments that use them, can be effective if the library has little control over usage rates. Charge-back systems are also effective if the services are of higher value to specific areas than they are to either the institution as a whole or to the library. The use of photocopy machines and transparency supplies are just two examples of types of costs often charged back to user departments. The librarian should decide if the cost can now be controlled, if the expense can be postponed, or if money budgeted for other purposes can be substituted. Are there ways to share, borrow, rent, or do without? Can income be obtained from another source? The librarian should try to assess needs and organizational objectives in order to clearly identify essential services and distinguish them from nonessential services. When budgets must be cut, it is necessary to be creative.

The goal of financial planning and control is the stability of quality library service. With practice and a clear grasp of objectives and responsibilities, a manager can learn to use budgeting as a tool toward this end.

READINGS

Alley B, Cargill J. Keeping track of what you spend: the librarian's guide to simple bookkeeping. Phoenix: Oryx Press, 1982.

Berman HW, Weeks LE. The financial management of hospitals. 5th ed. Oakbrook, IL: Health Administration Press, 1981.

Brown NB, Phillips J. Price indexes for 1982: U.S. periodicals and serial services. Libr J 1982 Aug;107:1379-1382.

Chen C. Zero-base budgeting in library management: a manual for librarians. Phoenix: Oryx Press, 1980.

Evans GE. Finance. In: Evans GE. Management techniques for librarians. 2d. New York: Academic Press, 1982.

Flandorf VS. Managing the library. In: Bloomquist H, Rees AM, Stearns NS, Yast H, eds. Library practice in hospitals: a basic guide. Cleveland: Case Western Reserve, 1972.

Gillespie JT. Budget. In: Gillespie JT, Spirt DL. Creating a school media program. New York: RR Bowker, 1973.

Grannis CB. Title output and average prices. 1982 preliminary figures. Publisher's Weekly 1983 Mar 11;223:44-47.

Hicks WB. Budget management. In: Hicks WB, Tillin AM. Managing multimedia libraries. New York: RR Bowker, 1977.

Kiritz NJ. Program planning & proposal writing. Expanded ed. (Reprinted from Granstmanship Center News 1979 May-June;33-79.) Los Angeles: Grantsmanship Center, 1979.

Koenig M. Budgeting techniques for libraries and information centers. New York: Special Libraries Association, 1980. (Professional Development Series, vol. 1)

Koenig M. Budgets and budgeting, Part II. Spec Libr 1977 July-Aug;68: 234-240.

Kok J. "Now that I'm in charge, what do I do?": Six rules about running a special library for the new library manager. Spec Libr 1980 Dec;71(12):523-528.

Lancaster FW. Cost-performance-benefits considerations. In: Lancaster FW. The measurement and evaluation of library services. Washington, DC: Information Resources Press, 1977.

Loucks C. Budgeting. Chicago: Medical Library Association, 1981. (MLA courses for continuing education; CE 246).

Mosher FC. The study of budgeting. In: Wasserman P, Bundy ML, eds. Reader in library administration. Washington, DC: Micro-Card Editions, 1968.

Prentice AE. Budgeting. In: McClure CR, Samuels AR. Strategies for library administration: concepts and approaches. Littleton, CO: Libraries Unlimited.

Randall GE. Budgeting for libraries. Spec Libr 1976 Jan;67(1): 8-12.

Sargent CW. Zero-base budgeting and the library. Bull Med Libr Assoc 1978 Jan;66(1):31-35.

Thompson JA, Kronenfeld MR. The effect of inflation on the cost of journals on the Brandon list. Bull Med Libr Assoc 1980;Jan;68:47-52.

Walch DB. Price index for non-print media. Libr J 1981 Feb 15;106: 432-433.

White HS. Cost-effectiveness and cost benefit determinations in special libraries. Spec Libr 1979 Apr;70(4):163-169.

Administration of Personnel

Lois Ann Colaianni
*Director, Health Sciences
Information Center*
Cedars-Sinai Medical Center
Los Angeles, California

*Currently:
Head, Biology Library
University of California
Berkeley, California

CHAPTER 14

Administration
of Personnel

Lois Ann Colaianni
*Director, Health Sciences
Information Center
Cedars-Sinai Medical Center
Los Angeles, California*

Appendixes

Figures

People are the most important resource of almost any organization. In large measure, the success of the hospital library depends on the staff's professional competence and attitude toward service. A competent staff that conveys a "go away—don't bother me" attitude is not likely to serve patrons well. A friendly, but incompetent staff may be a social success but will not provide library services in the most effective manner. The purpose of the hospital library is to provide information for patient care, continuing education, management, and research. Thus it is essential that the staff be competent to build an appropriate collection, supplement existing resources with those in the Biomedical Communications Network, and develop an environment that will encourage the dissemination of information. This chapter will deal with hiring, supervising, and developing a staff capable of meeting the information needs of the hospital.

All but the smallest hospitals have a personnel or human resources department. Its staff can be a valuable resource to the hospital librarian. Another resource is the large quantity of literature on the subjects covered in this chapter. A selected bibliography on administration of personnel is given at the end of the chapter.

LIBRARY PERSONNEL

The professional library staff is often the smallest department in the hospital. If the hospital library has only one employee, it is recommended that this person be a qualified medical librarian. The Joint Commission on Accreditation of Hospitals (JCAH) defines a qualified medical librarian as " . . . an individual who holds a graduate degree in library science from a school accredited by the American Library Association, and who is certified by the Medical Library Association, or an individual who has documented equivalent training and/or experience"(1:148).

When it is not possible to employ a full-time or part-time qualified medical librarian, the JCAH standards stipulate that the hospital should secure the services of such an individual on a regular consulting basis. More information on consultants can be found in Chapter 18. Of course, larger hospitals or those with more complex information needs and services will require a larger library staff.

Types of Library Positions

Three types of personnel are commonly employed in hospital libraries. These include professional librarians, library assistants or technicians, and clerical staff. Within each general classification there may be several levels of personnel. For example, the clerical staff may include a clerk, clerk-typist, and senior clerk-typist. When there is more than one librarian, one is usually designated as a member of the hospital managerial staff and has the title of chief medical librarian or library director. Special services in some libraries may require the hiring of specialized personnel, such as messengers or audiovisual technicians.

Determining Staffing Needs

The staffing needs of the hospital library can be determined by deciding how many and what types of positions are needed. These decisions can be made based on the tasks that must be performed, how much time each takes, and how often each task will be performed.

Analyzing Tasks

Task analysis is the process of determining both the tasks that must be performed and the average time needed to complete each one. Formal task analysis is a complex activity that takes into account unproductive time, vacations and holidays, and time off for illness. However, the general principles of task analysis can be used to determine whether the library needs additional staff members.

After the librarian lists the tasks to be performed, he or she must determine the average time each takes. Unfortunately, there are no national standards for the average time needed to perform library tasks. The librarian can use sampling or averaging for this purpose. For example, the average time for checking in a journal can be obtained by selecting a few journals and timing how long it takes to process each one. Or the librarian may time how long it takes to check in journals on a particular day and divide by the number of journals processed. This process should be repeated several times to obtain a fairly accurate estimate. The times given in Figure 14-1 may be used as a guide, although they may vary in each library.

Analyzing Workloads

Staffing needs also depend on the library's current or potential workload. The librarian must consider the number of (1) items circulated, (2) items reshelved after room use, (3) interlibrary loans requested and filled, (4)

Figure 14-1
Average Time for Performing Hospital Library Tasks

Task	Length of Time
Checking materials out and in, and reshelving each library item	5 minutes
Processing an interlibrary loan	15 minutes
Compiling a bibliography (5 years of literature)	30 minutes
Ordering a book	10 minutes
Processing a book	30 minutes

reference questions answered, (5) bibliographies provided, (6) books and journals ordered, and (7) library materials processed. This information should come from the library's statistical records and should reflect any changes in the number of tasks actually performed.

Evaluating Needs

Once the librarian has completed the task and workload analyses, he or she can evaluate staffing needs. For example, it may take an average of 15 minutes to process an interlibrary loan. A library that requests 100 loans each month would require 25 hours of staff time to process those loans (100 loans × 15 minutes per loan = 1,500 minutes, or 25 hours). If the volume of interlibrary loans were to double in a year, 25 additional hours of staff time would be needed each month to handle the increase. Conversely, if the number of interlibrary loans were to decrease substantially or the time required to process each loan were reduced, less staff time would be needed for this activity.

When increases in certain library activities are identified, the librarian should analyze whether such increases are worth supporting with additional personnel. If the number of gifts were to double in one year, it might be better to control the number of gifts rather than to add personnel. If the number of literature searches were to increase substantially, acquiring in-house access to computerized database searching might be the best solution. Increased circulation of journals may reflect a need for a photocopy machine in the library.

Determining Type of Personnel Needed

If the librarian determines that additional staff members are necessary, the next step is to identify the type of personnel needed. This may be done by reviewing the tasks done each day and analyzing which tasks must be handled by a librarian and which can be handled by clerical personnel. For example, filing catalog cards is primarily a clerical task. The librarian, however, must choose the type of catalog and the subject headings that will be used. After determining whether the tasks to be performed by additional staff are primarily clerical or professional, the librarian can formulate a job description.

Writing Job Descriptions

A job description details the duties and responsibilities of the position and qualifications needed to obtain it. Both hiring activities and performance evaluations are based on the job description.

A job description should accurately reflect what a person must do to perform the job satisfactorily. Tasks should be appropriate to the position and should require similar levels of skill or training. The qualifications listed must be necessary for satisfactory job performance. For example, shorthand might be helpful for taking interlibrary loan requests over the telephone. However, the job of library assistant does not require shorthand. Also, a job description should not be so detailed that there is no room for flexibility.

When writing a job description, the librarian should use the list of tasks to be performed and any information supplied by the hospital's personnel department as primary resources. Sample job descriptions from other hospitals or from textbooks can be secondary resources. The information usually included in a job description is listed below.

* Job title, classification, and code
* Summary of the key responsibilities of the job
* Major work activities, including how frequently each is to be performed
* Name of supervisor
* Supervisory responsibilities, if any
* Qualifications for the position, including education, training, and experience
* Special skills needed
* Statement of the contact required with various groups, including patients, the public, and physicians
* Description of any additional job responsibilities

Sample job descriptions for a librarian and a library assistant are found in Appendixes A and B. The United States Training and Employment Service is in the process of revising its 1970 job descriptions of hospital employees, including librarians (2).

Obtaining Approval for a New Position

Obtaining approval from the hospital administration for a new position in the library depends on a number of factors, but primarily on the availability of money. In most cases, a new position implies a financial commitment for an indefinite period of time. The hospital must consider the cost of the new employee's salary and fringe benefits. Unemployment benefits or workers' compensation payments are also a potential expense. Recently the number of new positions created in hospitals has come under the scrutiny of various regulatory bodies. Thus most hospitals not only have a limited amount of money for personnel costs but are often limited in the number of full-time equivalents (FTEs) that they may have. Positions involving patient care or revenue understandably take priority. Information services are valued, however, and most administrators will attempt to provide sufficient personnel to meet the information needs of the hospital, if those needs are documented.

HIRING NEW STAFF

With an approved job description and administrative approval to add or fill a position, the librarian is ready to begin the process of identifying qualified candidates and selecting a new staff member. The steps involved in this process are discussed below.

Recruiting

The first step is to contact the personnel department. Personnel practices vary, so the librarian should find out which hiring activities the personnel department will handle and which are the librarian's responsibility. Will the opening be advertised outside the hospital? Will advertisements be placed in newspapers and professional journals? Many hospitals require that an opening be advertised, while others feel that a two-week posting within the hospital is sufficient. Will announcements be placed in local educational institutions whose students or alumni might be potential applicants? Will the personnel department do screening interviews? What topics will they cover? Does the interviewer in personnel know which skills are needed for the position? Since interviewing takes time and costs money, résumés or applications can be screened, and the three or four best candidates can be invited for interviews.

A number of laws and executive orders affect hiring policies. Their purpose is to promote fairness in employment practices. The personnel department is an excellent source for current information on local, state, and federal requirements. Reviewing this information before interviewing applicants is often helpful.

The law states that employers shall not discriminate among applicants because of race, religion, color, age, national origin, or sex. Questions asked on written applications or during interviews should not elicit information that is not related to a bona fide occupational qualification. The interviewer should avoid asking questions about how an applicant would travel to and from work, or care for minor children. The applicant should not be asked about his or her marital status, other sources of income, or recreational activities. If an applicant is handicapped and the handicap would not interfere with job performance, the employer must not consider it when making the hiring decision. Often such information is volunteered in the interview. However, it must not be used when deciding among applicants, and it must not be solicited by the interviewer.

The issue of the validity of tests is often debated in personnel textbooks. The most common test given to library applicants is a typing test. It is sufficient to ask the applicant's typing speed and to indicate how much typing, if any, is required for the position.

Every librarian who has followed these employment practices only to have a new employee leave within a short time because of transportation problems, family commitments, or other problems, has experienced some frustration. However, it is a small price to pay for more equitable hiring practices. The employer should explain the job requirements to applicants and let them determine if they can fulfill them.

Interviewing

The process of evaluating the qualifications of applicants, both from written applications and from interviews, is time-consuming. It is vital, however, since a new staff member may have a tremendous impact on the library's services. Initial screening, based on the qualifications listed in the job description, will produce a group of several candidates to interview.

A job interview has two purposes: (1) to allow the applicant to determine if he or she can, and wants to, do the job, and (2) to allow the employer to assess the applicant's qualifications for successful performance of the job. Because the interview is such an important part of the selection process, the librarian should prepare for it well in advance.

Preparing for the Interview

The interviewer must have a clear idea of what tasks the new employee will perform on the job. The interviewer must also know the type of education and experience required and what kinds of training can be provided on the job.

A structured interview is recommended to make certain that all important points are covered with each candidate. Steps to follow include (1) greeting the applicant, (2) reviewing the application, (3) asking the prepared questions, and (4) discussing the job description and the salary. Each of these steps will be discussed separately below. By preparing in advance for each step, the librarian will be more comfortable during the interview and thus better able to assess the applicant's qualifications.

The list of questions to be asked of all candidates should be prepared in advance, typed with spaces between questions for recording notes, and duplicated so the same form can be used for each applicant. The questions should focus on the major tasks to be performed and should be phrased in such a way that applicants have to think and provide information about experiences they have had. They can also be asked how they would handle situations that may arise on the job. Sample questions are given below.

• If a patron is asking you a question and the telephone rings, what would you do? (How do applicants handle two or three tasks at once? How do they assign priorities?)
• What are some sources for verifying interlibrary loans? (Do applicants know the meaning of "verifying?" If not, do they ask? Do they cite sources for books and journal articles?)
• If a patron who received a bill for a long-overdue book says the book was returned and refuses to pay the bill, how would you handle the situation? (How do applicants enforce rules? When do they refer problems?)
• Describe how you would determine which tasks to accomplish each day and in what order. If there are too many things to do, how would you decide what is most important?
• What did you enjoy doing on your last job? What did you not enjoy doing?

Figure 14-2
Experience Table

Task	Frequency	Comment

Date _____ Applicant _____

Acquisitions:
    Did bibliographic checking _____
    Prepared order slips _____

Cataloging:
    Familiarized self with NLM classification _____
    Cataloged from copy _____
    Prepared card sets _____
    Filed card sets _____
    Labeled books _____

Circulation:
    Shelved materials _____
    Circulated materials _____
    Claimed overdues _____
    Billed for lost books _____
    Did shelf-reading _____

Equipment:
    Typewriter _____
    Mimeograph machine _____
    Tape recorder _____
    Videocassette player _____
    Slide-tape player _____
    Microfilm reader _____
    Photocopy machine _____
    Computer terminal _____

Interlibrary loan:
    Verified ILL _____
    Typed ILL _____

Journals:
    Checked in journals _____
    Claimed journals _____

Reference:
    Answered simple ref. questions _____
    Prepared bibliographies _____
    Answered phones _____
    Assisted patrons _____
    Operated MEDLINE _____

Other: _____
_____

Experience working in libraries: _____
_____
_____

• If a patron is looking for a book on stomach neoplasms by a particular author, how would you check to see if it were available in the library? What would you do if it were not?

An experience table like the one shown in Figure 14-2 can be useful for recording the applicant's experience in libraries. It should be prepared in advance and a copy made for use with each applicant. Although experience in all tasks is not required for each position, the table is useful in determining the extent of the applicant's library experience. It can be expanded to include more information on tasks related to the position being filled.

The librarian should also gather any materials to be given or shown to the applicant, such as a copy of the job description, the library service policy, or other library publications. The information that the personnel department will give the applicant concerning benefits should be determined so that the librarian can be prepared to provide any additional information.

Shortly before the candidate is due to arrive, the librarian should gather all the materials to be used during the interview. The candidate's application or résumé should be reviewed and any areas that need clarification or further discussion should be noted. Immediately before the interview, the librarian should arrange to have all calls and other interruptions held until the interview is complete.

Greeting the Applicant

The first step in the interviewing process is to put the applicant at ease. This may be done by explaining the format the interview will follow and encouraging the applicant to communicate freely. If the applicant arrives late and seems harried, the librarian might ask about any difficulties encountered, such as parking or bad weather conditions. The applicant will undoubtedly have some questions about the job even if only in regard to salary and hours. An explanation that there will be ample time for questions will reduce the applicant's anxiety. During this preliminary discussion, the librarian can assess the applicant's appearance, manner, method of self-expression and responsiveness.

Reviewing the Application

The next step is to discuss the applicant's work experience and education as presented in the application or résumé. If the applicant brings in these documents, the interviewer should take time to review them.

The discussion of the candidate's work experience should focus on type and level of employment, level of earnings, skills involved, length of time in previous jobs, and reasons for leaving. If the applicant has no work experience, the interviewer may ask about volunteer work or work with social or community groups. In addition to questions about the specific duties of each job,

questions such as the following are often useful.

• Which work experience did you like best? Least? Why?
• What qualities do you like best in a supervisor? Least?
• What are your career goals? How has each job helped in achieving those goals or modified them?
• How do you expect this job to help you achieve your goals?
• What life experiences have you had that might be useful preparation for this job?

When discussing the applicant's formal education, the interviewer should try to determine whether it is adequate for the requirements of the job. The applicant's ability to define and work toward goals and the level of achievement in course work relevant to the position are also important. Other types of educational experiences, such as workshops or continuing education courses, should also be considered. The interviewer might also ask the applicant how he or she approaches the task of learning about a new subject, such as personnel management or medical audiovisuals. Questions such as the following might also be asked.

• What subjects did you like best? Least? Why?
• What parts of your education do you expect to be relevant in this job?
• What are your future educational plans?

Asking the Prepared Questions

The type of questions to be asked was discussed in the section on preparing for the interview. The interviewer should note how the applicant handles different kinds of questions, and what the applicant does when he or she does not understand the question or cannot answer it. The way the applicant responds to questions may tell a great deal about his or her skills and thought processes.

Discussing the Job

The interviewer should show the applicant the job description and provide any additional information about the job or the hospital. It is best to be as candid as possible and not try to sell the job. Applicants are interested in information such as (1) salary, (2) kind and volume of work, (3) qualities the employer thinks are needed for success on the job, (4) type of supervision, and (5) any unusual rules and regulations. The librarian should also discuss hours, overtime, weekend work, any problems with handling patrons, and any special qualifications needed for the job. The applicant should be encouraged to ask questions or to comment on any training or life experiences that might prove useful on the job. The questions an applicant asks often indicate his or her level of interest in the job, knowledge of library functions, and degree of initiative.

Providing a Tour

Most applicants are curious about the prospective work environment. A tour of the library and part of the hospital is an appropriate way to end the interview. To allow the applicant to both ask questions about the interviewer and talk to another person who works in the hospital, someone other than the interviewer should conduct the tour. This person may also be given one or two questions to ask the applicant and may offer a second opinion when the selection decision is being made. Applicants should be told when the decision will be made and how they will be notified. Applicants should always be thanked for coming in and for their interest in the hospital.

Checking References

Useful information can be obtained by checking references. When possible, call the persons listed and review the applicant's employment in the organization. An assessment of the applicant's strengths and weaknesses may also be requested.

Evaluating Applicants

After interviewing the qualified applicants, the librarian must select the applicant to whom the job will be offered. Often one applicant will seem to be the obvious choice because of education, experience, and responses given during the interview. On other occasions, it is difficult to select among several candidates. In these cases, questions may be weighted and the answers scored. A method for doing so is described below.

The first step is to list the major areas of responsibility and assign a weight to each. The weight should be based on how important carrying out this responsibility is to successful performance of the job. The total of the weights is usually 100. If there are five major responsibilities or tasks, and they are all equal, the weight for each would be 20. Next, a raw score is assigned to each area. Usually ten is a good maximum score to use. Each candidate is scored in each area of responsibility based on information obtained in the interview and any reference checks. If, in your opinion, the candidate knows a great deal about processing interlibrary loans and has done it before, the score may be 9 or 10. If the candidate knows what an ILL form is and typed one once, the score may be 1. The raw score is multiplied by the weight for each task and a total weighted score obtained. A comparison of candidates' weighted scores should be used carefully, since such scores do not include all considerations. They do help to focus on job-related tasks. Figure 14-3 illustrates a comparison of candidates using weighted scores.

Orienting the New Employee

Careful preparation is needed to ensure that a new employee gets off to a good start. A general orientation

Figure 14-3
Weighted Comparison of Candidates

Area of Responsibility	Weight	Total Raw Pts. Possible	Total Weighted Pts. Possible	Candidate 1 Raw Score	Candidate 1 Weighted Score	Candidate 2 Raw Score	Candidate 2 Weighted Score
1. Answering telephones	10	10	100 (10 x 10)	5	5 x 10 = 50	5	5 x 10 = 50
2. Handling interlibrary loans	50	10	500 (50 x 10)	8	8 x 50 = 400	4	4 x 50 = 200
3. Staffing circulation desk	20	10	200 (20 x 10)	8	8 x 20 = 160	8	8 x 20 = 160
4. Filing	10	10	100 (10 x 10)	4	4 x 10 = 40	6	6 x 10 = 60
5. Photocopying articles	10	10	100 (10 x 10)	3	3 x 10 = 30	4	4 x 10 = 40
	100	50	1000	28	680	27	510

to the hospital and to the library's policies and procedures are essential. Using the job description, a checklist of tasks can be made, and dates on which the new employee should be reasonably competent at each task can be assigned. The librarian or other staff member will have to schedule training times for each task and possibly devise some practical ways to test the employee's newly acquired skills. If possible, the first few tasks the employee learns should enable the individual to begin working and contributing. A good procedure to follow is to have the employee read about a task, observe a staff member perform it, and then perform the task independently. Someone should always be available to answer questions or give assistance. A large amount of material to be assimilated in a short period of time is a source of frustration to most new employees, as is spending hours reading a procedure manual. Learning and working tasks should be alternated. Introducing the employee to patrons, employees from other departments, and hospital procedures can provide variety and make the employee feel more at home.

SUPERVISING PERSONNEL

Providing an environment in which employees can work together effectively takes time and thought. Fundamental to such an environment is a supervisor who is fair, empathetic, and focuses on competent job performance. Effective supervision also depends on the librarian's skill in the areas discussed below.

Communicating

Effective communication builds positive human relationships and is basic to any organization. Communication involves a sender, message, medium, and receiver. The sender must understand what is to be communicated. The message must be clearly stated in a manner the receiver is able to understand. It must also be communicated at the appropriate time. The medium used should be the most effective one for the message. Complex issues may be best communicated using several media. If the receiver does not understand the message, effective communication has not taken place. Chapter 15 discusses communication in more detail.

Motivating

Motivating people consists of getting them to do the work they are capable of doing. Setting an example is one way to motivate people. Some people are motivated by money. Others are motivated by job security, group acceptance, recognition, or their own sense of accomplishment. These motivating forces may change as a person's goals and values change. A successful supervisor makes an effort to determine what motivates each staff member. He or she attempts to motivate each employee to work as effectively as possible on an individual basis and also as a member of the library staff. Librarians working alone can determine what motivates them and can seek those rewards within the hospital or through professional associations.

Delegating

Management involves getting other people to accomplish certain tasks. Unless there is only one library employee, it will be necessary to delegate tasks. If the librarian delegates responsibility for sending out overdue notices, the employee and the librarian must both agree on how the task will be handled. They should discuss whether patrons will be contacted by telephone or mail, when the first notification and any follow-ups are to be made, and what exceptions the employee may allow. They must decide if an existing form will be used or if the employee may design a new one.

The limits of the employee's authority must be clearly defined. Most employees like to have responsibility for performing tasks and identify with tasks when they are done well. The supervisor's role is to provide the supplies, training, and encouragement necessary to do the job well while retaining ultimate responsibility for it. Librarians new to the supervisory role often do not delegate well. They are used to being rewarded for doing things, such as locating an obscure journal article or doing a literature search. Supervisors must learn to feel rewarded when their employees do jobs well.

Monitoring

An effective supervisor sets performance standards that indicate whether job responsibilities are being carried out effectively. If an employee is responsible for claiming missing journal issues within 30 days, the supervisor should periodicially check to see that timely claims are being made.

There are several ways of monitoring an employee's work. These include reviewing the quality of the product, consulting statistics on the volume of work done, and reviewing problems reported by the employee or others. Monitoring includes helping the employee correct problems promptly to avoid more serious difficulties later.

Appraising Performance

Employees need to know how well they are performing on the job and how to improve unsatisfactory performance. The supervisor should praise the employee when a task is done well. "You did an excellent job handling a very difficult patron. Offering the patron options was particularly good." Suggestions for improvement may be made just as spontaneously if offered in a helpful and constructive way. Many employees, however, prefer to hear suggestions privately. All lengthy discussions of performance problems should be conducted in private.

The annual performance appraisal is the time when the employee and supervisor meet to formally discuss job performance. A performance appraisal has four purposes: (1) to provide an evaluation of the employee's job performance since the last appraisal, (2) to review performance standards, (3) to set performance objectives for the coming year, and (4) to provide a basis for assigning a salary increase. Some supervisors also do informal career counseling and give employees an opportunity to suggest ways the supervisor might improve his or her performance.

A thorough performance appraisal takes approximately an hour. The supervisor and employee should agree on the time well in advance so each can prepare. The appraisal should focus on observable behavior and should result in positive motivation for the employee.

Most hospitals provide forms for performance evaluations. The supervisor should complete the form before the interview and be prepared to explain the ratings with examples. Some supervisors give the employee a blank copy of the form beforehand and ask the employee to think about his or her performance in each category.

The interview usually involves going through the appraisal form to identify areas of strength and weakness. Setting performance objectives is also a very important part of the interview.

The supervisor should work with the employee to set goals that are both realistic and measurable. The purpose of these objectives is to maintain or improve employee performance, or to allow the employee to assume additional responsibilities. Follow-up appraisals can be scheduled to determine if the employee is encountering any difficulty in meeting the objectives, and to help the individual if necessary. For example, the employee may be sending out interlibrary loan requests for items available in the collection. The performance objective would be to reduce to zero the number of interlibrary loan requests sent to other libraries for materials available in the collection. This objective should be reached within one year. To accomplish the objective, the employee could analyze why he or she could not identify these materials as being already available in the collection. In 30 days, the employee should meet with the supervisor to discuss these reasons and to determine if the employee now understands how to use the card catalog.

Another example might be an employee who is unable to locate statistical data requested by patrons. The performance objective would be to become familiar with five specific sources of statistical data used by health professionals. As a follow-up, the supervisor might develop a series of questions that would require the employee to use these tools.

There are many methods of conducting performance appraisals. However, the purpose of any performance appraisal is to let the employee know how he or she is doing and to help the individual improve.

Terminations

Termination of employment can be voluntary or involuntary. Voluntary termination may be a happy occasion if the employee is moving to a new location, taking a new job, or retiring. Involuntary termination is usually an uncomfortable situation for all involved.

Occasionally, an employee may do something that requires immediate dismissal. Hospital personnel policies usually define circumstances under which this might occur. However, termination most often occurs because an employee's job performance has been unsatisfactory over a period of time. During this period, the supervisor should document examples of unacceptable performance in writing. There should be frequent counseling sessions with the employee in which the supervisor sets objectives to help the employee improve. The personnel department should be consulted for advice on other ways the librarian might help the employee.

If it becomes necessary to terminate the employee, the personnel department may be able to suggest the best way to handle it. The actual termination may be painful, but like a tooth that needs pulling, it may be better to get it over with quickly. The questions below may be useful in deciding whether to terminate an employee

- Are the job performance standards reasonable?
- Was prior training or knowledge a prerequisite for employment, or was the employer to provide on-the-job training?
- Did the employee receive sufficient training on the job to be able to perform efficiently?
- Does the employee have the tools and the authority with which to do the job?
- Has the employee been notified in person and in writing that his or her performance is unsatisfactory? Were specific examples of unsatisfactory behavior included? Have the examples been thoroughly discussed with the employee? Were these discussions and the behavior that resulted from them documented?
- If other employees perform these same tasks, are the same performance standards expected and achieved?
- Are there extenuating circumstances to be considered?

In reference to the last question, the supervisor should recognize that health or family problems may temporarily affect job performance. Problems may be severe enough that the employee should seek professional assistance. Most supervisors prefer to help the individual work through difficult periods in order to retain a good employee. The most frustrating employee to deal with is one whose performance is marginal and whose life is a series of personal crises.

A supervisor is responsible for seeing that the hospital gets the best possible information services for each dollar spent. He or she should focus on job performance, establish reasonable performance standards, work with employees to achieve those standards, and tolerate temporary problems. If standards are not met, the supervisor should work with the employee on specific problems. Both should agree on the standard to be achieved and the time period in which job performance must be improved. The supervisor must keep the employee informed of his or her progress in person and in writing. If the employee does not achieve the standard, it will be no surprise when the employee quits or is terminated.

In the emotionally charged situation of termination, it is best to avoid negative comments such as "You'll never make it on any job unless you change your attitude." All people deserve to be treated with dignity. Some supervisors feel guilty for not having been more successful with an employee. Although a supervisor should learn from mistakes, he or she should not take too much responsibility for others' lack of success. It is best to look forward to recruiting, hiring, and working with a new employee.

Layoffs

A layoff is temporary or permanent interruption in employment usually for economic reasons. The hospital library, despite its relatively small work force, may be affected by layoffs. Although layoffs are unpleasant, the librarian should recognize that the fiscal viability of the hospital is usually essential for the continuing support of the library. The librarian must assume the responsibility to both support the hospital and protect the people working in the library. The librarian should also make certain the layoff of library personnel is necessary, and the economic benefits to the hospital are substantial enough to offset the reduction in information services.

Employees who are laid off need information about unemployment and health care benefits. They will also want to know when they may be called back to work. The possibility of a transfer to another department should also be explored. Of course, the librarian must be familiar with the hospital's policies on layoffs, seniority, and bumping. Regular communication with staff members regarding layoffs is essential.

In hospitals in which layoffs are a common occurrence, the librarian should prepare a general layoff plan in advance, including the services and staff to be cut. Despite a reduction in personnel, the library must continue to provide information services to patrons, who often expect service to be maintained as usual.

UNIONS AND STRIKES

In hope of obtaining a better negotiating position with management, workers in many libraries have joined or formed unions. If librarians are considered part of management, they are usually not included in the bargaining unit. However, other members of the library staff may be.

Union organizing campaigns, contract negotiations, and strikes may create tensions. During union organizing campaigns, the supervisor should recognize that employees have the right to choose to have a union represent them. He or she should respond to employees' questions in a candid and neutral manner and avoid making a big distinction between management and labor.

After all, all hospital employees are working together to assure quality patient care.

When a new contract is negotiated, representatives of the union and management discuss changes in the contract provisions. These changes usually involve not only salary and benefits but also personnel practices. If an agreement cannot be reached, the union members may strike. During a strike, minimal staffing in the library can free nonunion employees to be used in other departments.

The effects of a strike can last for years, not only by creating financial difficulties but also by polarizing employees. Once a strike is over, the librarian should try to heal any divisions among library staff members, or between the library staff and other hospital employees. This will help the staff to resume business as usual.

VOLUNTEERS

Many hospital librarians have the opportunity to use volunteers. The people working in the library, whether they are paid or not, are part of the library staff. Management of volunteers is as much a part of personnel administration as is the management of wage-earning employees.

Tasks

Volunteers, depending on their capabilities, may assist library staff by performing routine tasks or by providing special services. In hospital libraries volunteers are often assigned to (1) process the exchange of duplicate materials, (2) check in or claim journal issues, (3) answer the telephone, (4) photocopy articles, (5) mail new book lists, (6) inventory and acknowledge gifts, (7) file catalog cards, and (8) circulate library materials. Some volunteers have special abilities and can be very helpful in preparing exhibits or book displays. Others may be useful for special projects, such as organizing an oral history program, mending library materials or writing instructions for using audiovisual equipment.

Selection and Job Performance

Volunteers should be screened by the librarian to determine their expectations, abilities, and goals. The librarian should also discuss the duties and responsibilities that the volunteer would handle. A volunteer whose abilities and goals are not similar to those of the rest of the staff may not function as part of the team. He or she may also create a morale problem and may consume a great deal of the supervisor's time. Although it is tempting to accept "free" assistance, volunteers must be supervised, and supervision takes time. In order to justify "employing a volunteer," the benefits of the volunteer's efforts must be greater than the time required for training, motivating, and supervising the individual. Librarians with several volunteers may find job descriptions helpful. A prospective volunteer may decide after looking over the job description that the job is not suitable.

Volunteers need orientation and training as do other employees. A two-month probationary period will give the librarian and the volunteer time to see if the individual can do the job and is interested in doing it on a regular basis. If a volunteer is absent frequently, needs excessive supervision, or is a morale problem, the librarian should terminate the relationship. Frequently, a transfer to another department can be arranged by the volunteer services department.

Working with Volunteers

Although a volunteer cannot be expected to work at the same pace as paid employees and will usually not be available at holiday times, he or she can make a valuable contribution to the library. A volunteer, like any other employee, needs recognition. Since money is not a motivating factor, the volunteer must have other reasons for working in the library. Being aware of these reasons will help the librarian to motivate the volunteer.

Volunteers can be a valuable asset to the library. The head of the volunteer services department can be very helpful in encouraging capable volunteers or discouraging inappropriate ones, particularly if the department head understands the types of services the library provides.

Documenting Volunteer Activity

The number of hours contributed by volunteers and the tasks they perform should be recorded and included in the library's regular reports. The hours may be reported directly or in terms of FTEs, which are calculated by dividing the number of hours contributed by volunteers by the number of hours a full-time employee works each week. Thus the work of volunteers is counted when deciding the number of FTEs needed to staff the library.

Also, administrators should be aware that certain programs are supported totally or in part by volunteers, and that the library administers volunteer training programs.

STAFF DEVELOPMENT

One of the most rewarding aspects of personnel administration is staff development. The librarian may ask staff members to check with each other when they are unable to answer a patron's question. This will enable them to share knowledge and to discover areas in which additional training would be useful. Monthly staff meetings with time allocated for practical exercises can be informative and fun, particularly if each staff member takes a turn planning the educational part of the meeting.

The hospital may have training programs that employees can participate in, and many provide tuition reimbursement for formal education. Various schools and professional associations, such as the Medical Library Association (MLA), offer continuing education opportunities. Regional medical libraries often have training courses for library staff who do not have formal training in library science. Programs offered by the MLA and regional medical library groups provide numerous educational opportunities.

A policy developed in conjunction with the personnel and training departments will assist the librarian in administering an effective staff development program. Although continuing education in the area of reference is valuable, other topics such as medical terminology, management, and audiovisual equipment maintenance are useful. Documentation of continuing education activity provides a record both for the employee and for the hospital. Continued learning can keep the staff up-to-date, stimulate innovation, and lead to improved information services.

REFERENCES

1. Joint Commission on Hospital Accreditation. Accreditation manual for hospitals. 1983 ed. Chicago: Joint Commission on Accreditation of Hospitals, 1982:147-149.

2. United States Training and Employment Service. Job descriptions and organizational analysis for hospitals and related health services. Rev. ed. Washington, DC: Government Printing Office, 1970.

READINGS

GENERAL

Drucker PF. The practice of management. New York: Harper & Row, 1954.

Haimann T, Hilgert RL. Supervision: concepts and practices of management. Cincinnati: South-Western, 1972.

Strauss G, Sayles LR. Personnel: the human problems of management. 3d ed. Englewood Cliffs, NJ: Prentice-Hall, 1972.

Yoder D, Haneman HG Jr, eds. ASPA handbook of personnel and industrial relations. Washington, DC: Bureau of National Affairs, 1974-1979. 8 vol.

INTERVIEWING

Creth S. Conducting an effective employment interview. Acad Librarianship 1978 Nov;4:356-360.

Einstein K. Job interviewing: the art of hearing what the candidate would rather not say. Assoc Manage 1978 Nov;30:32-37.

Fear RA. The evaluation interview. 2d ed. New York: McGraw-Hill, 1973.

Lippin P. The delicate art of checking references. Admin Manage 1979 Aug;40:30-32.

Lopez FM. Personnel interviewing: theory and practice. 2d ed. New York: McGraw-Hill, 1975.

Peele D. Fear in the library. Acad Librarianship. 1978 Nov;4:361-365.

PERFORMANCE APPRAISAL

Allan P. Rosenberg S. Formulating usable objectives for manager performance appraisals. Pers J 1978 Nov;57:626-629,640,642.

Berkner DS. Library staff development through performance appraisal. Coll Res Libr 1979 Jul;40:335-344.

Henderson RI. Performance appraisals: theory to practice. Reston, VA: Reston Publishing; 1980.

Hilton RC. Performance evaluation of library personnel. Spec Libr 1978 Nov;69:429-434.

Kellogg MS. What to do about performance appraisal. Rev. ed. New York: AMACOM, 1975.

Levinson H. Appraisal of *what* performance? Harvard Bus Rev 1976 Jul/Aug;54:30-32,34,36,40,44,46,160.

Mager RF, Pipe P. Analyzing performance problems or "You really oughta wanna." Belmont, CA: Fearon, 1970.

Maier NRF. The appraisal interview: three basic approaches. LaJolla, CA: University Associates, 1976.

SPECIAL

Albrecht KG. Successful management by objectives: an action manual. Englewood Cliffs, NJ: Prentice-Hall, 1978.

Filley AC. Interpersonal conflict resolution. Glenview, IL: Scott, Foresman, 1975.

Kronick DA, Rees AM. An investigation of the education needs of health sciences library manpower. Part V; Manpower for hospital libraries. Bull Med Libr Assoc 1971 July;59:392-403.

Lorenzi NM. The art of planning for library personnel. Bull Med Libr Assoc 1976 Apr;64:212-8.

APPENDIX A
Sample Job Description: Medical Librarian

Medical Librarian—Job Code

Distinguishing Characteristics

This is the professional library position and reports to the Assistant Administrator. The medical librarian supervises library assistants and clerical personnel.

Duties Summary

The medical librarian is responsible for planning and administering the staff, budget, facilities, collection, and services of the hospital's library and information center.

Examples of Tasks

- Assesses information needs of library users
- Evaluates how well the library meets information needs
- Provides reference services, such as compiling bibliographies, doing literature searches, and answering reference questions
- Keeps statistics and prepares reports
- Selects and acquires new books, journals, and other library materials
- Instructs patrons in the use of the library
- Works with the library committee regarding library facilities and policies
- Supervises the circulation of library materials
- Prepares the library's budget
- Directs the expenditure of monies from the library's budget
- Attends educational programs and reads professional literature to learn of new developments in the library field
- Hires, counsels, disciplines, evaluates, and terminates library staff in accordance with hospital policy
- Performs other related duties as required

Minimum Education and Experience Required

Graduation from an ALA accredited library school with a master's in library science and one year experience, or an equivalent combination of course work and experience. MEDLINE training and certification by the Medical Library Association are desirable.

Other Qualifications

Management skills and the ability to communicate with various groups of people.

APPENDIX B
Sample Job Description: Library Assistant

Library Assistant—Job Code

Distinguishing Characteristics

The library assistant performs routine tasks necessary to the operation of the library. This position reports to the medical librarian.

Duties Summary

Under supervision, the library assistant is responsible for the clerical tasks necessary to support the activities of the hospital's library and information center.

Examples of Tasks
- Maintains circulation file
- Circulates library materials and sends out overdue notices
- Types, verifies, and receives interlibrary loans
- Checks in journals
- Claims unreceived materials
- Orders and receives new books, journals, and other library materials
- Prepares sets of catalog cards from cataloging copy
- Files catalog cards
- Prepares new library materials for circulation
- Orders supplies
- Answers the telephone
- Maintains records on volume of library activity
- Prepares materials for binding
- Answers routine questions for patrons
- Reshelves library materials
- Mends library materials
- Types library reports, correspondence, and bibliographies
- Performs related duties as required

Minimum Education and Experience Required

Graduation from college, clerical skills, and two or more years of experience in a library; or an equivalent combination of education and experience. Familiarity with medical terminology is desirable.

Other Qualifications

The library assistant interacts with members of the medical and nursing staffs, employees, and members of the public both in person and on the telephone. The position requires careful attention to detail and ability to handle a large number of varied tasks.

Managerial Communication

Jana Bradley
Director, Library/Media Services
Wishard Memorial Hospital
Indianapolis, Indiana

CHAPTER 15

Managerial Communication

Jana Bradley
Director, Library/Media Services
Wishard Memorial Hospital
Indianapolis, Indiana

Communication is a broad term for interactions between people involving the exchange of information. Hospital librarians should strive to communicate effectively, not only to exchange information but also to increase the hospital's understanding of library activities. In addition, librarians should consider communication a necessity because a library that operates in isolation cannot properly fulfill its users' needs. Knowledge of organizational communication, effective writing, and writing formats can assist the librarian in communicating effectively with library staff, library users and the hospital's administration.

COMMUNICATION IN ORGANIZATIONS

Each organization has its own patterns of communication. A good librarian must understand the organization in order to communicate effectively in it. In some organizations all communication traveling upward from a department must flow through the department head's immediate supervisor. In other organizations the content of the message determines the route. Size of an institution sometimes provides a clue to the formality of its communication system, but even very small hospitals can have highly structured, formal channels through which communication flows. Librarians should be aware of channels for different types of decisions and should develop a sense of which channels to use for specific situations.

Not only do institutions have their characteristic communication patterns, but individuals within an organization often have distinct communication preferences. Some people want immediate information over the telephone. Others prefer timely notes. Still others prefer regular meetings and some choose to communicate primarily through formal reports. Knowing the form of communication most likely to be effective in a given situation is essential to library success.

Directions of Communication

Communication in a library, a hospital, or any other organization can be analyzed by the direction in which it moves. Communication can move upward, downward, or laterally.

In general, information and recommendations for action move upward. Managers at all levels make decisions about operations in which they may not be directly involved. In order to make good decisions, managers depend on information passed upward in the form of memos, reports, and discussions. For example, hospital administrators rarely perform literature searches. They do, however, decide whether the hospital library will have access to online databases for bibliographic searching and information retrieval. Such a decision should be based on knowledge of the library's volume of search requests, the relative costs of manual and computer

searching, and the benefits of computer searching. If the administrator, however, does not have access to this information in an understandable format or if the information is incomplete, the decision could easily be based on misconceptions or misinformation. In upward communications the information itself, the way it is presented, the timing of the presentation, and the reputation of the sender all influence the ultimate decision.

Policies, procedures, and other instructional messages tend to move downward. The efficiency with which a job is performed and the quality of the results often depend on clear communication of both the reason for the assignment and the specific way to complete it. In addition, the attitude of employees toward assignments is often influenced by the tone of the directives or instructions they receive.

Lateral communications include messages to peers in the organization and colleagues outside the organization. They usually involve job-related information, requests, or services. Recipients of such messages usually do not report to the senders, and so compliance with these messages is frequently not required. Consequently, lateral communications must be clear and persuasive to produce results. For example, a flyer announcing the availability of reference services for hospital office staff must clearly state what these services are, who can use them, and how they will be helpful. Otherwise, the message may be received but probably will produce few actual calls to the library. As another example, a questionnaire sent to librarians must include a clear and persuasive statement about the need for such data, or librarians may not take the time to return the form.

Types of Communication

Communication can take place face-to-face, over the telephone, in writing, or in ways that do not involve words at all. Because each type of communication can work for or against the effectiveness of a message, librarians should give some thought to the choice of communication medium.

In addition to its individual characteristics, each medium of communication can be used with varying degrees of formality. Although face-to-face communication is usually considered more informal than written communication, the tone of each medium can be altered to fit a situation. A meeting chaired by the hospital administrator, for example, can be a more formal medium than a handwritten memo.

Face-to-Face Communication

Communication of a message in person can be a very effective means of achieving results. When talking to someone in person, the librarian can augment the message with inflection, tone changes, or nonverbal signals. Unscheduled meetings can provide opportunities to talk to people who are difficult to reach by appointment. The biggest advantage of face-to-face communication is that the librarian can judge the listener's reactions immediately and modify the message accordingly.

Face-to-face communication, however, does have drawbacks. Even if the message has been planned in advance, a conversation tends to be less organized than more structured forms of communication. Key points may be forgotten, or the speakers may stray from the topic. Usually no permanent record exists of face-to-face meetings. Often two people's perceptions of what took place will differ, perhaps without either realizing the discrepancy. Finally, success in face-to-face communication often depends on highly developed interpersonal skills. This is especially true when complex issues, personality clashes, or conflicting interests are involved.

When discussing face-to-face communication, it is useful to distinguish between social communications and job-related messages. While friendly interactions often make a workplace more pleasant, it is important not to expect too much from them. Being well liked is always an asset, but friendship alone will not necessarily bring the desired job-related results.

Social situations at work, however, provide excellent chances to communicate work-related messages in an informal way. Lunch conversations, coffee breaks, or rides to work can be very effective, particularly when the aim is to promote awareness of the library. Many hospital librarians have found that having lunch regularly with colleagues is one of their most productive communication techniques.

Librarians should be particularly alert for opportunities for unscheduled face-to-face communication, since often the people they most want to reach are those with the least time. Telling a physician about a new journal while standing in the cafeteria line or pausing in the hall to inform the director of nursing of an increase in use of reference services by nurses may be the best opportunity to convey this information. Librarians may reinforce such meetings with an appropriate follow-up, perhaps an article or a short memo.

Telephone Communication

On the telephone, it is still possible to react to the other person's responses, but fewer clues are available than in face-to-face communication. The spontaneous nature of the communication also means that the librarian should plan the message in advance so all the information is conveyed in an organized manner. A potential drawback of telephone communication is that the time of the call may not be convenient for the person on the other end of the line. The inconvenience may color his or her response. Determining the best time to call someone takes a little ingenuity, but it is usually worth the effort.

Finally, there is usually no permanent record of telephone calls. Depending on the situation, librarians often follow a telephone call with a short memo that summarizes the outcome of the call.

Nonverbal and Indirect Communication

Communication takes place not only through words but also nonverbally through body posture and movement. Nonverbal communication has received much attention in recent years, helping librarians to be aware that their facial expressions, gestures, and random movements send messages.

Hospital librarians can do much to communicate their philosophy of service through actions and nonverbal behavior. Pleasant responses, willingness to help, and prompt action all communicate user-oriented service. Businesslike attire, adherence to requests and deadlines, professional communication, and efficient operation of the library communicate effective management.

Nonverbal communication is not as precise as verbal communication and is open to the subjective interpretation of the recipient. Nevertheless, all librarians should be aware of the possible implications of their actions and to use them to their best advantage.

Written Communication

Writing is the least spontaneous form of communication. It also can be one of the most expensive. The format is the most formal, although the tone of any communication can do much to establish its formality. Writing does have powerful advantages, however, especially in the situations listed below:

- When sending the same message to more than one person
- When a permanent record is desired
- When the message is complex
- When careful organization and phrasing of the information is important
- When the recipient prefers to read the message at his or her convenience
- When a thoughtful response is desired

To transact most business, organizations depend on written communication. Although face-to-face and telephone communication often precede written documents, eventually the most important information is recorded on paper.

EFFECTIVE WRITING

Effective writing helps accomplish a desired goal. Conversely, ineffective writing interferes with the achievement of that goal. Interference can occur in several ways. The reader may not understand what has been written or, if vital information has been omitted, may only partially understand the message. The recipient of a poorly written report may skim it or not read it at all because it looks too long, too boring, or too complicated. Even if read, poorly written material may fail to convince its readers, or worse, may antagonize them. When a piece of writing fails to achieve the purpose for which it was written, it becomes a waste of energy and money. Indeed, poor writing may even prejudice future efforts to achieve the same objective.

Effective writing is a skill. Although most librarians learn writing skills as part of their education, that knowledge is sometimes forgotton as other concerns become more important. The following section provides a quick review of basic writing skills used in organizations.

Planning the Message

Unclear writing is often a result of unclear thinking. For an idea to be clearly expressed, it must be clearly and logically conceived in the writer's mind. Developing an idea does not have to be a lengthy process, but some planning of content often makes the difference between clarity and confusion. When planning a piece of business writing, four areas should be considered: (1) the purpose, (2) the audience, (3) the format, and (4) the content.

Purpose

The purpose for writing usually falls into one or more of these categories:

- To give information
- To influence attitudes
- To produce action

A librarian should be able to state precisely the desired outcomes of a piece of writing in terms of information, attitudes, and action. Then the message can be consciously tailored to achieve those results.

Audience

Before writing, the librarian should consider the characteristics of the potential audience. General characteristics include position, profession, and education. Perhaps less obvious and vastly more important are the readers' attitudes toward the subject of the message. What previous knowledge or experience do they have? What preconceptions or beliefs might influence their reactions and decisions? What possible vested interests do they have, both positive and negative? The answers to these questions can help the librarian see the subject as it appears to the readers. The librarian can then compose the message in a way that addresses the readers' interests, concerns, or misgivings.

Format

Choosing the format that best suits a message is usually a straightforward decision. It is based on the length and complexity of the message, the formality of the subject or occasion, the general practice in an institution, and common sense. In-house forms are available for many types of messages, and they should be used if appropriate. When in doubt about the format to use for a message, locating a similar message written under similar circumstances can help. Judgment should be used, however, to be certain that the model is a good one. In business, the most commonly used formats include memos, reports, proposals, letters, policies, procedures, and forms. These formats will be discussed in detail later in the chapter.

Content

Probably the most important part of planning the message is deciding on the points that will be made and the order in which they will be presented. For a longer piece of writing, content should be organized in outline form, which is an almost indispensable aid to organizing complex thoughts. For most shorter pieces, simply written phrases provide an adequate tool for developing the idea. Decisions about content should be based on the analysis of purpose and audience, on the requirements of the format, and on the subject matter.

One of the most effective ways to organize material is for the librarian to think in terms of main sections, main ideas, and supporting details. Every topic or subject can be broken down into main sections. These natural divisions come from the subject itself. Within each of these sections, main ideas can be identified. Main ideas usually form the structural skeleton of the message and often serve as topic sentences. Each main idea is supported or developed by more specific information.

In expository writing, information is often presented in order of decreasing importance, from most important to least important. This principle can apply to the ordering of main sections, main ideas, and supporting details. Another useful application of this principle is to begin each piece of writing with a summary of the most important information. In longer reports, a brief summary of major points or a statement of the conclusion can precede the introduction. When it is not feasible to put a summary first, a statement of a major point or a statement of purpose is a good way to begin.

Writing the Message

Poor writing is usually not the result of one dramatic error but rather the cumulative effect of small stylistic problems that interfere with clear communication. The best way to improve writing skills is to learn to identify the most common causes of poor writing and then practice correcting them through revision. Developing the habit of reading handwritten drafts for possible revisions will provide continual practice in strengthening writing skills.

Before leaving the subject of writing, the use of specialists' terminology, or jargon, deserves some attention. Most disciplines, including librarianship, have a specialized vocabulary used to denote concepts for which there is no plain equivalent. Jargon has many valid uses, but it obstructs communication when the audience does not understand the term. Common sense dictates that if specialists want to be understood by nonspecialists, they should use plain language. Two assumptions cause this seemingly practical advice to be ignored. First, many people tend to assume that everyone in the profession as a whole speaks the jargon of a particular specialty. A technical services librarian familiar with automated cataloging may assume that all librarians know what a "check tag" is. Audiovisual librarians may assume that "cluster carrel" is a universally understood term in librarianship. Second, specialists often use a term for so long that they do not realize it is unfamiliar to nonspecialists. Terms like "ready reference," "bibliographic retrieval," and "reference question" may not be fully understood by people outside the library profession.

Inappropriate use of jargon affects communication between librarians and administrators. The use of terms that are unfamiliar to administrators not only decreases their understanding of the message but also increases the impression that library activity is different from other hospital activities. Administrators may not feel they encounter many "reference questions" during a typical day, but they know that they frequently need addresses, facts, and statistics. Obviously, librarians can teach others their vocabulary. However, that time can be used more effectively by teaching the value of the concept rather than the specific word to express it.

Planning the Layout

Layout involves the position of words, titles, paragraphs, graphic elements, and the overall visual effect. Almost everyone pays attention to layout when designing a printed brochure. Yet people often do not recognize that the same considerations can apply to designing typewritten messages.

Using short paragraphs, liberal spacing, headings, lists, and outlines increases the readability of a message. Underlining, capitalization, indentations, asterisks, and dashes can be used for highlighting. When using these devices, a librarian should consider the total effect and make sure that the layout reinforces the central idea of the message.

The impact of a written message is also affected by its overall appearance. A poorly spaced, smudged memo typed with a faded ribbon and containing spelling errors and handwritten corrections adds little to the credibility of the sender. Although many librarians have to do most or all of their own typing, the extra time needed to produce a crisp, professional-looking message is well worth the effort.

FORMATS IN ORGANIZATIONAL WRITING

The principles of effective writing apply to all formats. In addition, specific considerations apply to each of the following writing formats.

Memos

Memoranda, or memos, are the most frequently used form of internal written communication. Most hospitals have printed memo forms. If the forms are unavailable, the librarian can adapt letterhead stationery by typing the word "memorandum" in capital letters centered and several spaces below the letterhead. The three-part heading is illustrated in Figure 15-1.

Memos are useful for short messages, when a record is

needed, when the recipient is not available in person, or when more than one person is to receive the message. In many institutions, however, memos are overused, resulting in a virtual avalanche of paper, much of which is unread. Using memos for the reasons listed above, observing hospital routine, and applying common sense will help determine when a memo is needed.

Recipients of memos are usually extremely busy people who appreciate memos that are direct, clear, and short. On the other hand, many memos deal with potentially sensitive topics, so judgment, tact, and logical persuasion are equally necessary. Often the way a request is phrased influences the attitude with which it is received and acted upon. Compare the two memos in Figure 15-1.

Figure 15-1
Memos: Importance of Careful Phrasing

MEMO A: Blunt Phrasing

July 2, 1982

TO: John Smith, Assistant Administrator

FROM: Jane Doe, Librarian

SUBJECT: Replacing the Library's Typewriter

Please approve the attached request for replacement of the library's typewriter. It is over 10 years old, and it needs repairing on the average of once a month. This severely interrupts library routines.

Your cooperation in this matter is appreciated.

MEMO B: Rewritten to Strengthen Tact and Persuasion

July 2, 1982

TO: John Smith, Assistant Administrator

FROM: Jane Doe, Librarian

SUBJECT: Request for Replacement Typewriter

The library's only typewriter has exceeded the normal useful life of hospital machines (10 years) and is now requiring repairs on the average of once a month. On his last visit, the serviceman recommended replacement.

I have attached the completed Request for Replacement form, including the serviceman's recommendation, for your consideration.

Please let me know if you would like further information or documentation of need.

Thank you for your help.

In addition to the conventional heading already mentioned, a memo generally contains an opening statement, the body of the memo, an action statement, and a courtesy close. Of these elements, the opening sentence is in many ways the most important. After reading the first sentence, a reader will unconsciously decide whether to continue. The first sentence in a memo must catch and hold the reader's attention.

Although the nature of the first sentence depends on the content, several common kinds of beginnings can be identified. In reports and proposals, the first sentence is often a summary. For requests and short memos, the first sentence may state the reason for the request. The memo's most important fact may appear in the first sentence, or the memo may begin with a summary of its contents. Beginning a memo with information that is already known or is of secondary importance makes a weak start. It is better to begin with significant information and then provide necessary details.

The information in the body of the memo is usually arranged in order of decreasing importance. Librarians can use headings and layout techniques such as lists, underlining, and indentations to both emphasize important points and make them clearer to understand. To keep memos short and clear, supplementary information can be attached separately.

When action is desired, the librarian can make a request directly or indirectly. A direct request states the expected action and any requirements such as deadlines. Direct statements are less likely to be misunderstood. Librarians may use indirect requests as in memo B, Figure 15-1, when a direct request is too blunt or when the decision to act rests solely with the recipient of the memo. In such cases, a persuasive statement of the reasons for the action is often more effective than a direct request.

The courtesy close in a memo is largely a question of style. Phrases such as "Thank you for your help" are always acceptable but librarians will benefit from tailoring a phrase to suit a particular situation such as "Thank you for your help in organizing the 1983 Book Fair."

Reports

Any organization's administrative staff regularly needs reports from middle managers concerning the operation of their areas or departments. These may include monthly or annual reports as well as reports on special projects or topics. The purpose of these reports is to inform management of the levels of activity in the department, the significant trends that may affect the operation of the department, and the areas where problems may arise.

Submitting reports regularly offers the librarian the opportunity to inform management about the nature and value of the library's activities. For these reports to be read, however, they must be concise, understandable, and above all, relevant to the concerns of hospital administrators.

Monthly Reports

Through statistics and narrative, monthly reports should provide an accurate picture of library activity. The librarian probably keeps monthly statistics for internal use and may submit them along with a narrative to administration as a monthly report. Although this procedure saves time, it has disadvantages. Monthly statistics are designed to monitor library operations and information meaningful to the librarian. The information that will be useful to an administrator may be entirely different or may require different, jargon-free wording. To be most effective, the monthly report should be written with the needs of management in mind. Librarians should consider designing a monthly report format, including a statistical form, specifically for communicating to their supervisors. The advantages gained in an administrator's understanding of library functions far outweighs the extra time required.

The report to the librarian's supervisor should be designed to describe clearly and briefly the major library activities and indicate the levels of those activities. In addition, the librarian may tell how hospital staff members benefited from using the library. An effective way to communicate this information, and one that is already familiar to hospital administrators, is to list "significant indicators" of library service. Significant indicators are statistics that reveal major services or activities. Indicators stated in plain language rather than jargon make library activity more understandable to nonlibrarians.

Significant indicators and the language used to express them should be tailored to each institution. Opinions vary on what information is important to management and what terms will best convey this significance.

Section I of Appendix A lists some possible significant indicators, and Section II illustrates how these categories might be broken down to provide more information, perhaps in an attachment to the report.

Section IIB is a category that not all librarians may want to include. It analyzes types of library activity by user group. Not all librarians will feel it necessary to keep user group records. Some librarians keep them only for selected activities. Such statistics are generally used when the librarian is concerned with demonstrating that the library provides a valuable service to the entire hospital staff. The initial planning for monitoring user groups involves providing a place for that information on all forms and then determining a collection procedure. If book cards are used, user status for circulated materials must be recorded when the material is checked out.

Section IIC, which lists purposes of library use, is another category not all libraries may want to include. Hospital librarians have long been attempting to find ways of quantifying the value of library services. In the absence of empirical studies, purpose of use might be a way to indicate the importance of these services. At the very least, purpose of use relates library use to a wide range of hospital activities. It also provides a way of documenting the user's perception that information was sought for patient care.

So far the discussion of reports has focused on the statistical review. Most reports include a narrative summary organized by topic. Topics can include service areas, program areas, or items of concern during a particular month. The amount of detail included should be determined by the subject, its importance, and the preference of the supervisor. The librarian should be extremely careful in choosing details that are meaningful to an administrator. Because the monthly report is an official document, significant events should be mentioned for the record as well as for the supervisor's information.

Encouraging administrative supervisors to read monthly reports begins by providing them with reports that are short, relevant to their needs, and easy to read. Then the librarian should try to ensure that the reports are actually read by reinforcing the concepts, trends, and issues in face-to-face meetings. Most administrative supervisors will be interested in information about the library's performance, productivity, and impact on the hospital if that information is concise, understandable, and related to their management concerns.

Annual Reports

An annual report has two major purposes. In some ways, they tend to work against each other. As the official record of yearly activity, the report must completely document all major areas of library activity. It will be filed in the library as well as in the administrative offices, and therefore it is the primary source of information about library operations. As such, the report must contain all statistical information used for and relevant to internal library operation.

The annual report also is a public relations and educational tool. This tool will be effective if the report clearly and concisely sums up major library achievements.

One way to accomplish both objectives is to begin an annual report with a summary of significant indicators, preferably ones that are already familiar to administrators from monthly reports. Then, within the body of the report the librarian can include all statistical data relevant to each category.

Many institutions have forms or guidelines for annual reports. If none exists, Appendix B can provide ideas for appropriate categories. Within each category, operations can be summarized, highlights presented, and problems discussed. Institutions treat annual reports with varying degrees of availability and confidentiality. The librarian's supervisor can be helpful in determining the advisability of discussing sensitive issues in the annual report.

Special Reports

Reports are often prepared on special topics, such as the merits of manual versus automated cataloging or the value of joining a consortium. Special reports are often prepared in memo format. In general, special reports include a summary of the report's topic, a statement of a problem or need, criteria for effective solutions, an analysis of alternatives, and a recommendation.

The emphasis in the report will depend on its objective. If the purpose of the report is primarily to show that a problem exists, then the statement of the problem or need will be lengthy. If, however, the report's purpose is to present an alternative solution to a commonly acknowledged problem, then the problem statement may be only a brief summary and the emphasis will fall on the criteria and the solutions.

Statistical Reports

Since statistics are often a part of other types of reports, a brief discussion of the purposes and methods of collecting statistics will be useful. Information on the types of statistics most useful to collect for various activities can be found in other chapters.

The management questions regarding the collection of statistical records concern the purpose of the statistics, the time involved in record keeping, and the benefits derived from the use of statistics. Statistics should be kept for a specific purpose, not merely to keep statistics. As mentioned earlier, statistics are useful both for internal monitoring and for reporting to the administration or the library committee.

Although librarians collect different types of statistics, some categories are commonly used (Figure 15-2). It should be emphasized that the categories in Figure 15-2 are merely examples. Each library should choose categories based on its own need.

Procedural questions regarding statistics concern the methods for collecting statistics. Generally, four levels are possible: daily, monthly, annually, and by transaction. Although the librarian can use separate forms, much time can be saved by counting and tabulating several methods on one sheet. The efficiency of combination forms depends on the source and the amount of information and the number of categories. Usually some trial and error will be involved in determining the most effective forms and procedures to keep needed statistics. Once an efficient procedure is established, however, collection should proceed easily.

Proposals

Proposals are plans for projects, programs, or other activities. They vary in length and format from a short memo to a long report or application.

Proposals Submitted Within an Institution

At some point in the process of suggesting a major change in library services, staffing, or other activities, it is often useful to submit a written proposal. Such proposals are usually brief, written in memo format, and submitted to the librarian's supervisor. The librarian may attach more lengthy documentation. Proposals might be submitted to the administration for the following activ-

Figure 13-2
Statistical Summary for Internal Library Management

Category	Sub-category	Item	(blank data columns)
USERS		Walk-in	
USERS		Telephone	
USE OF MATERIALS	Circulation	Books	
USE OF MATERIALS	Circulation	Journals	
USE OF MATERIALS	Circulation	AVs	
USE OF MATERIALS	Photo-copies	Books	
USE OF MATERIALS	Photo-copies	Journals	
USE OF MATERIALS	In-library use	Books	
USE OF MATERIALS	In-library use	Journals	
USE OF MATERIALS	In-library use	AVs	
INTERLIBRARY LOAN	Loans	Books	
INTERLIBRARY LOAN	Loans	Jrnl. art.	
INTERLIBRARY LOAN	Loans	AVs	
INTERLIBRARY LOAN	Borrows	Books	
INTERLIBRARY LOAN	Borrows	Jrnl. art.	
INTERLIBRARY LOAN	Borrows	AVs	
REFERENCE		Fast answer	
REFERENCE		Info. search	
REFERENCE		Bib. (manual)	
REFERENCE		Bib. (computer)	
REFERENCE		SDIs	
REFERENCE		Other alerting	
REFERENCE		Orientations	
COLLECTION	Books	Books added	
COLLECTION	Books	Bk. coll. (TOTAL)	
COLLECTION	Jrnl. vols.	Jrnl. vol. added	
COLLECTION	Jrnl. vols.	Jrnl. vol (TOTAL)	
COLLECTION	Jrnl. subs.	Jrnl. sub. added	
COLLECTION	Jrnl. subs.	Jrnl. sub. (TOTAL)	
EX-CHANGE		Items sent	
EX-CHANGE		Items rec'd	

Note: Adapted with permission from L.A. Colaianni and F.I. Lyon Hospital Library Management. Chicago: Medical Library Association, 1982. (MLA Courses for Continuing Education, CE-129).

ities: adding a half-time clerical position, providing MEDLINE services, joining a consortium, adding additional database services, providing information services to patients or the community, or initiating audiovisual services.

A proposal generally includes a title; a summary; a statement of need; a project statement, including an overview of what will be done, objectives, and specifics of proposed actions; a breakdown of costs; and a summary of the projects' impact.

The statement of need should clearly and forcefully present the problem that will be solved by the proposed project. The librarian should also document the statement of need. If lengthy documentation is necessary, the librarian may summarize the main points and attach full documentation.

The project statement will vary according to the amount of detail necessary for approval of the plan. The criteria for effective operation of the proposed activity, or the objectives, should be included, but depending on the circumstances these formal terms are not always necessary. The impact statement predicts the benefits of the project. It should stress benefits to the organization but should also mention benefits to the library.

Proposals Outside the Institution

The format for proposals submitted for outside funding is by no means uniform. Government agencies and large foundations usually have extensive forms. Small foundations and local or regional groups may require only a detailed letter or a short proposal similar to the type already discussed. The librarian may request application procedures or forms in a brief letter to the funding agency. It is helpful to include a summary of the proposal in the letter.

A multipurpose outline for a proposal is impossible to provide. Most proposals, however, cover the following topics: a summary of the proposed project, a history of the applicant, the objectives of the project, specific details of the project's organization and operation, costs during the grant period, funding after the grant period, plans for evaluating the project's effectiveness, and the qualifications of the project personnel. More information on writing proposals for grants can be found in the reading list at the end of this chapter.

Policies

Policies are the guidelines that direct library activity; they define what the library does and under what conditions. Well-designed policies balance the requirements of all users, an individual user, and the library itself. All three elements need to be fairly provided for in a successful policy.

Good policies are user-oriented and provide ways to meet users' reasonable, job-related information needs. In designing policies, librarians may want to recall situations in which they have been users and to anticipate the

kinds of needs their users will have. When a policy infringes on a user need, even for a valid reason, alternative ways should be available to meet that need. The alternatives may not be as attractive to the user as the initial request, but if flexible compromises can be developed most users will be satisfied. For example, in most reference collections basic textbooks do not circulate and are available for use at all times. If a staff physician wants to photograph an illustration available only in a noncirculating book, the librarian might allow the physician to borrow the book for a two-hour photography session. If a library's policies are genuinely structured around users' needs, if limitations and restrictions have clear and valid explanations, and if the librarian is flexible and tries to solve conflicts, then most users will be understanding.

Policies have no fixed format. Many hospitals have policy manuals set up according to a prescribed, in-house format. Some hospitals require that all policies affecting more than one department be documented in a manual. Major library policies that might be submitted for such a manual might include a statement of goals, general objectives, user group statements, policies on use of the library and responsibility for materials, policies about services to patients, and policies concerning departmental or unit libraries. General policies affecting users can also be summarized in a special handout or brochure and distributed to users.

When the format for library policies is not prescribed by the hospital, the librarian can choose the format for the policy manual. There are a number of different ways of organizing policy statements, depending on the amount of detail desired and the use of the manual. Some libraries have a combined policy and procedure manual. Others keep the two separate. Either method can work well as long as the distinction between policies and procedures is maintained. Policies are general rules governing activity, and procedures are specific instructions for the performance of that activity. An advantage of having a separate policy manual is that, because it is usually shorter and more management-oriented than a combined manual, it is often easier to involve hospital administrators in its formulation and review.

Appendix C presents an outline for a hospital library policy manual. Further details about specific policies can be found in relevant chapters. The topics and the depth of the statement depend on the individual library; some topics require only a generalized, all-purpose sentence. If desired, the outline can be expanded to include procedures under each topic. Alternatively, the procedures can be classified separately by task responsibility or job descriptions. Procedures are written in basically the same way wherever they are kept.

Procedures

A procedure is a set of step-by-step instructions for the performance of a specific task. Good management requires a set of written procedures for major library routines: to organize activity, to establish standardization, and to ensure continuity. Sometimes librarians tend to avoid writing procedures, perhaps because they feel that procedures are difficult or time-consuming to develop. In fact, writing a procedure can be a natural extension of either planning or performing an activity. If new routines are being developed in conjunction with a new project or policy, the procedure can be used as a planning tool or a way of thinking out the necessary steps. When procedures are developed before the activity is initiated, they must be tested and revised as necessary. Writing procedures for an activity that is already established gives the librarian an excellent chance to analyze the way an activity is performed and make improvements.

To be useful, procedures must be up-to-date and reflect current practice. Any change in the way a routine is performed should be noted on the procedure. Whenever a procedure is revised, the date should be noted. For both writing and revising procedures, it is a good idea to deal with one routine at a time at regular intervals, such as one procedure a week, rather than to attempt to cover all the library's activities in one effort.

A procedure or any set of instructions can be broken down into parts. They are a purpose; an overview of main steps; materials and equipment; instructions; and comments. Not all the parts are needed for every procedure. They should be used whenever they are applicable to the purpose, the intended audience, and the subject matter. Each part will be discussed in detail below. A sample procedure appears in Appendix D. Since there are no fixed rules governing the writing of procedures, the sample is intended as a guide. It can be modified to suit specific situations. In particular, the length and detail of the procedure should be adapted to individual tasks.

Title and Purpose

All procedures should be titled. They may be part of a larger grouping and may be numbered.

A brief statement of the reason for performing the procedure is useful to clarify objectives. In the sample, the real purpose of the procedure is not to send out overdue notices but to get the books back.

Overview

All but the shortest routines can be divided into major activities or steps. An overview of these steps may be listed, as shown in the sample, or presented in a flow chart. Listing the major steps at the beginning provides an introduction to the entire process, plus a structure for organizing the individual smaller steps. If the sample procedure shown in Appendix D were not broken down into three major sections, the procedure would have more than eighteen steps. Generally, people find instructions easier to follow if they are presented in units of less than ten steps each.

Materials and Equipment

This section identifies needed materials and equipment and can include their location. Just as recipes do not mention kitchen stoves, instructions do not need to mention obvious office equipment and supplies.

Instructions

Instructions may be written in block narrative or in numbered steps. Numbered steps are generally considered clearer and easier to follow. Use of steps also tends to result in a more organized progression of separate activities. Generally, each step should represent one complete action. An action can be defined narrowly or broadly depending on the level of detail. Steps may then be broken down into substeps. Information needed to perform the steps may be handled in several ways:

- In an introduction to the steps
- Within the step itself, either introducing it as part of the step, or following it
- In a note

The required activity is usually clearer if steps are phrased in the active voice, often in the imperative, and if the verb is placed near the beginning of the sentence.

Forms and Form Letters

Any situation in which standard information is required repeatedly is an opportunity to use a form or a form letter. Forms and form letters can save time both in composition and in preparation. In addition, they ensure that the same information is transferred in all situations.

Forms

Although designing good forms takes time, a form that suits its purpose exactly will save time by providing all the necessary information in a convenient format. Forms can be designed to be used by patrons, library staff, or a combination of both. Forms can also be combined with publicity and information. For example, a flyer announcing awareness services can also include a sign-up form.

A good form has a clear purpose and is easy to understand and complete. It also provides standard information in a format suited to the efficient use of that information.

The content of a form should be based on a clear understanding of what information is needed and how it will be used. The following questions can be helpful in deciding what the form should contain.

- What is the purpose of the form?
- What information is needed to accomplish the purpose?
- How will the information be used?
- How will it be tallied and stored?

Questions on the form may be phrased in many ways. The format of the answers should be chosen carefully to match the use of the information. A basic choice involves whether to use open or closed questions.

An open question allows the respondent to choose the phrasing of the answer, thus providing a much wider range of answers. Answers to an open question tend to provide more information, particularly more subjective information, but are less easy to quantify and summarize.

A closed question offers the respondent a series of choices. It usually includes the catch-all choice, "other." Answers to closed questions are easy to tabulate, but unless the categories are chosen very carefully, they may not represent the full range of possibilities. Another pitfall of answers to closed questions is that they tend to reflect the questioner's view of the subject, which may not necessarily correspond to the respondent's viewpoint or understanding.

Other choices include whether to use qualitative (descriptive) terms or a quantitative scale; whether to use blanks, boxes, or items to circle; and whether to arrange choices vertically or horizontally. In choosing the physical layout of the form, the librarian should consider the amount of information needed, the length of the form, the general impression it gives, and the way the form will be used.

Form Letters

The advantages of form letters are obvious. The disadvantages stem from the fact that a general message may not be specific enough to meet the needs of a given situation. This disadvantage can be overcome in several ways. The tone of the form letter can be friendly and natural. Blank spaces may be left for specific information, such as dates or book titles. Notes may be handwritten or typed, although any modification lessens the time-saving value of the form. Finally, the message may be typed according to a standard form and modified as needed. This modification process is particularly easy if the librarian has access to a word processor.

Librarians, in their constant efforts to streamline operations, should be alert for all possible uses of form letters. Well-written form messages can save much time and increase the amount of communication without sacrificing the atmosphere of service that is the trademark of so many hospital libraries. Topics that are suitable for form letters include:

- Notification of availability of books, articles, or information
- Request for review of book for purchase

- Sign-up sheets for services such as SDIs
- Form attached to search, providing information on how to get articles
- Library welcome for new physicians or hospital staff members
- Notice of copyright
- Notice that material is being supplied by interlibrary loan
- Notice that material is being supplied by a consortium, network, or shared services group

Of course, a form letter does not have to be in letter form. It can be duplicated on slips of paper, card stock, or standard-size paper in any color. For special purposes, a logo or a letterhead from a transfer or a large-size typing element can be used for the master form. In fact, using graphics or other special effects is often more feasible in form letters because it need be done only once.

Letters

To complete the review of the types of organizational communication, letters should be mentioned briefly. Letters, perhaps even more than memos, should be written with an understanding of the reader's point of view. In addition to tone, language should also be appropriate for the intended reader, free from jargon, and suited to the purpose of the letter.

The organizational structure of a letter is suited to the individual situation. Generally, letters that present positive or neutral information begin with the most important information. Next the letter states any required explanations, necessary details, the action required, and closes in a positive way.

Letters containing negative information are usually more effective if they begin not with the bad news but with a statement that is pleasant, neutral, or noncontroversial. The reasons or justification for the negative action should be given, starting with the most acceptable and noncontroversial first and leading to the most important. The negative information is then stated. The librarian should attempt to close the letter on a positive note by offering alternatives or stating a sentiment that both parties can share.

A letter intended to persuade can follow the same pattern used for negative letters. The persuasive letter begins with a mutually acceptable statement, proceeds logically to more controversial subjects, and culminates in a logical statement of the position. Any action that is required should be stated. The closing should be friendly and respectful(1).

REFERENCES

1. Bowman JO, Branchaw BP. Successful communication in business. San Francisco: Harper & Row, 1980.

READINGS

Bernstein TM. Miss Thistlebottom's hobgoblins. New York: Farrar, Straus & Giroux, 1971.

Brusaw CT, Alred GJ, Oliu WE. The business writer's handbook. New York: St. Martin's, 1976.

Burne KG, Jones EH, Wyler RC. Functional English for writers. 2d ed. Glenview, IL: Scott, Foresman, 1978.

Haggblade B. Business communication. New York: West, 1982.

Pocket Pal. A graphic arts handbook. New York: International Paper Company, 1974.

Strunk WS Jr, White EB. The elements of style. 3d ed. New York: Macmillan, 1978.

University of Chicago Press. The Chicago manual of style. 13th ed. Chicago: University of Chicago Press, 1982.

APPENDIX A
Sample Statistical Categories for Monthly Reports

I. Summary: Significant Indicators of Library Services   Number

    Information Services   _____

    Awareness Services   _____

    Use of Library Materials   _____

    Document Delivery   _____

    Audiovisual Services   _____

    Technical Processes   _____

    Library Collection (total volumes)   _____

    Cooperative Activities   _____

II. Significant Indicators of Library Services: Breakdown by Category

    A. Library Activity

Category	Total Number	% Inc. (Dec.) Previous Month	% Inc. (Dec.) Same Month Previous Year
1. Information Services	_____	_____	_____
Fast Answers	_____	_____	_____
Information Searches	_____	_____	_____
Literature Searches	_____	_____	_____
Research Requests	_____	_____	_____
Research Requests	_____	_____	_____
2. Awareness Services	_____	_____	_____
Journal Scans	_____	_____	_____
Updated Bibliographies	_____	_____	_____
Newsletters Routed	_____	_____	_____
Newspaper Clipping file routed	_____	_____	_____
3. Use of Library Materials	_____	_____	_____
Books	_____	_____	_____
Journals	_____	_____	_____
Audiovisuals	_____	_____	_____
4. Document Delivery	_____	_____	_____
Borrowed	_____	_____	_____
Lent	_____	_____	_____
5. Audiovisual Services	_____	_____	_____
Information Searches	_____	_____	_____
Media Searches	_____	_____	_____
Equipment Used	_____	_____	_____
Programs Obtained	_____	_____	_____
Purchase	_____	_____	_____
Rental	_____	_____	_____
Borrow	_____	_____	_____
Preview	_____	_____	_____
Software Loaned	_____	_____	_____

6. Technical Processes
    Materials received
    Materials ordered
    Materials cataloged
    Materials processed

7. Library Collection
    Books
    Journals (Bound Volumes)
    Journals (Subscriptions)

8. Cooperative Activities
    Materials Borrowed
    Materials Lent
    Information requests referred
    Information requests answered
    Cooperative meetings
    Other

B. Library User Groups

	Information Services	*Document Delivery*	*Awareness Services*	*Audiovisual Services*
1. Medical Staff				
2. Housestaff				
3. Nursing Staff				
4. Administrative Staff				
5. Other Hospital Staff				
6. Students				
7. Patients				
8. Other				

C. Purposes of Library Use

	Information Services	*Document Delivery*	*Awareness Services*
1. Patient Care Decisions			
2. Management Decisions			
3. General Knowledge			
4. Continuing Education			
5. Student Use			
6. Teaching/Training			
7. Speeches/Presentations			
8. Cooperative Activity			
9. Other			

APPENDIX B
Sample Annual Report Outline

I. Summary (Significant indicators or highlights of year)

II. Review of objectives (Optional)

III. Review of current year's operation

    A. Book, journal, and audiovisual collection
    B. Information and awareness services
    C. Document delivery services
    D. Audiovisual services
    E. Patient library and health information services
    F. Technical services

IV. Statistical summary of operations

V. Review of administrative and program changes

    A. Assessment of needs for services
    B. New services
    C. Policy changes
    D. Changes in operations
    E. Staffing changes

VI. Budgetary review

    A. Summary
    B. Budget and expenditures
    C. Grant activity
    D. Funding equivalents
        1. Gifts
        2. Volunteer staff
        3. Cooperative services

    E. Revenues
        1. Fines
        2. Photocopying
        3. Service fees
        4. Miscellaneous

VII. Continuing education, committee membership, and participation in professional activities

    A. Continuing education/In-service education
    B. Committee membership
    C. Professional activities

VIII. Cooperative services activities

IX. Objectives for the following year

APPENDIX C
Hospital Library Policy Manual: Topical Outline

I.   Administration

   A.   Goals and objectives of library service

   B.   Organization chart of hospital (with library included)

   C.   Library personnel

      1.   Organization chart of library
      2.   Job descriptions
      3.   Volunteers

   D.   Library standards

      1.   JCAH standards and related documents
      2.   Other applicable standards
      3.   Documents for compliance (either documents or index to location)

   E.   Financial information

      1.   Sources of support
      2.   Budget
      3.   Library accounts
      4.   Funding equivalents

   F.   Reporting and recordkeeping

      1.   Reports: frequency and forms
      2.   Statistical records: forms

   G.   Needs assessment, evaluation, or quality assurance mechanisms

   H.   Library committee

   I.   Departmental libraries

   J.   Cooperative arrangements and networking

   K.   Professional development

      1.   Professional organizations: institutional memberships
      2.   Continuing education and staff development

   L.   Brief history of library

II. Use of the Library

   A.   User groups

   B.   Hours (also after-hours access)

   C.   Circulation policies

      1.   Borrowing periods
      2.   Circulating and noncirculating materials
      3.   Loan periods; fines; renewals

III. Services

   A.   Information services

      1.   Objectives
      2.   User groups (priorities and limitations)
      3.   Types of services available

   B.   Document delivery (interlibrary loan)

      1.   Borrowing policy
         a.   Objectives
         b.   Relationship to collection development
         c.   User groups
         d.   Network participation and borrowing channels
         e.   Copyright law
         f.   Cost support sources

      2.   Lending policy
         a.   Objectives
         b.   Network participation
         c.   Material eligible for loan
         d.   Copyright law
         e.   Cost support

   C.   Photocopying arrangements

   D.   Audiovisual services

      1.   Objectives (definition of program within library and relationship to other hospital departments involved with audiovisuals)
      2.   User groups
      3.   Services
         a.   Software services
         b.   Equipment services (if any)
         c.   Production services (if any)

   E.   Patient Services

      1.   Objectives
      2.   User groups and conditions of use
      3.   Selection responsibility
      4.   Special programs and services

   F.   Special services (eg. archival services, community health information services, publication services)

IV. Selection of Materials

   A.   Objectives

   B.   Selection responsibility and mechanisms

   C.   Subject coverage/levels of coverage

   D.   Selection criteria

E. Gifts and duplicates

F. Currency of collections

   1. Criteria
   2. Retention periods
   3. Weeding
   4. Historical materials

G. Cooperative agreements

H. Departmental collections

V. Technical Services

  A. Acquisitions

    1. Books: sources and conditions
    2. Journals: sources and conditions
    3. Audiovisuals
      a. Purchase
      b. Rental
      c. Preview

  B. Cataloging and processing

    1. Classification system
    2. Subject headings
    3. Mechanism for obtaining cataloging
    4. Cataloging procedures
    5. Producing and filing cards
    6. Processing
      a. New Materials
      b. Binding
    7. Cataloging/Processing of special materials
      a. Journals
      b. Government publications
      c. Audiovisuals
      d. Patient education materials
      e. Staff publications
      f. Vertical file material
    8. Departmental collections

APPENDIX D
Sample Procedure

CIRCULATION PROCEDURES

OVERDUES

Purpose: The purpose of processing overdue materials is to secure the return of outstanding material as quickly as possible.

Overview: Processing overdues consists of three major steps:

1. Determining which materials are overdue

2. Confirming that overdue materials are not in the library

3. Notifying users of overdue materials

Materials and Equipment: The following materials and equipment are needed to process overdues.

1. Circulation file

2. Preprinted overdue postcards (supply cabinet 2)

3. Invoices (supply cabinet 2)

Instructions:

Introduction: The library assistant is responsible for processing overdues every Friday, if possible. The following instructions offer a guide for easy reference.

1. Determine which materials are overdue.

   a. All materials with due dates *before* the cutoff date are overdue. Determine the cutoff date by counting back four Fridays, starting with the Friday in the current week as one.

   b. Go through the circulation file card by card and pull all cards with dates earlier than the cutoff date.

2. Confirm that overdue materials are not in the library.

   a. Arrange the cards in shelf-list order.

   b. Check the shelf for each item.

   - If an item is found, cross off the borrower's name and return the book card to the pocket. Notify the librarian when materials are found on the shelf.

   - If the item is not found, write "s.c." for "shelf check" and the date lightly in pencil next to the borrower's name on the book card.

   Note: Be sure that the book card and the item, if found, match exactly, including copy number or accession number.

   c. Check the following additional areas in the library for overdue items:

   - return truck or return box
   - tables and carrels
   - reserve and hold shelves
   - one-day signout sheet

3. Notify users of overdue material.

Comment: Maintaining a good relationship with the user, while getting our material back, is the primary objective in all overdue transactions!

Planning Library Facilities

Jacqueline Bastille
Director, Treadwell Library
Massachusetts General Hospital
Boston, Massachusetts

CHAPTER 16

Planning
Library
Facilities

Jacqueline Bastille
Director, Treadwell Library
Massachusetts General Hospital
Boston, Massachusetts

Appendixes

Figures

The physical environment of the library significantly influences both library use and library service. Inconvenient space discourages use; poor arrangement of the stacks and furniture makes the user overly dependent on library staff; and inadequate working space for staff results in inefficiency. Conversely, adequate space, easy access to materials, and an organized and clearly marked arrangement of materials contribute to effective library service.

Since existing space in most hospitals is often limited, and new construction is not always possible, competition for space is intense. In order to make sure there is adequate space for the library, librarians must convince hospital management that library services are essential and that adequate space is vital for providing good service. The process of demonstrating the necessity for adequate space and designing the effective use of that space are the subjects of this chapter.

RESPONSIBILITY FOR SPACE PLANNING

The process of obtaining library space takes a great deal of time and involves many people in addition to the librarian. Because procedures vary for planning and developing space, librarians should learn what the appropriate channels are for their own institutions. Talking with representatives of administration and with departments that have recently moved into new space is a good starting point. A general description of the roles and responsibilities of the people involved in planning and constructing library space follows.

The Librarian

The hospital librarian should be the central figure throughout the planning process. Because librarians are responsible for the effective use of the space given to the library, they must become experts in planning library space. This expertise can be developed and maintained by reading, talking to librarians who have recently planned new space, and visiting other libraries. The readings listed at the end of this chapter can provide much information.

In addition to becoming an expert on library space, the librarian should assume a leadership role in the planning process. This role includes initiating the study of space requirements, planning a solution to space problems, acquiring administrative approval for plans, and working with the building team to translate plans into a functional library. To succeed, the librarian must be attuned to political dynamics and continually analyze the situation to determine effective ways to initiate action or remove blocks to progress.

Planning Teams

Planning new space for a hospital department is rarely done by one individual alone. Sometimes space planners or architects work with departments to determine space requirements. Many institutions organize planning teams for a particular project, either in place of or in conjunction with planning staff. The library committee, usually representing various user groups, is often very effective in this role because it is familiar with library problems. Another approach is to appoint a special committee of interested, committed, and influential users. Frequently, one or two nonusers are also appointed to the committee to provide insight into why people do not use the library. The purpose of the planning team or committee is to explore and express user needs and desires, react to all aspects of planning, and apply pressure to bring about an effective outcome.

Hospital Management

The administrative officer to whom the librarian reports can be the most effective advocate for the development of a good library. Therefore, the librarian should involve the administrator in assessing space needs. Through this process the administrator can gain a clear understanding of how the library functions and how it contributes to the quality of patient care.

If committed to the essential role of the library, the administrator will participate actively in the preparation of the space proposal, often to the library's advantage. When the completed proposal is referred to the committee or board responsible for decisions on space, the administrator can be a knowledgeable advocate for the space proposal. Depending on the circumstances, money to finance the project may be sought before or after final approval. When finances are secured, specialists are appointed to implement the approved plans.

Design Professionals

An architect, engineer, hospital space planner, or hospital draftsman provides assistance in space planning by preparing schematic drawings, floor plans, construction documents, and specifications. The architect, hospital engineer or planner will also check state and local code requirements and confer with mechanical, electrical, and structural engineers. This person can also assist in selecting furniture, color schemes, carpeting, wood finishes, and stack materials. Sometimes a hospital will employ an interior designer or ask the advice of a designer on the staff of a large furniture supply firm. This specialist can prepare a layout for library areas, select furniture, decor, colors, carpeting, wood finishes, and so forth. Commercial shelving companies can also be a useful source for advice on placement of shelving.

The range of services provided by these professionals and the overlapping of abilities make it essential that librarians have some knowledge of every aspect of design. With such knowledge, librarians can make more informed decisions on design, furniture, and aesthetics.

The Library Consultant

A consultant can be hired to assist the librarian with a building or renovating project. The consultant should have strong experience and knowledge in planning libraries so that he or she can help analyze needs, prepare the written plan for use of library space, and recommend whether to remodel the existing area or provide new space.

Because an outside consultant is not familiar with the day-to-day operation of a specific library, a consultant's services are more effective when reviewing and critiquing the space plan or program. This expert opinion may influence the revision of the program or add support to the planning team's recommendations. In some areas, the staff of the Regional Medical Library (RML) can give advice and assistance on planning new or remodeled facilities.

Builders and Contractors

Construction work can be done by the hospital maintenance department or by a hired contractor. If a contractor is hired, he may also use subcontractors for special jobs such as electrical or ventilation work. Usually a contractor agrees to do all the work indicated on the final plans for a fixed price. Any changes or additions to those plans are charged as extras. Therefore, it is extremely important for the librarian to plan all the details carefully so that all necessary work is covered in the original agreement.

PLANNING FOR ADDITIONAL SPACE

Responsibility for initiating the planning process usually rests with the librarian. He or she should begin the planning process by evaluating the existing library space.

Evaluating Existing Library Space

New space in a hospital is both expensive and scarce. Before a request for new space is made, the librarian should evaluate the existing space to determine its limitations and identify specific needs for new space.

Data should be gathered on the use of existing space, user populations, and standard or typical library space needs. The analysis of the use of the existing space includes the size of the total space in square feet, the collection size, annual growth rate, seating capacity, and staff size. The librarian should also determine both present and potential user populations by job category: staff physician, resident, nurse, pharmacist, and so forth. The projections of library use should be based on actual hospital programs or projected new ones.

Using Standards for Projecting Space

Few specific guidelines or standards for hospital library space exist. A planning guide has been prepared for United States government hospital libraries, but it is of limited use for community hospitals(1). Suggested guide-lines have been proposed and adapted by regional groups with limited success(2,3,4). The standards published by the Hospital Library Standards Committee of the American Library Association (ALA) are also of limited value (5). The first edition of the syllabus for the Medical Library Association continuing education course for planning hospital library facilities contains an adaptation of various library space standards for use by hospital libraries(6). The standards developed for Canadian hospital libraries provide minimum standards for planning space(7). Currently, the Hospital Library Standards and Practices Committee of the Medical Library Association is developing standards for hospital libraries, including space requirements.

Considering Alternatives to New Space

By evaluating existing library space, the librarian or a consultant can identify areas that are overcrowded or no longer functional. They should examine these areas thoroughly and look for solutions that may alleviate the problem without requiring additional space. The size of the collection should be reviewed first. The following methods of reducing its size should be assessed: (1) studying the use of materials to determine the most cost-effective size, (2) withdrawing or storing infrequently used items, (3) exploring the use of microforms, (4) increasing the use of interlibrary loans, and (5) considering cooperative collection-sharing arrangements with other libraries. If the library is located in the basement, compact shelving can be considered. It is not an option for many libraries, however, because it requires a floor capable of supporting 300 pounds per square foot.

After reviewing the collection size, the librarian should analyze the use of floor space to determine if any additional space can be gained by any of the following methods: (1) reducing the width of the aisles between stacks, tables, or carrels, (2) replacing bulky furniture with smaller pieces, or (3) rearranging the entire layout to make optimum use of tight space. Finally, space outside the library can be considered. Sometimes the librarian can find rooms available on the same corridor as the library, or areas in the basement that are also adequate for storing backfiles and special supplies, for accommodating a photocopier, or for other special purposes. If changes are made to accommodate the need for space, the librarian should document them. This may strengthen any future proposal for acquiring additional space.

Once all reasonable avenues for alleviating space shortage have been explored and documented, the librarian or consultants can begin plans for creating additional space. Additional space can include space in a new building, space in an area vacated by others, or renovation of the existing space. All these options require the same planning process. The decision about which option to choose depends on individual circumstances within the institution.

Developing Support for Library Space

Competition for physical space can be as intense as competition for monetary resources. Therefore, the librarian needs to develop influence that can be effective in convincing the administration to support the library's need for space. By studying the hospital's power structure, especially in relation to space decisions, the librarian can identify special interest groups and individuals in positions of authority. The librarian may also wish to interview influential members of various user groups, informing them about the condition of the library and assessing their views, interests, and willingness to support the library's bid for space. In addition to identifying supporters, the librarian should also identify those people who might create obstacles for the library because their interests are in conflict with the library's need for space. Of all the methods librarians use to develop support for library space, two are essential. Librarians must discuss needs and strategies with the hospital administration and with the library committee. They must also get to know the people who are concerned with space planning, while keeping informed of projected space plans for the hospital. With the assistance of the planning team, the librarian can prepare a well-documented space program and use it as a marketing tool when requesting space from influential committee members and the administration.

ESTIMATING GENERAL SPACE REQUIREMENTS

Obtaining additional space is expensive. Therefore, when requesting space, the librarian should project future needs as well as the present needs of the library. To plan for a flexible facility, the space needed to accommodate future growth must be estimated. Rapid technological change has made it impractical to attempt to project growth for more than ten years. Using the completed evaluation of the existing space, the librarian can estimate space requirements by their function and their relationship to one another. The librarian can identify the areas to be accommodated and determine the numbers and types of materials, furniture, equipment, and people to be placed in each area.

After existing space has been evaluated and alternatives have been considered, a general estimate of required space should be calculated. The librarian should have a realistic target figure, based on projected growth, to cite early in the process of selling the need for larger space. For example, although a 50 percent increase in present space may seem reasonable at first, growth projections may show that such space would only alleviate the problem temporarily. Therefore, the librarian must not only calculate realistic figures at the start of the planning process but also demonstrate the cost-effectiveness of arranging for flexible space that can be used effectively for a period of ten years.

The librarian can make a general estimate of the total amount of space needed for all library activities by calculating the number of seats needed to accommodate users during peak periods. This number is based on 10 percent to 25 percent of the number of potential users. The percentage of potential users may divide into primary users (those who use seats regularly) and secondary users (those who use the library infrequently). For many hospital libraries, seating 10 percent of primary users and 1 percent of secondary users provides adequate seating(8). For hospitals with extensive teaching commitments, seating 15 percent to 25 percent of heavy users such as students, 10 percent of moderate users such as residents, and 1 percent of light users such as social workers or dieticians, may be more realistic. For a sample profile of potential users in a teaching hospital, see Appendix A.

After the number of seats has been determined, the total is multiplied by 100 to 120 square feet(9:288). This estimate usually provides an adquate amount of space for all the furniture, equipment, and materials needed for the entire facility. Appendix B provides several space formulas for determining needs. The formulas for determining the general estimate of total library space follow:

$$\begin{array}{lll} \text{Number} & = & 10 \text{ percent to} & + & 1 \text{ percent} \\ \text{of Seats} & & 25 \text{ percent} & & \text{Potential} \\ & & \text{Potential} & & \text{Secondary} \\ & & \text{Primary} & & \text{Users} \\ & & \text{Users} & & \end{array}$$

$$\begin{array}{lll} \text{Total Space} & = & \text{Number of} & \times & 100 \text{ to } 120 \\ \text{for Library} & & \text{Seats} & & \text{Square Feet} \\ \text{in Square} & & & & \\ \text{Feet} & & & & \end{array}$$

ESTIMATING SPACE REQUIREMENTS BY AREA FUNCTION

Another type of space estimation involves calculating space needed for broad functions, such as the stack area, seating area, staff area, and core areas. This type of estimate can be prepared fairly quickly using standard formulas. It provides backup for the general estimate, documentation of actual space required, and guidance for the architect or space planner. Management may be more receptive to space estimates based on area functions than to the undifferentiated estimate based only on a number of seats.

Stack Area

On the average, 8½ medical periodical volumes can be housed in 1 square foot of floor space in 7½-foot high stacks, accounting for both stack and aisle space(9:306). From 9 to 9½ monographs may be shelved in 1 square foot of floor space. It is a good idea to use the smaller figure (8½ volumes) when calculating space for books and journals to compensate for unestimated growth.

The number of volumes should be calculated based on ten years growth. There are several methods for determining this figure. The simplest is to multiply the number of volumes added during the present year by ten and add this figure to the current volume count. Space needed for the collection is then estimated as follows:

$$\text{Stack Area in Square Feet} = \frac{\text{Collection Size (ten-year projection)}}{8\frac{1}{2}\text{ volumes}}$$

Seating Area

On the average, 30 square feet per user-seat will provide adequate space for various types of seating, including aisle space around each chair(9:303). The librarian should use the number of seats calculated in the general estimate and figure the amount of space needed for seating users as follows:

$$\text{Seating Area in Square Feet} = \text{Number of Seats} \times 30\text{ Square Feet}$$

Staff Area

The formula of 175 square feet for the librarian and 150 square feet for other staff members includes space for desks, aisles, equipment, storage and work counters (9:299-300). Space for the staff is then estimated as follows:

$$\text{Staff Area in Square Feet} = \text{Number of Staff} \times 150\text{ to }175\text{ Square Feet}$$

Central Core Areas

Calculating the amount of space needed for central core areas such as the information desk, the card catalog, and the reference section is more involved. For each of these areas, the librarian should make a list of the furniture, materials, and equipment that must be accommodated, omitting seating and working surfaces for users that may be provided in the reference and index area or the journal display area. Then a drawing should be made of each area. Areas should be drawn independently of each other. To draw to scale, the librarian should use graph paper and a scale of 1:48 (¼ inch = 1 foot) or 1:24 (½ inch = 1 foot). To accommodate a walkway, one-half of a three-foot aisle space should be allowed on at least two sides of each area. The space needed for core areas can be estimated as follows:

$$\text{Core Areas in Square Feet} = \text{Sum of Square Feet for Each Core Area}$$

Trade-offs and space saving may occur later when the librarian makes a detailed estimate of allocated space.

Entrance and Information-Circulation Desk Area

The librarian can include entrance space or "traffic" space for users in the estimate of space needed in front of the information desk. Usually six to eight feet is allowed for this "milling room." The size of the information desk, space for staff seating behind the desk, as well as shelving should also be included. Figure 16-1 shows a sample layout of the area.

Current Journal Display Area

If the librarian is using standard 90-inch high steel stacks with 36-inch wide sections 10-inches deep, 25 issues can be displayed on 5 slanted display shelves (9:302). A maximum of five shelves is recommended for easier reach. The librarian should also allow for one-half of a 4-foot aisle, or 2 feet in front of each display, for standing and passing.

Card Catalog and Dictionary Area

The number of books projected for the collection, and therefore the number of cards to be filed determines the size of the catalog case needed. A standard 17-inch tray will provide 14 inches of net filing space. If filled to 72 percent capacity, such a drawer will hold 1,000 cards averaging 1/100 inch in thickness (10:397). The librarian should figure an average of five cards per title. A collection of 1,000 books would require five drawers. Additional space can be added for a consulting table, a large dictionary on a stand, and space for standing and passing. Figure 16-2 shows a sample arrangement of a card catalog and dictionary area.

Reference and Index Area

Shelf space for reference books and indexes is based on using shelves 10 inches deep. Since aisle space is usually shared, the librarian should provide one-half of a 3-foot aisle, or 1½ feet to these sections. All growth projections should be based on the number of volumes added to the collection each year plus any additions which may be under consideration. Seating estimates for this area are included in the previous estimate for seating.

Audiovisual Area

Audiovisuals should be kept in an area near the circulation desk. Many librarians consider standard stack sections comprised of shelves 10 to 12 inches deep the most flexible space for software. Since library holdings of these materials are so varied, as is the format and the method of storing them, no standard measures have yet been developed. Growth projections can be based on present growth rates. Seating estimates are included in the previous estimate for seating.

Figure 16-1
Entrance and Information-Circulation Desk Area

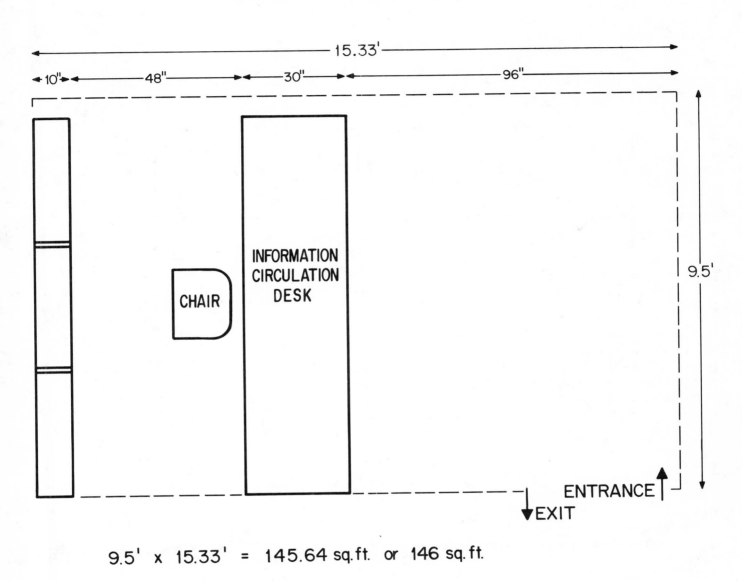

9.5' x 15.33' = 145.64 sq. ft. or 146 sq. ft.

NOTE: This sample was developed for the requirements of an active library in a 200-bed community hospital.

Figure 16-2
Card Catalog and Dictionary Area

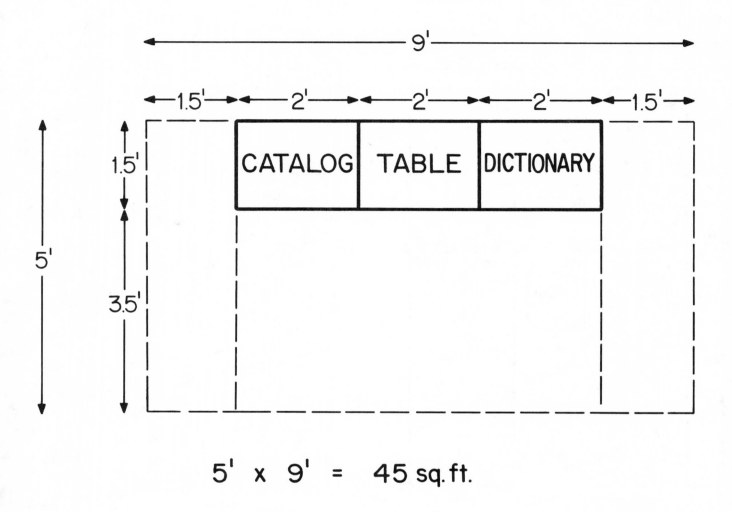

5' x 9' = 45 sq.ft.

NOTE: This sample was developed for the requirements of an active library in a 200-bed community hospital.

Photocopy Area

When estimating space for the photocopy area, the librarian should include the following items: the photocopy machine, additional work space on either side of the machine, a book truck, a counter for stapling and cutting copies, a supply cabinet, and space for a large wastebasket. A sample layout of the photocopy area is shown in Figure 16-3.

Computer Terminals

Space for a computer terminal, a chair, and shelves also needs to be estimated. The drawing, such as the one in Figure 16-4, should represent "ideal space." Later on, the librarian should locate this function in the most convenient place for staff and users, such as at the information desk or in the librarian's office.

Book Trucks

Finally, the librarian should estimate the number of book trucks needed and calculate the space required to park them when not in use. Small trucks are about 1½ feet wide by 2½ feet long. Large trucks are 3 feet long by 1½ feet wide.

Totaling Area Estimates

After space requirements have been estimated for the stack area, the seating area, the staff area, and core areas, the estimates should be totalled and compared with the general estimate of space. The results should be fairly similar. If not, the librarian should examine both estimates to make sure that the projected requirements have been analyzed thoroughly. To compensate for wasted space that may be caused by the idiosyncracies or the configuration of the actual assigned space, the librarian can add a 6 percent configuration loss to the estimate (11:81). If the general estimate remains much larger than the estimate by area function, the formula chosen for the general estimate may be more generous than is appropriate for this facility.

MAKING A DETAILED SPACE ESTIMATE

The two general estimates discussed above are useful in the initial stages of planning, especially for selling the idea of additional library space. When approval of new space becomes certain, the librarian will want to make detailed calculations of the space needed for materials, furniture, equipment, and people. This estimate should include space for each activity and each item to be accommodated in the new space. Specific space allocations for types of seats, such as lounge chairs or a chair at a carrel, should also be included. Appendix B can be referred to for information on space formulas.

The librarian must be very precise when making a detailed space estimate, since an architect or space planner will be using it to design a floor plan. When the floor plan is completed, the architect will check it against the detailed space estimate for errors or overlooked items.

Central Core Areas

For each of the central core areas, the librarian should first describe the function and list all materials, furniture, seats, and equipment that will be needed. Then specific measurements should be determined for each item and the total calculated. At this point, possible placement and spatial relationships should be considered. Figure 16-8 can be helpful in this regard. Figures 16-5, 16-6, and 16-7 provide samples of how to draw to scale the areas that require seats, such as reference and indexes, current journal display, and audiovisuals. Space estimates for the entrance and information desk area, photocopy area and the card catalog area can be taken from the previous estimate by area function.

To develop minimum space requirements for these areas, the librarian should consider needs for the next few years only. Sometimes, trade-offs have to be made, such as doing without a current journal display or lounge-type seating to provide space for user terminals, microforms, or expanded audiovisual capability.

Stack Area

The function of the stack area should be described in the detailed estimate. The librarian should also list the number of materials, furniture, and equipment needed, such as bound journals and number of carrels for users. If audiovisuals are to be stored in the stacks, they need to be included, as well as the special carrels to accommodate equipment. The area required to house the stacks, aisles, and carrels should be drawn to scale and also estimated in number of square feet.

Shelving

The number of linear feet of shelving required must be determined. Since many journal volumes measure as high as 12 inches, only 6 of the 7 shelves in a 90-inch stack section may be usable. With 36-inch shelves, this provides 18 linear feet per stack section. In order to allow space for shifting, Metcalf considers shelf space at full capacity when it is 86 percent filled (10:155). Therefore, in a section for journals with 18 linear feet, 86 percent reduces the space to 15 linear feet and accommodates about 75 volumes at 5 per linear foot. If 84-inch high stacks with six shelves are used, then only 5 may be usable. At 13 linear feet, 65 journal volumes can be accommodated at 5 per linear foot.

When calculating the linear feet of shelving required, the librarian should use the standard of five volumes per linear foot for books and bound journal volumes. This provides a flexible estimate to accommodate unforeseen changes in the growth of the collection. If space is limited and a trade-off is necessary, space for books only may be successfully calculated using seven to eight volumes per

Figure 16-3
Photocopy Area

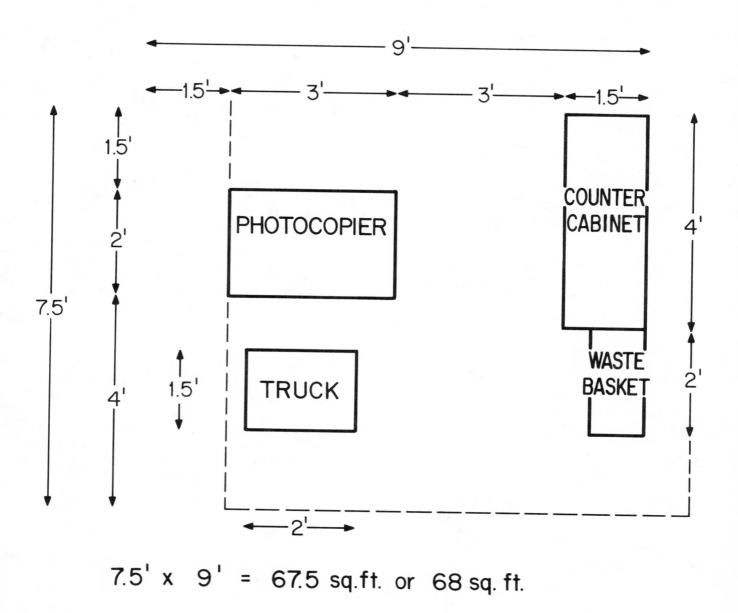

7.5' x 9' = 67.5 sq.ft. or 68 sq. ft.

NOTE: This sample was developed for the requirements of an active library in a 200-bed community hospital.

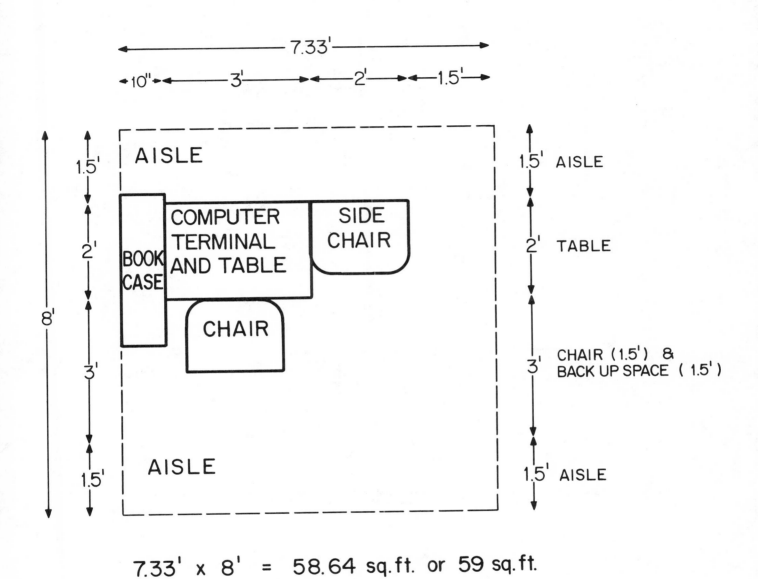

Figure 16-4
Computer Terminal Area

7.33' x 8' = 58.64 sq.ft. or 59 sq.ft.

NOTE: This sample was developed for the requirements of an active library in a 200-bed community hospital.

Figure 16-5
Reference Books and Index Area

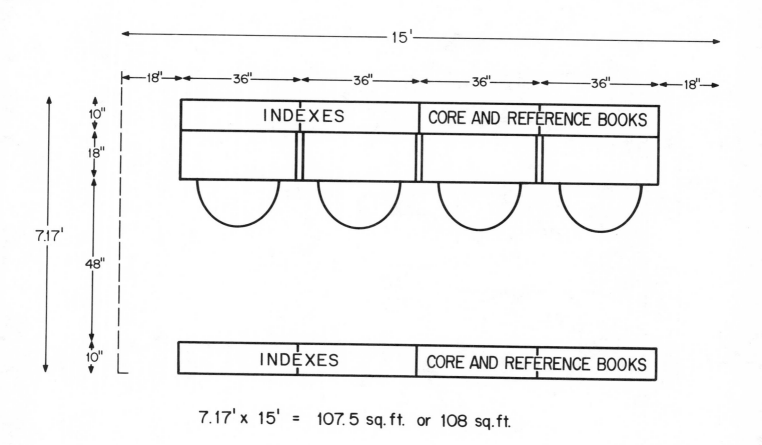

7.17' x 15' = 107.5 sq. ft. or 108 sq. ft.

NOTE: This sample was developed for the requirements of an active library in a 200-bed community hospital.

Figure 16-6
Current Journal Display Area

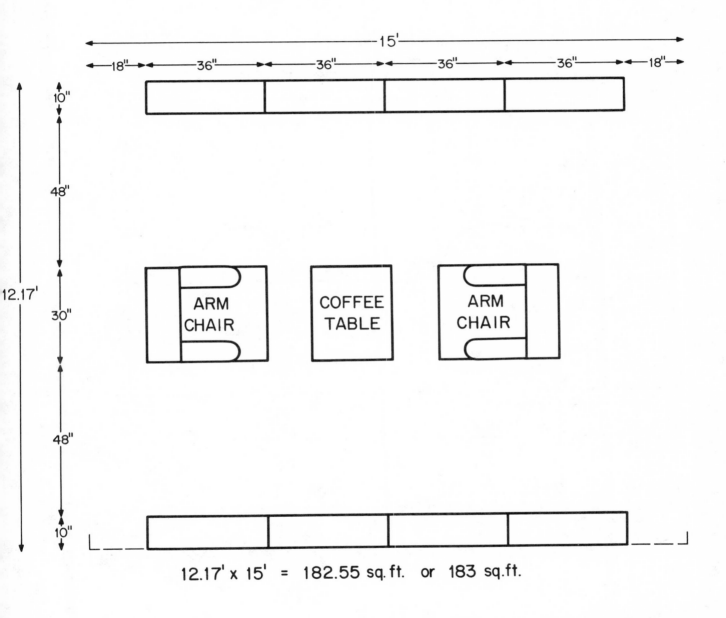

12.17' x 15' = 182.55 sq. ft. or 183 sq. ft.

NOTE: This sample was developed for the requirements of an active library in a 200-bed community hospital.

Figure 16-7
Audiovisual Area

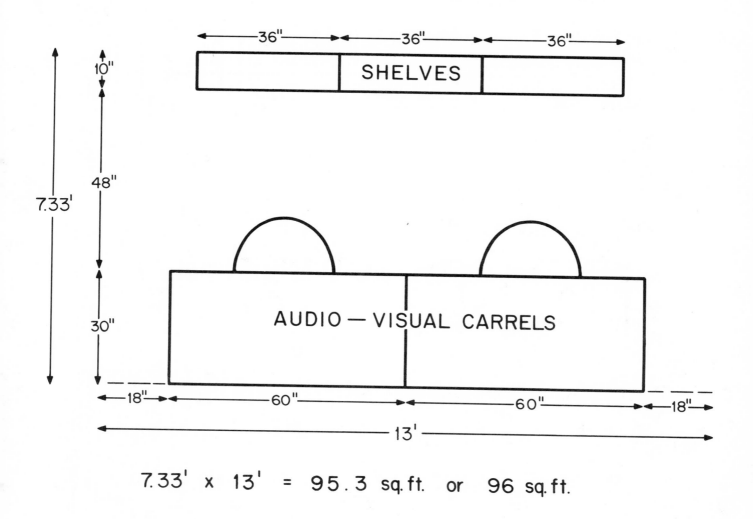

7.33' x 13' = 95.3 sq.ft. or 96 sq.ft.

NOTE: This sample was developed for the requirements of an active library in a 200-bed community hospital.

Figure 16-8
Sample Library Diagram Illustrating Spatial Relationships

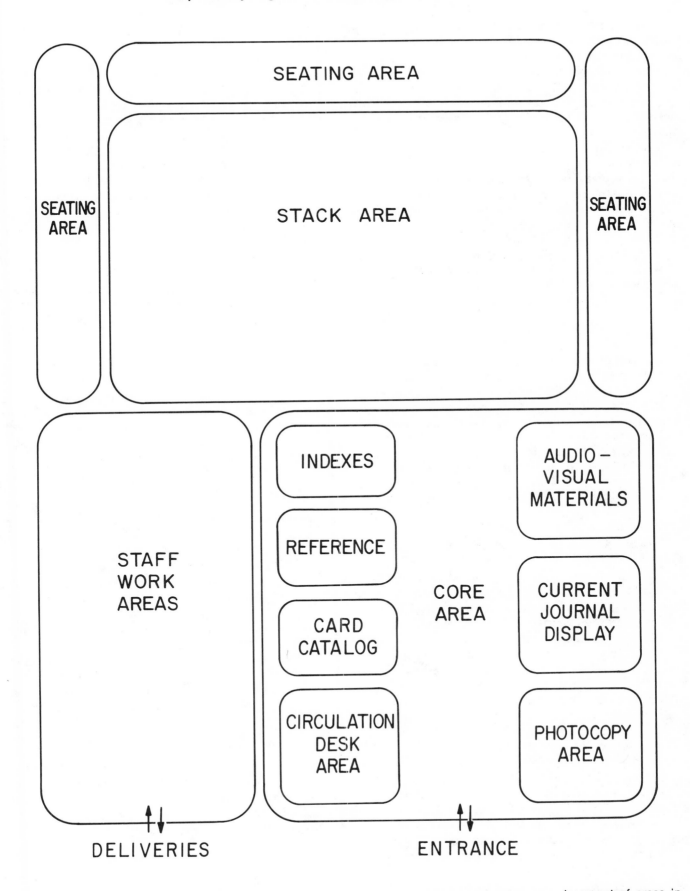

This floor plan for an active library in a community hospital illustrates the most advantageous placement of areas in

linear foot. Journal space should still be calculated using five volumes per linear foot.

Stacks usually measure 12 inches in depth for a single stack or 24 inches for a double. A stack 10 inches in depth is sufficient for both journals and books and can save four inches of aisle space. A 36-inch aisle between stacks is a comfortable width and allows wheelchairs to enter and exit but not turn. Minimum stack aisle width for wheelchairs is 33 inches(10:221). A stack using 12-inch shelves and a 36-inch aisle is often described as measuring "5 feet on center." This is the dimension from the center of one double stack across the aisle to the center of the next. Such measurement reveals the depth of both the shelves and the aisle. A stack using 10-inch shelves with a 33-inch aisle is described as measuring "4 feet 5 inches on center"(11:80). A range of stacks longer than five sections (15 feet) is awkward and time-consuming for users. Four or more sections in a row require an entry from either end for quick access, particularly for users in wheelchairs who cannot turn in normal width aisles. Wheelchairs need a space 63 inches by 56 inches for turning(10:221).

Carrels

Carrels should be 48 inches wide and 24 inches deep to accommodate bulky materials. Using a carrel 42 inches wide to save space is acceptable, but using a carrel only 36 inches wide is not. Backup space for chair and user requires three feet for comfort. Carrels for audiovisual equipment should be 30 inches deep and 60 inches wide. Aisles between the carrels and stacks should be a minimum of 36 inches. If the librarian is faced with the choice between a narrower aisle or a narrow carrel, he or she should choose a 48-inch carrel and narrower aisles.

Floor Specifications

The capacity of the floor to bear the weight of the stacks filled with heavy volumes is the most important determinant in the effective use of space in a hospital library. Floors must be able to support 150 pounds of live load per square foot. Because most hospital floors are built to support a live load of about 70 pounds per square foot, this requirement often presents a problem for hospitals and may severely restrict suitable locations for the library. A building must be able to suport dead load and live load. Dead load refers to the weight of the elements in the structure, such as steel, wood, and concrete. The live load refers to the elements that can be moved around in the building, such as furnishings and people.

The ability of the floor to bear the weight of stacks can only be determined by a structural engineer. The formulas presented for space assume 3-foot aisles between stacks that require a live load capacity of 150 pounds. Compact shelving requires 300 pounds. Reinforcing the weight-bearing capacity of the floor is very costly, but it provides a more flexible use of the space. Using wider aisles between the stacks reduces the amount of weight per square foot, but it will increase the amount of total space needed. For a more detailed discussion of floor load capacity, librarians should read Metcalf and Cohen (10, 11).

Staff Work Area

The librarian should give the staff work area a high priority when determining adequate space. Each work station should have two work surfaces 30 inches by 60 inches and 24 inches by 60 inches, spanned on one side by a counter for a typewriter or computer terminal. If there is to be a separate librarian's office, it should have space for two visitor's chairs and perhaps space for a terminal with necessary work surface and a user's chair. Office shelving should be generous. Storage cabinets should be no deeper than 24 inches over work counters of the same depth.

Special space in work areas should also be designated for receiving and processing mail, for holding cartons of books or bound journals on the floor, for a large waste basket, for an exit door to the corridor, for book trucks, for a sink and a refrigerator, and for a coat closet.

Comparing Estimates and Making Trade-offs

When totaling the space estimated in detail for core areas, stack area and work areas, the librarian must add a 6 percent configuration loss to it. The detailed space estimate should be compared to the two other estimates already prepared. The librarian can now examine trade-off possibilities and decide if cutting or adding is necessary. This process of calculating and estimating space is time-consuming but it offers many advantages. It assures that the new space will be an improvement and that it can be adjusted to meet changes over the ensuing years. It also helps to achieve a well-balanced allocation of space. Furthermore, it prepares the librarian to work productively with the architect as the plan is being applied to a specific site. Finally, estimating helps a librarian to accept trade-offs, such as narrower aisles in order to provide for a wider carrel.

Prior to actual approval of additional space, a librarian may be asked to prepare an estimate of the minimum amount, medium amount, and maximum amount of space required for a workable library. An administrator may request this in order to make the best decisions on location and funding. The formula for a general estimate by number of seats can be used as a maximum figure. The minimum and medium figures can be derived from the detailed space estimate and can represent various space-saving trade-offs. Well-documented estimates of space may prompt the administration to allocate the maximum amount needed but develop only the minimum amount for immediate use. The undeveloped space should be adjacent to the new space and maintained so that the library can expand into it later with a minimum of cost and effort.

When estimating for new space, the librarian should

not skimp. Skimping is only appropriate when making the best use of inadequate existing space. However, allotting too much space should also be avoided. Space must be adequate, reasonable, and based on standard specifications, such as those listed in the space formulas in Appendix B.

The three types of space estimates are illustrated in Appendix C as applied to an active library in a 200-bed community hospital. A possible floor plan for this new library is also presented. (See Figure 16-9).

PREPARING PLANNING DOCUMENTS

At some point in the process of planning for additional library space, the librarian may want to prepare written documents detailing space needs. These documents are often developed with the help of the administration, the library committee, influential user groups, or a specially appointed planning team. A number of different formats are possible for planning documents, including in-house space request forms, memos detailing space needs, and formal space programs.

Purpose of a Library Space Program

The space or building program is the standard document used in planning libraries. It is often useful in lobbying for hospital library space. This document can vary in length, depending on the detail necessary in a given situation. Whatever its length, the document can be used for the following multiple purposes:

- To assist in developing initial planning concepts
- To help in the process of analyzing space needs
- To organize all the details throughout layout, construction, and moving
- To provide an excellent reference source for all planning details
- To determine the essential needs of the library and encourage all concerned to acknowledge them
- To provide a persuasive document for all to read and evaluate
- To form the basis on which the architect can plan a satisfying facility

The space program document functions as an outline of space requirements as well as a planning and marketing tool throughout the entire process.

Elements of a Library Space Program

The space program presents objective facts and figures about users, staff, services, and the collection, as well as specific estimates of space required. These elements should be related to the philosophy of the library and its environment. The program should be well organized and succinct so that it can be read easily and quickly. If the document is more than a few pages, the highlights should be summarized on the first page. A table of contents

should also be provided. The following elements may be addressed in the library space program:

- *Goals and objectives.* These should relate to the goals of the hospital.
- *Setting or environment.* This section describes the hospital user groups, the library programs, the library's role in the community, cooperative arrangements with local libraries, and participation in library networks.
- *Present conditions.* This section describes space problems, action taken to alleviate problems, and changes in use of library services. It also provides statistics to indicate increase or decrease in use.
- *Changes needed.* This section describes what needs to be done, and why, to support changes in projected increase of users and services, or changes in hospital programs.
- *Consequences if changes are not implemented.* This section includes a description of reductions in collection size, services to be limited, or number of users who won't be seated.
- *Profile of potential users.* This section lists the number of projected users by category of job status and by level of use. The profile may analyze and list users as primary and secondary users, or as heavy, moderate, or light users. It also calculates the number of seats required for users and estimates the general space required. Appendixes A and C provide additional information on this topic.
- *Estimate of space required.* This section provides the general estimate of space based on a percentage of potential users, as well as a detailed estimate with capacity for users, collection, furniture, and staff in each area of activity.
- *Location.* This section describes factors to be considered, such as an open square or rectangular shaped space with no interior weight-bearing walls; floor load capacity per square foot of weight (150 pounds for libraries as compared to 70 pounds for patient care areas); quick and easy access; future expansion possibilities; and protection from water damage and excess noise and odors. Also included are discussions of feasible locations and possible trade-offs.
- *References.* This section cites sources for standards and formulas, and adds credibility and authority to the document.
- *Appendixes.* The final section includes reports or documents that help to illuminate the problem, such as a chart of comparative data on libraries in similar hospitals, or space formulas used.

CHOOSING BETWEEN NEW CONSTRUCTION OR REMODELING

Once a detailed space estimate has been developed, the librarian should consider whether remodeling the existing space provides a feasible alternative to space in another

Figure 16-9
Sample Floor Layout for Library in 200-Bed Community Hospital

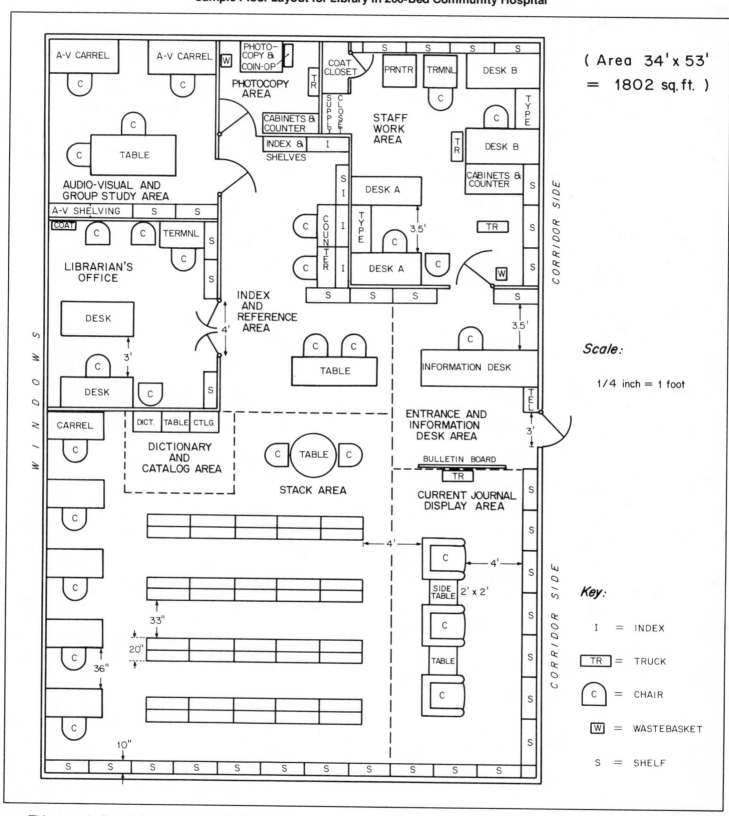

This sample floor layout has been designed as a part of the space planning process for an active library in a 200-bed community hospital. The area functions, and the equipment and space measures for this plan are detailed in Appendix C.

location. Remodeling existing space may be a particularly attractive option if adjacent space is available, or walls can be altered to allow the most flexible use of the space.

Remodeling requires the same planning process as does new space. The librarian must check the existing space for the following features: (1) the new, estimated space requirements, (2) the floor load capacity, if a new stack configuration is planned, and (3) space-stealing structural problems, such as weight-bearing walls, hidden clumps of plumbing pipes, dumb waiters, and numerous other unusual features that may not be included on the hospital engineer's structural plans.

For the best remodeling results, the librarian should work with a design professional, such as a space planner, architect, engineer, or interior designer. Such professionals can provide a more effective concept for utilizing space and better solutions to the problems caused by structural idiosyncracies. If old furniture must be retained, for example, design professionals can measure the furniture to ensure compatibility or suggest cost-effective alternatives.

When planning to use the existing space to better advantage, the librarian may have to make compromises or trade-offs to achieve overall improvement in the quality of the physical facility. The conditions that rate the highest priority for excellence and the lowest priority for compromise include staff working space; ventilation, heating, and air-conditioning; lighting and noise reduction; and one monitored entrance/exit.

The cost of remodeling or enlarging existing space should be compared to the estimated cost of new space, if both options are possible. A final consideration should be whether the remodeling can be done while the library continues to operate. This can become a major factor, especially when good space is available elsewhere. If the existing site is preferred, however, the several months of dirt, noise, and disorganization in the library may be an acceptable cost for a remodeled facility.

DESIGNING AND CONSTRUCTING LIBRARY FACILITIES

When the project moves into the design or construction phases, the librarian must continue to be involved. Although design and construction professionals are responsible for the project, the librarian should understand the design and construction process and be active in the planning, approving, and monitoring phases. The remainder of this chapter considers various aspects of hospital library design. Additional information may also be found in the readings at the conclusion of this chapter.

General Design Considerations

Design influences people's behavior, and thereby, affects the use of space. Planning major alterations of space requires knowledge of how people feel about space, how much distance between people is needed for comfort and security, and how people react within a given space. Application of these principles contributes to the effective design of space for different activities.

Private, secure, and quiet work space encourages concentration. To provide this kind of space, the librarian can place individual carrels at right angles to the wall so that the user is enclosed on three sides. This offers privacy and also reduces noise. To encourage group participation, and still maintain a quiet environment, the librarian may place round tables in a conference room. To control the noise level in a lounge area, lounge chairs can be placed facing away from each other.

The way people use space or behave in it is also governed by the appearance or the aesthetics of the space. This principle is easily observable in restaurants. Fast food restaurants use bright, sharp colors, hard surfaces, and small immovable furniture to discourage lengthy conversations and leisurely meals. French restaurants, on the other hand, are more apt to use soft colors, comfortable chairs, and individual lighting to provide a feeling of comfort, privacy, and leisure. The same ideas can be applied to the library. Bright colors around the information desk will draw people to it, while subdued colors in the study area will provide a quiet, soothing environment.

A library should be functional, comfortable, and attractive. Ideally, these three elements should be in balance. For example, a current journal display area should have seats adjacent to the display shelves. Lounge-type chairs are often used for this seating area to provide comfort, and designers frequently group a sofa with chairs to make the area attractive. Unfortunately, library users do not like to sit next to each other on sofas. Although the bulk of the sofa is pleasing to the eye in the overall design of the area, it is not functional because it may accommodate only one person in space large enough for two or three. It is also not comfortable for the two or three people who must sit elbow-to-elbow. The solution lies in choosing individual chairs to provide an attractive, comfortable grouping within a limited amount of space. Such a workable compromise is attainable if the librarian and the designer balance function, comfort, and attractiveness as they work together in solving design problems. Cohen provides a substantive discussion of the behavioral aspects of space(11).

Design, Furniture and Flooring for Specific Areas

Library space should be flexible and should allow for the adequate operation of primary library functions. Nonassignable space—such as rest rooms, janitor's closets, stairs, or corridors—should be located outside the library space. Heating, ventilation, lighting, floor load capacity, and ceiling heights should remain consistent throughout the space. In furnishings, the librarian should avoid built-in cabinets or bookcases, decorative walls, and planters in order to maintain the greatest flexibility for future change. The ideal shape for library space is the square or rectangle. It is the most workable and space-saving. If this shape is not possible, the librarian can apply the concept of the central square to the areas of heaviest user activity, the core areas, and the places most likely to change. This makes the central square the focal point of the library where people and activities converge (11). Although an architect or designer designs the floor layout, librarians should review these decisions to be sure that they are functional.

Spatial Relationships

The arrangement of areas and how they relate to each other is an important consideration in the design of the floor plan. The librarian and the designer should discuss the function of each area, the relationship of each area to other areas, and the traffic flow of users and staff from area to area. This is essential before any floor layout for new space is planned. The librarian may also consider illustrating spatial relationships in outline form, in diagram form such as the one in Figure 16-8, or in a rough floor plan before a designer makes the actual floor plans.

Areas that are frequently used for a short period of time and are monitored by staff should be located in the central core. In libraries managed by one person, it is best to arrange the core areas in a sequence to facilitate efficiency and quick service to users. Activities that require concentration for longer periods of time should be placed away from the busy center core area.

Entrance and Exit Areas

The layout of the library should be visible as the user steps through the door. For purposes of control, there should be only one door that serves as both the entrance and the exit. Fire exits are necessary, but they can be fitted with special locks so the doors can be opened easily in emergencies.

Information and Circulation Desk

The information and circulation desk should be adjacent to the entrance for both convenience and control of library materials. The most comfortable desk for both users and staff has a counter at standing height on the user's side and a desk of seating height on the staff side. The desk can be bought commercially or can be designed by the architect to fit a particular situation. Working surfaces should be covered with a synthetic, nonshiny laminate for durability. Bookcases can be constructed from sections of the same steel shelving used in the stacks and can be placed behind the desk. Uniform shelving used throughout the library provides greater flexibility for future changes.

Card Catalog

The card catalog should be located close to the information desk so that the staff can easily consult it or assist users with it. Catalog drawers should be purchased with a guarantee on construction. A flat surface on or next to the catalog should be provided for the placement of tools, such as the MeSH, journals holdings list, and scrap paper. The surface can also be used for the placement of the catalog drawer when referring to the cards at greater length.

Reference Books and Journal Indexes

Reference books and journal indexes are usually located near the information desk on steel shelving. A flat or slightly sloped counter hung on shelving at seating height is useful for consulting current indexes or reference sources. Because indexes are consulted for a short time only, stools or typing chairs on casters make good seats for this activity.

If the volume of library use warrants a reference desk for the librarian as well as an information-circulation desk, a conventional office desk can be placed at a right angle to a section of the reference shelving. This forms an adequate reference center. A computer terminal for bibliographic searching can be placed here also if electrical and telephone outlets are available. Locating reference activity in full sight of users encourages the use of these services and is more convenient for a small staff.

Journal Display

The display of current journal issues should be located in the central core or square, visible from the information desk. Steel shelving with fixed slanted display shelves is most appropriate because it allows users to recognize the issue quickly by its cover. It also displays only the most current issues. Keeping the other unbound issues on the shelves with the bound issues is less confusing and more convenient for the user. Carousel type display stands can be used if the shape of the space available is square rather than oblong. Carousel racks do not display the journal cover well, and because they rotate, it is harder to determine where the alphabetical sequence of titles begins. Lounge chairs and low tables for newspapers are also useful in this area.

Photocopy Area

The librarian may find it helpful to set up the photocopy area close to the information desk so that staff can assist users and quickly service the machines. Special sound absorbing divider panels can be used along with book shelves to muffle the noise. The area should be well ventilated and equipped with special electrical outlets. Other items essential to the area are counter space for collating and stapling copies, a book truck for library materials, storage for machine paper and toner, and a very large wastebasket.

Audiovisual Area

The audiovisual equipment and software should also

be located near the information desk so that staff can easily help users with equipment. Special carrels with high privacy screens, earphones, and electrical outlets are essential for using portable equipment efficiently. Built-in audiovisual equipment cores in these carrels are not practical. They restrict use and in time become obsolete. If space is available, the librarian can set up small rooms for group use of audiovisuals.

The audiovisual area can be part of the stack area, or it can be screened off with shelving. If it is included in the stack area, software should be stored on the shelves closest to the information desk. The carrels should also be placed near the desk.

Miscellaneous Items in Core Area

The following items should be considered for the core area: a dictionary stand, a wall telephone with a small shelf, a pencil sharpener, bulletin boards, book trucks, wastebaskets, coat racks, a book return, clocks, step-stools, and fire extinguishers.

Seating Facilities

The librarian will want to provide a variety of seating facilities to accommodate an assortment of library activities: quick consultation, relaxed reading, group study, and concentrated study. Although a variety of seating should be provided, about 60 percent of all seating should be in carrels for concentrated study (12). To facilitate study, several components should be included in carrels—a shelf, a lamp, and a writing surface with a light-color matte finish to reflect the light.

Arrangement of carrels is important. The placement of carrels in a row at right angles to the wall, facing in the same direction, helps to maintain a quiet area free of distractions. Back-to-back or clover leaf arrangement of carrels can become congested at times and may not be conducive to concentration. Carrels placed facing the wall are often the last to be used. This arrangement exposes the user's back, reducing privacy and visual control of the space around the user.

Tables absorb space in the library and should be used sparingly. A four-chair table may only seat one or two people when the chairs are also used for belongings, or when books and papers are spread out over the entire surface of the table. Therefore, only a few tables should be provided for consultation or short-term study. Group study rooms are a wise alternative to group study at tables. They can accommodate four to six people. If the room is equipped with outlets, audiovisuals can be used. A bare white wall makes an effective projection screen.

Chairs should be sturdy enough to withstand tipping. The librarian should sit in the chair before approving a selection. Chairs with arms must fit under tables and carrel surfaces. Often it is better to pay more for a chair that guarantees durability. Sturdiness, fit, and comfort are more important than look or design. Lounge chairs add to the comfort and look of the library. They are appropriate as long as their size is proportional to the space available. Sturdy coffee tables provide a place for newspapers or journal issues and are a practical accompaniment to lounge chairs. Sofas are not practical at all. People do not like to rub shoulders while reading the *American Heart Journal* or even the newspaper.

Shelving

Standard steel shelving provides versatility, especially when supplementary components are added, such as slanted journal display shelves, working surfaces for carrels or index consultation, slotted shelves with dividers for audiovisual software or journal issues, and coat racks that fit the standard brackets. The base of the steel shelving stack may vary in depth from 10 inches to 24 inches; the wider base prevents tipping of a free standing stack. The 10-inch base saves aisle space. The stack ranges can be braced to provide stability. It is best to avoid built-in shelving or alcoves of counter-height shelving. Freestanding, braced, double-faced stacks are preferred. They provide a uniform, clean, and simple shelf arrangement for users and make an effective sound barrier for study carrels.

Staff Work Area

The best location for the work area is behind the information-circulation desk. The work area should be enclosed by sound proof walls and a door with a glass panel. A panel is preferable to a glass wall because the wall exposes too much activity and makes it too tempting for staff to work in the offices rather than at the information desk.

The work area should be furnished with standard office furniture. Each work station should have at least two work surfaces and special counters or tables for typewriters and computer terminals. Steel shelving sections and a counter for preparing journals for binding are necessary items. Near the workroom exit to the main corridor an area should be established for receiving mail, books, and supplies. Floor space should also be available for holding and receiving cartons of binding. Other important items that should be included in the work room are a small sink, counter space for a coffeepot, a coat closet, and large wastebaskets.

Staff work areas and offices should be comfortable, well-organized, and well-ventilated to support effective, productive performance. The librarian should plan for generous work surfaces, storage areas, and shelving space. To be prepared for future changes, extra space should be planned for at least one additional staff member.

Carpeting

Carpet is the best material for sound absorption. It can be cleaned cheaply, and it is easy to maintain. If possible, carpet should be placed in every area of the library. Nylon or another synthetic with a low cut or loop pile and antistatic qualities is preferable to wool, which is very expensive. Carpet should be glued to the floor without padding. This gives the carpet longer wear and allows book trucks to roll more easily. If new space is planned, it is easier and cheaper to lay the carpet first and then place the stacks over it. If new carpet is to be placed in the existing space, it is easier to cut the carpet to fit around the stacks than to remove the books and the stacks to lay the carpet. Cohen presents an extensive discussion on carpeting (11).

Color Considerations

Selecting a color scheme is important in the design of a new library. People are affected by color, but their reactions are diverse. The use of primary colors, for example, attracts some people and repels others. Conversely, subdued tones may be oppressive to some people and soothing to others. Therefore, it is important to create an environment comfortable for most.

Choosing colors for the most effective impact requires an expert—an architect, an interior designer, or furniture salesperson. The librarian can exert influence on the outcome by expressing preferences, discussing the psychological effect desired, or reacting to the selections of the expert. If no expert assistance is available, the librarian should coordinate the color scheme. Color design by committee does not work well, since people may have conflicting tastes. Staff and other members of the planning team can participate in the selection by reacting to the effect of the overall scheme, thus supporting or helping to amend the choices.

When selecting colors, it is best to start with the color of the largest area first—the walls. The choice of an off-white color for the walls is the most popular solution to the problem of various color tastes. The next area, the carpet, should have color variations. Tweed provides such a variation and will hide dirt or lint. The ceiling should be white or a light shade so that light can be reflected effectively. Bright splashes of color can be used on small walls or on stack ends as long as the colors are kept uniform throughout the library. A mild color should be selected for areas of concentrated study. In areas of high activity, such as the information desk, the librarian can use stronger colors.

Color selections for fabrics, paints, carpets, and wood finishes should all be matched under the light and on the surface where they are to be used. For a more extensive discussion on color, librarians should read Cohen (11).

Lighting, Power, Acoustics, Heating and Cooling Systems

Adequate lighting, heating and cooling systems, and acoustics are not the major responsibility of the librarian.

However, some knowledge of these areas is essential. A librarian must work with the electrical engineer and the architect or hospital engineer to make sure that library requirements are satisfied by the systems they design. For a more technical discussion of lighting, power, and acoustics, librarians can read Metcalf(10) and Cohen (11).

In the past libraries were lighted above the level of 100 foot candles. The term "foot candles" describes the amount of light produced by one plumber's candle at a distance of one foot. Today, it is used as a measure of the level of lighting available. The present level for overall lighting is about 30 foot candles. Table and desk top lighting requires a higher level of illumination, from 50 to 100 foot candles depending on the detail of the work and the duration. For concentrated tasks, desk lamps provide more flexible lighting to satisfy the variations in users' needs. These lamps are more expensive to install but save energy in the long run. It is important that lighting be well diffused and that sharp contrasts be avoided.

The rapid increase in the use of microform readers, slide-tape machines, photocopy machines, and computer terminals in hospital libraries has created the need for many electrical outlets and separate telephone lines. The most flexible arrangement is to install conduits through which cables can be run to provide electrical, telephone, and communication outlets as the needs arise. This capability is particularly important if the library is to have long-range flexibility in its power systems.

Tolerance for noise in a library varies. In general, intermittent noise can be masked by constant noise or "white sound" at a level of 40 to 50 decibels. This sound is more easily tolerated than even complete silence. It provides a measure of accoustical privacy, and is often provided by the heating-ventilation-air-conditioning system (HVAC). The absorption of sound by books, soft materials, and acoustical panels should be considered, as well as user and staff traffic patterns, in reducing noise levels. Walls and ceilings can be constructed to minimize sound transmission, and carpeting can be used on the floor to provide a 50 percent quieter environment than other types of flooring.

The same HVAC system that serves the hospital proper should serve the library. If the building is old, the HVAC system may have to be supplemented by heaters and electric fans. Providing adequate ventilation for any small offices or the photocopy area and any electronic equipment should be carefully considered.

Construction Concerns

The librarian is responsible for monitoring construction, watching carefully for deviations, and working with architects to eliminate problems. He or she should realize that during construction unexpected problems can crop up, such as delayed delivery of materials or unexpected structural barriers.

The librarian should obtain permission to visit the building site daily but should avoid instructing or criticizing workers. He or she should check all final drawings for changes, particularly in cabinet measurements. For help in reading blueprints, librarians can consult the books by Wallach or Huth at the end of the chapter.

Graphics

A new or refurbished library requires new and well-designed graphics to guide users in their search for resources. Signs should be posted to identify particular areas in the library, indicate direction, provide "how to" information, and mark contents of stack sections and reference shelves.

The librarian can enlist the aid of staff to plan for signs and their locations. The administration may suggest in-house help and advice on making the signs. The librarians can also consult an architect for assistance or refer the work to a firm. If signs must be made by library staff, the following suggestions should be helpful.

Establishing a Consistent Format

Consistent size and color of signs presents a unified appearance and enables users to recognize them as location and informational aids throughout the library. In printing signs the librarian should make sure that ample border space is left with a margin on at least two sides of the design. The size of the left-hand margin should be consistent on every sign. The placement of the first letter of the sign should be measured from the left-hand border and from the top.

Keeping the Message Simple

All messages should be kept clear and concise. If a service is being advertised, the sign should explain why the service is being offered, to whom the service is available, and how the service can be obtained. Paragraph format should be avoided in information signs. Brief statements are easier to read and require less space.

Designing for Emphasis

Librarians should keep the number of signs to a minimum. Too many signs clutter the library and are ineffective. The use of strong contrasting colors—light and dark or warm and cool—on an off-white or neutral background will draw attention to the signs. Maps, on the other hand, provide more information in less space and inform the user of the relative locations of the rest of the collection.

Lettering

Keeping the same simple typeface for all signs creates consistency. All signs read better with upper- and lower-case letters. When printing small signs, the first letter of each word (excluding articles and prepositions) should be capitalized. In narrative signs, only the first letter of the first word of each sentence should be capitalized.

Lettering kits are efficient and provide a professional appearance. Even among commercial artists, hand lettering is a specialty requiring long hours of study and practice. Stencil letters should be avoided. The results are often neither precise nor attractive.

Although some people do not read signs, the majority of people do find signs useful. Clear, helpful signs reflect the library's service-oriented attitude. Librarians can refer to Cohen for more information on signs(11).

MOVING THE LIBRARY

Careful planning, organizing, and effective delegation of responsibility will make the library move a success. Planning the move and executing it should be a team effort. If there are fewer than three library staff members, the librarians should request additional help from the administration. Although several people are needed on the planning team to develop procedures and time frames and to help make decisions, the librarian should supervise and coordinate all moving activities. This includes delegating tasks, documenting assignments and procedures, and organizing the entire process.

Preparing for the Move

The librarian should prepare for the move by weeding the collection, taking inventory, and then measuring the collection for total current linear feet. A diagram should be made of how the collection will be arranged in the new expanded shelving space. The current linear feet of volumes and the total linear feet of new shelving will make a ratio that may be used to determine how much empty space should be left on each shelf. For example, if the total new linear shelf space is double the existing dimensions of the collection, the ratio is 1:2. That means that 50 percent of each shelf may be filled, or the top and bottom shelf may be left empty in each section allowing the five shelves in between to be filled two-thirds full. The amount of empty space that should be left for journals can be figured by adding the measurements of each title, its projected growth, and space for potential new titles. If the manipulation of the journal collection is complex—such as sending some volumes to storage, discarding others, and integrating new titles and volumes—a special working file should be prepared with a separate card for each title indicating linear measures and instructions for shelving, storage, or disposal.

The librarian should mark the location of both new and old items on the floor plan. The placement of the collection in the new stacks should also be marked, indicating direction of the alpha-numeric arrangement with arrows.

Preparing for the move also involves arranging to have the following items taken care of:

- Equipment disconnected in the old location and reconnected in the new location

- Telephones connected in the new location at the start of the move so service is available in both locations
- Mail held in the mail room until the move is completed
- Carpenter service contacted for projects at the old and the new locations
- New keys turned over on the first day of the move

Assigning Responsibilities to Movers

If professional movers are hired for the move, they should do the following:

- Provide cartons or special carts with shelves for moving volumes
- Provide color-coded labels for furniture, stack sections, and cartons
- Pack up the collection
- Unpack the collection in the new location, shelving all books and journals according to coded labels
- Provide special equipment to move furniture and equipment
- Arrange for controlling the elevators
- Provide for trucks if the move is to another building

More typically, hospital or volunteer help is organized to move the library. The librarian then must arrange with the administration to have the above tasks performed. In addition, the following should be done:

- The color codes for each area should be noted on the floor plan, such as reference area, workroom, or stack area. Each section of stacks should be numbered, and the floor plan posted for consultation in the new location.
- Each piece of furniture should be color coded.
- Card markers should be placed in the collection to indicate the area color and the section number of the stack to which items are being moved. All volumes following a card marker and up to the next marker should be packed in boxes or cartons and labeled with the area and stack section where volumes are to be shelved. After the move, rearranging the collection will simply entail shifting within each section.

- Staff should be assigned to supervise the packing, unpacking, and shelving by movers or helpers.
- Helpers should be assigned to shift the collection, read the shelves, and revise the shelving as needed.
- The work area should be organized for reopening.
- The closing and reopening dates of the library should be publicized throughout the hospital.

When the library has reopened, the librarian may want to host a social event to display the new facility and to acknowledge everyone who participated in the project. The invitation list should include members of the planning team, the administration, hospital employees who assisted with the construction and the move, and department heads, as well as all potential user groups.

PLANNING FOR THE FUTURE

Rapidly changing technology and the subsequent increases in library services can cause a carefully organized ten-year plan for space to be inadequate within five years. Automation requires more space for equipment and necessitates an increase in staff as the service grows in sophistication.

To accommodate change, new space should be evaluated within one year. The librarian should collect staff opinion on the working effectiveness of the space; conduct a brief survey of users' opinions; and document all opinions, details on problem areas, and suggestions for improvement. As service grows, space problems can be documented and reviewed periodically for necessary solutions.

At the end of a five-year period the space can be re-evaluated again. The librarian can present the results as a report to members of the hospital's organizational structure. Thus, planning for the use of space becomes a continuous process that ensures effective use of space and secures the availability of new or additional space when needed.

REFERENCES

1. Medical library unit. In: U.S. Health Care Facilities Service. Administrative services and facilities for hospitals: a planning guide. Rockville, MD: Government Printing Office, 1973: 39-45. (DHEW publication No. (HSM) 72-4035).

2. Postell D. Planning the hospital library. Hosp Prog 1963 Feb;44: 84-85.

3. Cramer A. Hospital library development. Salt Lake City: Network for Continuing Education. Intermountain Regional Medical Program, 1972. (Hospital Library Handbook No. 2.)

4. Greenfield M. Hospital libraries: focal point in the continuing education crisis. Bull Med Lib Assoc 1970 Oct;58(4):578-583.

5. American Library Association. Hospital Library Standards Committee. Standards for library services in health care institutions. Chicago: American Library Association, 1970.

6. Mayden P. Planning hospital library facilities. Chicago: Medical Library Association, 1975. (MLA courses for continuing education; CE 22).

7. Canadian standards for hospital libraries. Canad Med Assoc J 1975 May 17;112:1271-1274.

8. Suggested minimum guidelines for Connecticut health science libraries. New Haven: Connecticut Regional Medical Program, 1970.

9. Fry A. Library planning, furniture and equipment. In: Annan GL, Felter JW, eds. Handbook of medical library practice. 3d ed. Chicago: Medical Library Association, 1970.

10. Metcalf KD. Planning academic and research library buildings. New York: McGraw-Hill, 1965.

11. Cohen A, Cohen E. Designing and space planning for libraries: a behavioral guide. New York: RR Bowker, 1979.

12. DuVal MK, Alpert S. The health sciences library: its role in education for the health professions. Report of the Library Study Committee of the Association of American Medical Colleges to the National Library of Medicine. J Med Educ 1967 Aug;42(8pt2): 1-63.

READINGS

Alley B. A utility book truck designed for moving library collections. Libr Acquis 1979; 3:33-37.

Ambrose K, Ambrose L. Improving library effectiveness through a sociophysical analysis. Bull Med Libr Assoc 1977 Oct; 65:438-442.

Bell JA. Microforms: uses and potential. Bull Med Libr Assoc 1978 Apr;66:232-238.

Committee on Institutions of the Illuminating Engineering Society. Subcommittee on library lighting. Recommended practice of library lighting. Journal of IES, 1974 Apr;3:253-281.

Daghita JM. A core collection of journals on microfilm in a community teaching hospital library. Bull Med Libr Assoc 1976 Apr;64:240-241.

Duva AM. From closet to library in the community hospital: remodeling a hospital medical library. Bull Med Libr Assoc 1971 Jan;59:71-74.

Ellsworth RE. Academic library buildings: a guide to architectural issues and solutions. Boulder, CO: Colorado Associated University Press, 1973.

Fry A. Writing the building program: the significance of "AND." Bull Med Libr Assoc 1971 Jan 59:77-81.

Hayne F. Planning hospital library quarters: a bibliography. Bull Med Libr Assoc 1970 Jan;58:30-36.

Huth MW. Basic construction blueprint reading. New York: Van Nostrand Reinhold, 1980.

Kamenoff L. Retention of journals in a community hospital library. Bull Med Libr Assoc 1977 Oct;65:446-447.

Klein MS. Space utilization in hospital libraries with space shortages. Bull Med Libr Assoc 1977 Jan;65:63:65.

Long JB. A journal use study in a VA hospital. In: Chen, CC. ed. Quantitative measurement and dynamic library service. Phoenix: Oryx Press, 1978:95-102.

Lyles MA. Environmental design applications. Spec Libr 1972 Nov;63: 495-501.

Meiboom ER. Conversion of the periodical collection in a teaching hospital library to microfilm format. Bull Med Libr Assoc 1976 Jan;64: 36-40.

Miller JD. Health sciences libraries in hospitals. Bull Med Libr Assoc 1972 Apr;60 Suppl:19-28.

Mount E, ed. Planning the special library. New York: Special Libraries Association, 1972.

Pings VM. Building precepts and library programs. Bull Med Libr Assoc 1968 Jan;56:24-31.

Pings VM. Planning and designing hospital health science libraries. Bull Med Libr Assoc 1971 Jan;59:82-86.

Robeson CA. Planning and maintenance of library facilities and resources. In: Bloomquist H, Rees AM, Stearns NS, Yast H, eds. Library practice in hospitals. Cleveland: Case Western Reserve University, 1972:147-171.

Rouse R. Within-library solutions to book space problems. Libr Trends 1971 Jan;19:299-310.

Sommer R. Personal space: the behavioral basis of design. Englewood Cliffs, NJ: Prentice-Hall, Inc., 1969.

Strain PM. Efficiency and library space. Spec Libr 1979 Dec;70: 542-548.

Tenhundfeld EL, Lorenzi N. A hospital library building program. Bull Med Libr Assoc 1976 Jan;64:41-44.

Testa SN. Journal use in a community hospital. In: Chen, CC. ed. Quantitative measurement and dynamic library service. Phoenix: Oryx Press, 1978:129-135.

Wallach PI, Hepler, DE. Reading construction drawings. New York: McGraw-Hill, 1979.

Williams JF, Pings VM. A study of the access to the scholarly record from a hospital health science core collection. Bull Med Libr Assoc 1973 Oct;61:408-415.

APPENDIX A
Sample Profile of Potential Users in a Teaching Hospital Library

Primary—Heavy Users	Current	10-Year Projection		Current	10-Year Projection
			Nursing staff development	9	15
			Nurse clinical specialists	3	25
Students			Nursing staff (25%)	161	175
Nursing, Diploma	346	360			
Nursing, University	60	60	Total	652	743
Allied health	111	140			
Medical	48	125			
			Secondary—Light Users		
Total	565	685			
			Active medical staff (50%)	136	150
			Nursing staff (RN,LPN) (75%)	483	525
Primary—Moderate Users			Administrative staff	18	20
			Pharmacy	4	5
Students—Practical Nursing	110	125	Pharmacy students	18	22
Faculty			Dieticians	21	23
Nursing, Diploma	45	47	Social service	22	24
Nursing, University	13	15	Respiratory therapists	2	3
Practical nursing	16	16			
Allied health	14	15	Total	704	772
Housestaff	136	150			
Active medical staff (50%)	136	150			
Bioscientists	9	10	*Grand Total*	1921	2200

APPENDIX B
Space Formulas

The following formulas may be used in determining space estimates for the library.

1. Formulas for Collection Space

Volumes per linear foot	4½ to 5
Books per linear foot	7 to 8
Volumes per 3 foot single faced section, 6 shelves high	75*
Volumes per square foot of floor space	8½*

    *This estimate satisfies the Metcalf formula that complete working capacity of shelves is reached when they are 86 percent full.

2. Formulas for Seating Space

At 4-place tables	20 to 25 square feet each
At individual carrels	25 to 30 square feet each
At AV carrels	30 to 45 square feet each
In lounge chairs	30 to 40 square feet each
Enclosed studies	50 to 60 square feet each

3. Formulas for Staff Space

Librarians at desk in enclosed office	175 square feet each
Assistants at desks	150 square feet each

4. Formulas for Determining the Number of Seats

    For the United States:

    - Seat 10% of all potential users, or
    - Seat 10% of primary users and 1% of secondary users, or
    - Seat 15% -25% of heavy users, 10% of moderate users, and 1% of light users.

    For the United Kingdom:

• Undergraduates and trainees	1 seat for 4
• Student nurses and other students	1 seat for 8
• Graduates and medical staff	1 seat for 6
• Trained technicians	1 seat for 10
• General practitioners, dentists, nurses	1 seat for 20

    For Canada:

    - Seat 1/6 of all potential users

5. Formula for General Estimate of Library Space

    Total number of square feet to house all library activities =

    Number of seats × 100 square feet to 120 square feet

APPENDIX C
Sample Space Estimate
for a Library in a 200-Bed Community Hospital
(Ten-Year Projection)

I. Profile for Community Hospital Library

A. Potential Users

Primary Users	Current	Projected
Active Medical Staff	75	83
Nursing Staff (RN)	25	28
Pharmacists	4	4
Social Workers	4	4
Dietitians	2	2
Lab Technicians	6	7
Respiratory Therapist	4	4
	120	132

Secondary Users		
Visiting Medical Staff	95	105
Dentists	12	13
Nursing Staff (RN & LPN)	150	165
Physical Therapists	4	4
Respiratory Therapists	5	6
Lab Technicians	18	20
Medical Records Administrators	2	2
Radiologic Technicians	6	7
Administrators	6	6
	298	328

B. Collection

		Current	Projected
1.	Books	1,500	2,000
2.	Journal Subscriptions	130	160
3.	Journal Volumes	1,250	1,600
4.	Indexes	300	350
5.	Reference Books & Core Texts	120	150
6.	Audiovisual Titles	150	250

C. Staff

	Current	Projected
Librarian—Director	1	1
Assistant	1	2
Volunteers	.5 FTE	0
	2.5	3

II. Space Estimates for 10-Year Projection

A. General Estimate = 2,040 square feet

1. Total Seats: 17
    Seat 10% of potential primary users: $132 \times .10 = 13.2$
    Seat 1% of potential secondary users: $328 \times .01 = 3.2$
    Total = 16.4 or 17 seats

2. Total Space for Library: 2,040 square feet
    17 seats $\times$ 100 - 120 square feet =
    1,700 - 2,040 square feet

B. Estimate by Area Function = 1,927 square feet

1. Stack Area: 424 square feet
    3,600 volumes $\div$ 8.5 volumes = 424 square feet

2. Seating Area: 510 square feet
    17 seats $\times$ 30 square feet = 510 square feet

3. Staff Area: 475 square feet

Librarian	175 square feet
2 Assistants	300 square feet
	475 square feet

4. Core Areas: 409 square feet

    a. Entrance and information desk area =
        9.5 feet $\times$ 15.3 feet or 146 square feet
        (See Figure 16-1)
    b. Card Catalog and Dictionary Area =
        5 feet $\times$ 9 feet or 45 square feet
        (See Figure 16-2)
    c. Photocopy Area = 7.5 feet $\times$ 9 feet
        or 68 square feet
        (See Figure 16-3)
    d. Reference Books and Index Area =
        24 feet $\times$ 2.5 feet or 60 square feet
        This refers to 8 sections of shelving plus aisle—no
        seats.
        (See Figure 16-5)
    e. Current Journal Display Area =
        24' $\times$ 3' or 72 square feet.
        This refers to 8 sections of slanted shelves
        plus aisle. (See Figure 16-6).
    f. Audiovisual Area = 9 feet $\times$ 3 feet or 18 square
        feet. This refers to 3 sections of shelving plus aisle,
        no seats
        (See Figure 16-7)

7. Configuration Loss of 6% : 109 square feet

C. Detailed Estimate = 1762 square feet plus 6% configuration
    loss: 106 square feet = 1,868 square feet

This estimate was calculated by designing an ideal floor
layout for an area 34 feet $\times$ 53 feet or 1,802 square feet to
show how many items can be accomodated in an area providing less space than the general estimate. (See Figure 16-9.)

The space is close to ideal and will likely never occur in
practice for the following reasons:

1) The bays used in buildings vary in size so no allowance
    has been made for the space loss of construction col-
    umns.

2) The shape of the space determines how effectively space
    can be used. A narrower rectangle would not accomo-
    date all the areas in this plan.

3) The measures for the rooms and areas do not allow for
    the space losses caused by the thickness of walls, heat-

ing and ventilating ducts, and other idiosyncracies which exist in all buildings—old or new.

Therefore, it is important to add the 6% configuration loss suggested by Cohen (11). Also, the space accommodates 18 chairs instead of the estimated 17. To take into account the building's possible idiosyncracies, an area closer to the size of the estimate by area function (1,920 square feet) would be more appropriate. However, it is also possible to accommodate this library's needs in less space by making a trade off: for example, cutting seats back to 16 instead of 18, or narrowing traffic aisles. To save space in the work area on this floor plan, the exit door, the sink, and the refrigerator were omitted in order to place the index area near the information desk.

Core area and seats	809.5	square feet
Stack area and seats	536	square feet
Staff work area	416	square feet
	1,762	square feet
6% Configuration loss	106	square feet
TOTAL	1,868	square feet

1. Stack Area: 536 square feet

   a. Function:

      The area provides shelving for 3,600 volumes of books and journals.

   b. Equipment:

      48 sections of 90-inch high, 10-inch deep, 36-inch wide steel shelving on 4 feet 5 inch centers to house 3,600 volumes (75 volumes per section)

      5 study carrels—48 inches $\times$ 24 inches

      1 round reading table—36 inches in diameter

      7 chairs

   c. Space allocated:

      Stacks = 370 square feet
      20 feet $\times$ 18.5 feet

      Carrels = 100 square feet
      4 feet $\times$ 25 feet

      Table = 66 square feet
      11 feet $\times$ 6 feet

2. Staff Work Area: 416 square feet

   a. Function:

      A private soundproof area is needed for organizing and processing materials and for conferring with users and library staff. It accommodates 1 librarian and 2 library assistants.

   b. Equipment:

      1. Librarian's office
         desk with 2 work surfaces,
         each 30 inches $\times$ 60 inches
         1 typing chair
         1 desk chair
         Table for computer terminal—2 feet $\times$ 3 feet
         3 visitors' chairs
         3 sections of 90 inch-high, 10 inch-deep, 36 inch-wide steel shelving
         1 coat tree

      2. Library assistants' office
         2 work stations, each with 2 work surfaces, each 30 inches $\times$ 60 inches
         2 typewriters
         1 table for computer terminal, 2.5 feet $\times$ 3 feet
         1 printer, 2.5 feet $\times$ 3 feet
         3 typing chairs
         1 visitor's chair
         7 sections of 90 inch-high, 10 inch-deep, 36 inch-wide steel shelving
         1 receiving counter on cabinet 2 feet $\times$ 4 feet
         2 book trucks
         1 large wastebasket
         1 supply closet
         1 coat closet

   c. Space Allocated:

      1. Librarian's office: 168 square feet
         12 feet $\times$ 14 feet

      2. Library Assistants' office: 248 square feet
         7 feet $\times$ 15 feet or 105 square feet
         11 feet $\times$ 13 feet or 143 square feet

3. Core Areas: 809.5 square feet

   a. Entrance and Information Desk Area: 130 square feet

      1) Function:

         The area controls and provides information to users. It houses circulation records and protects special materials.

      2) Equipment:

         Space for entrance traffic at door and in front of information desk, 6 feet $\times$ 10 feet

         Information Desk, 2.5 feet $\times$ 8 feet
         1 desk chair
         1 section of 90 inch-high, 10 inch-deep, 36 inch-wide steel shelving
         1 free standing bulletin board, 4' X 1'
         1 wall telephone for users

      3) Space allocated: 13 feet $\times$ 10 feet = 130 square feet

b. Card Catalog and Dictionary Area: 45 square feet

  1) Function:

    The area provides a place for card references on the collection of books, journals, and nonprint media, and the unabridged dictionary. It also provides space for consulting the items.

  2) Equipment:

Card Catalog	2 feet × 1.5 feet
Table	2 feet × 1.5 feet
Dictionary Stand	2 feet × 1.5 feet
Space for Users	4.5 feet × 7.5 feet

  3) Space allocated: 7.5 feet X 6 feet

c. Photocopy Area: 49 square feet

  1) Function:

    The area provides a soundproof section for duplicating library materials.

  2) Equipment:

    A coin-operated photocopy machine (Xerox 4000), 40 inches × 28 inches
    Space for service maintenance and machine, 70 inches deep × 64 inches wide
    Counter and cabinet for machine supplied, 1.5 feet × 4 feet
    1 book truck
    1 large wastebasket

  3) Space allocated: 7 feet × 7 feet

d. Reference Books and Indexes Area: 209.5 square feet

  1) Function:

    The area provides housing and use of 500 volumes of reference sources and indexing services.

  2) Equipment:

    8 sections of 90 inch-high, 10 inch-deep, 36 inch-wide steel shelving
    2 seating high counters, each attached to a section of shelving 18 inches × 36 inches
    1 table—2 feet × 6 feet
    4 typing chairs

  3) Space allocated:

    Reference books: 118 square feet
    13 feet × 8.5 feet = 110.5

    Indexes = 99 square feet
    9 feet × 11 feet

e. Current Journal Display Area: 220 square feet

  1) Function:

    The area provides a display and reading section for current issues of 150-200 current journal titles.

  2) Equipment:

    10 sections of 90 inch-high, 10 inch-deep, 36 inch-wide steel shelving with 5 slanted display shelves in each section
    2 side tables, 2 feet × 2 feet
    3 lounge chairs, 3 feet × 3 feet
    1 book truck

  3) Space allocated:

    22 feet × 10 feet = 220

f. Audiovisual Area: 156 square feet

  1) Function:

    This area provides a soundproof section for housing and using 250 titles of nonprint media, and for group study.

  2) Equipment:

    4 sections of 90 inch-high, 10 inch-deep, 36 inch-wide steel shelving
    2 audiovisual carrels, 2.5 feet × 5 feet
    1 table, 3 feet × 6 feet
    4 chairs
    Audiovisual equipment

  3) Space allocated:

    12 feet X 13 feet

4. Configuration Loss

Space actually assigned	1,802
Total estimated space allocation	1,770
6% configuration loss	106
	1,876 square feet

Promoting Library Services

Judith Messerle
*Director, Educational Resources
    and Community Relations*
St. Joseph Hospital
Alton, Illinois
and
Sara I. Hill
*Director, Library Services
 St. Luke's Hospital
 Kansas City, Missouri

*Currently:
 Marketing Support
 Dataphase Systems, Inc.
 Kansas City, Missouri

CHAPTER 17

Promoting Library Services

Judith Messerle
Director, Educational Resources and Community Relations
St. Joseph Hospital
Alton, Illinois
and
Sara I. Hill
Director, Library Services
St. Luke's Hospital
Kansas City, Missouri

Appendix

Figures

The phrase "hospital library" carries a variety of meanings for hospital and medical staff members. Images of a hospital library often relate to past educational experiences and to personal interactions with specific libraries. Since no two personal experiences are ever alike and no two hospital libraries identical, there is a continuing need to promote the hospital library and its changing services, both to longtime users and to potential patrons.

PROMOTIONAL GOALS

The first step in working out a promotional plan is to establish goals. In hospital libraries, these goals often include increasing the use of the library's services and enhancing the image of the library as a professional service. Achieving these goals usually involves increasing the hospital and medical staff's awareness of the role of the library within the institution.

One promotional technique the librarian can use to increase public awareness is to disseminate information about the library. Library hours, conditions of use, and special services available are all items of information that potential users need in order to have access to the library's services. Some library activities tailored to meet the needs of a specific user group will also increase user understanding of the library's role.

The imaginative librarian can develop promotional activities in numerous formats that focus on a variety of general or specific aspects of the library. These activities could target new user groups or focus on current library patrons. Whatever the focus or the format, the librarian should remember that the promotion will always be much more effective if part of an overall strategy. This chapter will discuss in detail how to develop a promotional strategy for a library and the activities that can make up such a strategy.

STRATEGY DEVELOPMENT

Staff members of most hospital libraries have only a limited amount of time to devote to promotional activities, so the activities carried out must be chosen carefully to produce maximum results. Once promotional goals have been defined, a systematic strategy for achieving those goals can be developed by defining objectives, choosing promotional activities that will accomplish the objectives and evaluating the results(1).

Defining the Objectives

An effective approach to promotion requires determining who the current users of the library are and how they use the library. The librarian can refer to circulation and reference records to determine which user groups need more encouragement to use the library and which library services are underused(2). Having made an analysis of the current situation, the librarian will be able to decide on specific promotional objectives. These ob-

jectives should be documented in writing so that they can be referred to throughout the design and implementation of the promotion. Objectives that are measurable facilitate evaluation of the promotion at the conclusion of the activity.

Formulating a Plan of Action

Having defined the objectives, the librarian can next develop a plan of action. This is the opportunity for the librarian to be creative in the selection of the most appropriate formats and types of promotion. Several considerations should be kept in mind, however.

Audience

In developing an action plan, the librarian should begin by reviewing the audience, or target group, in terms of needs, interests, and educational level. A needs analysis is an essential first step in order to avoid wasting energy promoting services that are not relevant to the target audience. Needs analyses are discussed further in Chapter 12. The librarian should also study the interests of the target audience. Are the targeted physicians more research-oriented or more clinically-oriented? What topics are currently important to the administrative staff? Even if the librarian does not wish to build an entire promotion around a few specific interests, the astute librarian can use those special interests to intrigue the various audiences.

Approach

Most promotions have both a "hard" and "soft" approach. The "hard" approach refers to promotional tools such as brochures, balloons, newsletters, and cable television spots, while the "soft" approach means working on a person-to-person basis. The most successful action plan should include elements of both.(3)

Input and Advice

In determining the approaches to be taken, the librarian may wish to discuss options with members of the target group. The potential audience usually has a good understanding of what will and will not be most effective. This group can provide ideas for timing and can identify current interests that might bring in new patrons. Once members of a target group have provided advice, they usually become advocates, helping support the library's promotional effort among their colleagues. Useful advice on promotion can also come from other hospital departments, such as the public relations, audiovisual, education, communications, or printing departments.

Timing

Timing is also important to the success of a promotion. Before scheduling an event, the librarian should check to see if other important events will overshadow or conveniently coincide with the planned library promotion. The time of day events take place is also critical. If the target audience includes staff members who are involved in providing direct patient care, then some times of day will be clearly better than others.

Promotions are most likely to succeed when they are timed to coincide with the target audience's need for a particular service. Students about to begin an extensive research paper are more receptive to an orientation session on how to use an index than students who are ready to leave for Christmas vacation. Similarly, notifying the administrative staff of the library's ability to track a bill through the legislature will be most effective when there is a bill in process that is of particular interest to the administration.

Evaluating Results

When considering the overall strategy of a promotional plan, the librarian should build some type of evaluation into the plan. Evaluation is important because it provides the librarian with feedback on what was and was not effective. The librarian can then use this information to refine and improve future promotional activities.

BASIC PRINCIPLES OF PROMOTION

Any promotional activity can benefit from the application of a few basic advertising principles. For example, advertising depends heavily on creating recognition of a name or product. The librarian can apply that same principle to the library by establishing an identifiable logo or letterhead for all library promotional efforts. The library logo could be a symbol, involving books or audiovisuals, combined with the departmental name. Or if using a separate symbol for the department does not seem feasible, then the library might adopt a distinctive design that incorporates the hospital's symbol and the library or department name.

Having determined the concept for the logo, the librarian will find some professional assistance from a designer invaluable. If the institution has a graphic artist on the staff, the artist can assist with instant lettering systems and ready-made art. Public relations or audiovisual department staff members can also give useful advice. The same logo should then be used to identify all library publications, messages, and products.

A second advertising principle to bear in mind is: keep it simple. The best promotional efforts are those that are aimed at a specific audience and that are simple in design. Too much information provided in shotgun fashion will miss the mark and serve little purpose.

PUBLICATIONS

Publications are a common and effective way for libraries to bring their services to the attention of their users. Such publications might be aimed at long-time users, potential patrons, or newcomers to the hospital.

Before embarking on any publication, the librarian should consider what purpose the publication is intended to serve, who will use it, how much staff time and money can be allotted to it, how it should be produced, and how distributed.

Types of publications

Libraries typically design and produce many types of publications serving different purposes. These range from printed, semi-permanent users' guides, to one-page photocopied fact sheets, and include also fliers, brochures, leaflets, newsletters, lists of newly acquired titles, and bibliographies.

Guides to Library Services

Most hospital librarians will give high priority to producing a guide to the library's policies and services. To determine what type of guide to produce, the librarian will need to answer certain key questions:

• Who will the guide be for? Will one guide be aimed at all library users or will separate publications be produced for each major user group, such as the medical staff, nursing, management, and students?
• What will be the guide's content? Will the guide include only such general information as policies, services, and hours, or will the publication contain more detailed information on how to use the library?
• What will be the guide's format? Will the guide be a simple one-page information sheet, a photocopied brochure, a printed brochure, or a printed booklet?

The answers to these questions will depend on user needs, the way the librarian intends to use the guides, and the amount of time and money available. Benefits should be carefully weighed against the costs and staff time involved. One general photocopied fact sheet may be less expensive to produce than a printed brochure or booklet but may contribute less to the overall professional image of the library. In a hospital with many diverse user groups, one general booklet, however slick, might be less effective than a series of carefully designed, photocopied fact sheets or brochures targeted to specific user groups. Secretaries, for example, may find very little in a general library services brochure that applies to them. A fact sheet that details services available to them, such as routing of secretarial newsletters, supplying address and zip code information, providing answers to factual questions, and assisting with verifying references will seem more relevant. To give another example, a brochure containing only general information might be easier and cheaper to produce than a detailed user's guide, but if a library is used frequently without a staff member present, the guide with detailed instructions might be worth the extra effort and cost.

Figure 17-1 shows a sample topical outline for a guide to library policies and services. A more detailed user's

Figure 17-1
Guide to Library Policies and Services: Topical Outline

```
I.    Library mission

II.   Library policies
      A.  User groups
      B.  Circulation
      C.  After-hours use

III.  Library services
      A.  Book and journal collection
      B.  Information services
          1.  Fast answers
          2.  Information searches
          3.  Literature searches
          4.  Alerting services
      C.  Document delivery
      D.  Orientations
      E.  Audiovisual equipment and programs
      F.  Photocopying

IV.   Library facts
      A.  Location
      B.  Hours
      C.  Staff members
      D.  Telephone numbers
```

guide could also include the library floor plan, a description of the classification system, information on available indexes and how to use them, and more detailed descriptions of services.

Fliers

A flier is a leaflet that is widely distributed, either by mail or from pick-up points either outside or inside the library. A library flier might describe a specific service, such as computer or manual literature searches, interlibrary loan, or ready reference. The flier should include a clear description of what the service is, who is eligible to use it, how it is used, and any conditions of use, including fees. Fliers for services that involve registration should include a deadline registration date and possibly a registration form to be completed and returned. A general flier can be designed to announce ongoing services such as a monthly management film. The information for a particular month can be typed in before duplication.

Newsletters

Hospital library newsletters are a popular form of promotion. The content of a newsletter will depend on its purpose and its target audience. If one newsletter is de-signed to be sent to all user groups, a variety of topics and subject areas should be covered. Targeting a particular user group and tailoring a newsletter to the interests of that group might be more effective than attempting to reach all groups in one publication, but time and fiscal constraints usually dictate one newsletter for all.

Depending on the audience targeted, newsletters might contain any combination of the following information:

• *New acquisitions.* The newsletter might list newly acquired books, journals, and audiovisuals, once the materials are ready for use. The newsletter might highlight gift materials by use of a special symbol or by providing information about the donor.

• *Book and audiovisual reviews.* By printing reviews of books and audiovisuals, the newsletter can call attention to new items or emphasize material already in the collection. Such reviews should point out to hospital staff how the material can be used. The librarian may wish to include short quotations from book reviews that have appeared in the journal literature. Uncopyrighted reviews may be reprinted, either in part or in totality.

• *Library activities.* Articles on library activities highlight new services, vacation hours, or the arrival of new staff members. Information on activities should be selected with the audience in mind. For example, publicity for an open house for medical students might not be appropriate in a newsletter that goes to the entire hospital staff, but reporting the event after it has happened might be of general interest. Occasionally library newsletters might include news about the library staff and volunteers. Information of this sort should be carefully screened to be certain that it is of general interest to the library newsletter's readers. Often, the general hospital newsletter is a more appropriate vehicle for staff news.

• *Schedules of upcoming education and audiovisual programs.* Depending on its target audience, a library newsletter might list audiovisual showings and educational programs. Times and places should be included, as well as a person to be contacted for more information. Coordination with the education department or department responsible for the event is, of course, essential.

• *"How-to" articles.* The newsletter might incorporate "how-to" articles, which subsequently could be reproduced separately and made available in the library or at orientations. For example, a newsletter article might highlight a new piece of audiovisual equipment, identify the software that goes with it, and explain how it is to be used. The same information could then be attached to the piece of equipment or distributed to first-time users of that equipment.

• *Statistics.* Newsletters sometimes include statistics on library activities. The librarian should be selective about the use of statistics and make certain that the information is genuinely of interest to the readers.

• *Profiles of library services.* A newsletter might highlight a particular service, such as one that is underused. Focusing on a narrow aspect of a broad service area will give the librarian a chance to explain the service in detail. The newsletter could, for example, highlight selective dissemination of information or the library's film rental service. Examples of other topics for service profiles include providing addresses of hospitals and physicians; searching the literature, either manually or by computer; obtaining government documents; and scanning the *Federal Register*.

Production of a quality newsletter takes considerable time and effort. A newsletter requires planning and consistency of publication and should be well thought out before initiation. Often a library will do better to start with a quarterly publication rather than a monthly one. The news might be less recent, but the library staff will find it easier to meet deadlines.

Lists

Lists of newly acquired books and journals, bibliographies on popular topics, and lists of journals and audiovisuals are all potential library publications. Such lists usually can be developed easily and inexpensively yet receive wide circulation. If new book and journal lists are extensive, they might be divided into subject categories. Adding the call number helps the user locate the book in the library.

The librarian can produce bibliographies on popular topics whenever there is sufficient demand. A computer-generated bibliography can be used as the basis for the publication, and the format adapted to make the bibliography more attractive and interesting to users. Short annotations are particularly helpful. The librarian will wish to carry out some selective editing with scissors and tape to remove from a computer-generated bibliography information irrelevant to the user, and to include a cover sheet explaining symbols and abbreviations. Some libraries use microcomputers to "capture" online searches and reformat the information into more legible bibliographies for distribution.

Some libraries produce lists of available journals and audiovisuals to distribute to users. Lists by general subject are helpful for new users who wish to review what is available in their particular subject area. As mentioned earlier, the time involved in producing these materials must in every case be weighed against their projected usefulness to library patrons.

Piggybacking Information

Piggybacking on the publications of other departments is a double-barreled approach to library promotion. Not only does this method ensure a different readership for library information, but it also links the library and the other department as partners. Prime departments for such cooperation are education, which can insert a statement on its program fliers about the availability of additional information in the library; public relations, which

can include notes from the library in the hospital newsletter; personnel, which can include a word about the library in recruitment brochures; patient education; and audiovisuals. By exploring options for this type of promotion, the librarian raises the visibility of the library and stresses the library's cooperative role.

Bookmarks and Table Tents

Many hospital libraries have successfully used bookmarks and table tents for promotional purposes. Bookmarks, which are usually produced on card stock, offer an opportunity for creativity in both content and design. A bookmark can echo a major promotional theme or highlight a service. Table tents are folded pieces of card stock with a brief thematic message on both sides. They can be placed in meeting rooms, lounges, and in the cafeteria. The library staff should remember to seek the permission when necessary of the administration or the person responsible for the location where the tents are placed. As is the case with other publications discussed, the message on a table tent should be applicable to those who read it. A table tent in the cafeteria might announce an open house, while table tents in the physicians' lounge or nursing report rooms might more appropriately announce the availability of MEDLINE searches.

Production

Production of a library's publications might involve nothing more than typing and photocopying, or it might include more elaborate design and production techniques. Whether simply or elaborately produced, a publication will be made more interesting and attractive by paying attention to the content and design(4).

Content

When selecting the content of a publication, the librarian must keep the audience's needs, interests, and educational level clearly in mind. Clear, simple, vigorous writing will communicate to a wide range of readers. Even publications aimed at well-educated readers do not need jargon, polysyllabic words, and complex sentences in order to be effective. The librarian as editor should maintain consistency within a single publication of the style, level of writing, and level of formality. If the publication is part of a larger promotional effort, the overall theme should be clear and the overall tone consistent. More information on writing can be found in Chapter 15.

Design

A small amount of time spent in planning the design of a publication will pay large dividends in its final appearance. The expertise available in the public relations department, the audiovisual department, or the print shop has already been mentioned. Additional information on the design of publications can be found in the references at the end of the chapter. Among the design considerations to explore are the final image to be projected, the type of layout to be featured, the paper stock and ink color to be selected, and the production method to be used.

The image projected by library publications is critical to their effectiveness. If the librarian can identify exactly what image to convey, design decisions can be evaluated accordingly. For example, if the library wishes to promote itself as a highly professional information center, a sophisticated contemporary graphic might be an effective logo. In laying out a publication, the librarian should coordinate the size of type, spacing both within and between articles or paragraphs, and graphics to catch and hold the readers' attention. The librarian as designer should relate the titles of each individual publication to the logo or permanent masthead in a way that is consistent and attractive.

The publication can feature headlines typed in capital letters or underlined to provide emphasis. Typewriters with large-type elements or transfer lettering that is rubbed on can be used to produce larger title type. For a change of pace, headlines can be offset into the margins. Designers stress that white space is as important to the total effect of a publication as the actual print. Other ways of making information easy to understand are using short paragraphs, short sentences, wide margins, special symbols, outline form, and lists. Many in-house publications use two columns on a 8½-inch by 11-inch page with a white space between, because research has shown that this format is easy to read. The two-column format includes sufficient white space and gives the publication eye-appeal.

The librarian can use graphics and line drawings to enhance the visual appeal of publications. Often a simple technique such as drawing a box around an item or around an entire page adds a special flair. Public relations and audiovisual departments may have prepared graphics on various themes that can be incorporated into the design.

Having determined the format of the publication, the librarian may wish to move blocks of typed copy and graphics around on an empty sheet to find a balance pleasing to the eye. More important than a perfectly symmetrical layout is a balance between the heavy and light elements on a page. Good visual balance in a publication comes with practice and by observing other publications. The librarian-designer should try for an overall well-balanced effect that looks planned instead of thrown together haphazardly. The librarian can choose a variety of paper stocks with different rag content and weight. These variables contribute to the texture and appearance of each paper stock.

Color draws attention to publications and adds variety. If materials are photocopied, a colored paper can be used. If materials are printed, an ink in a color other than black can be used without adding much to the cost. A single color of ink can be "screened" to produce a lighter and a darker shade, giving the impression of more expensive two-color production even though only one color is actually used. Combining an unusual paper color with a non-black ink can create some effective combinations. Some hospital libraries develop a consistent image by using not only the same logo for each publication but also the same color combination, such as maroon ink on buff stock.

Hospital libraries can produce publications on a copy machine or a duplicating machine. They may also have them produced by the hospital print shop or copy center or by a commercial firm. The librarian should choose a production method on the basis of the hospital's in-house production capability, the intended use of the publication, and the available budget. If the publication is intended to be ephemeral but widely distributed, a librarian may choose to use photocopying, relying on the design and perhaps a colored paper stock to give the publication a professional appearance. Professional typesetting and printing may be justified for important pieces, such as the library brochure in which the content will not have to be updated frequently.

Distribution

The method of distributing a particular publication may depend on the purpose and audience intended. The librarian may choose to have a particular publication mailed, posted, available on a countertop, or distributed by hand.

Mailing

The library can compile a mailing list by combining lists that already exist in the offices of administration, personnel, medical staff secretary, medical education, and others. Often such lists are maintained on computers and updated regularly. Printouts may be available on labels, or a special master can be typed manually for easy photocopying onto labels. Updating such a list only involves pulling off an outdated name or address and replacing it with a corrected label. An extensive and accurate mailing list and an efficient method of addressing mailers, such as using photocopied labels, can be a boon to a library's promotional program. Using mailing lists from other departments facilitates targeting mailings to particular interest groups. The library can also request users to sign up to receive a specific type of publication. This ensures that the material is sent to library users who want to receive it.

Mailings can be time-consuming, but they are a primary means of library publicity. With a little ingenuity the librarian can streamline the process and can often locate volunteers who are willing to assist.

Distribution Within the Hospital

An obvious point of distribution of library publications is in the library itself. Fliers and brochures can be conveniently placed on a table or counter with a sign inviting users to take one. Similar arrangements can also be placed, with permission, near hospital bulletin boards or in hospital lounges. In some institutions, the librarian may be able to arrange for fliers to be included with employee pay checks.

Brochures and other publications also can be handed out during library orientations or at special events. Special fliers might be distributed in conjunction with a departmental meeting or to students as they receive an assignment that involves library work.

Posting

Posting fliers in high traffic areas is an effective means of disseminating information. Next to employee time clocks, near cafeteria lines, and on departmental bulletin boards are all likely locations for posting library fliers. The librarian should remember to request permission of the department in charge before posting materials and to remove the fliers after about two weeks or when the event is over.

DISPLAYS

Displays on bulletin boards or in table or wall cases are another popular means of library promotion(5). Exhibits, involving the use of more than one display case or board, may be accompanied by a simple catalog or list of items shown. Displays and exhibits have special design and production considerations.

Bulletin Boards

Bulletin boards in central areas, lounges, or departmental offices might be used for library displays. Most institutions have policies regulating what can and cannot be posted on hospital bulletin boards. In addition, most bulletin boards come under the jurisdiction of specific departments that may have their own rules governing the boards' uses. The librarian should remember to check with the department or individual in charge before planning a bulletin board display.

The library bulletin board is a good place to start with promotional displays. The librarian should make certain that the bulletin board is in a highly visible location and cleared regularly of outdated postings. The librarian can use the library's own bulletin board for periodic displays, highlighting a disease, a new book, a new piece of equipment, the library staff, or a new service. When arranging a display, the librarian should remember that color and variety are essential. Color captures the viewers' attention, but people will stop looking at something that is static. Pieces of construction paper in various colors can be used as mats for plain white paper, and thin strips of contrasting paper can tie one area to another. Transfer letters, if carefully used, give the work a neat and professional appearance. Display-size letters also can be pur-

chased or cut out of paper. If the hospital has a graphics department or print shop, the librarian may wish to consult them for other means of providing lettering.

The library may wish to maintain an informational bulletin board only, for posting announcements of workshops, educational activities, and lectures. Such an announcement board is most useful if divided into clearly marked topical sections, by type of activity or broad subject, and if weeded frequently. Each item can be stamped with a clearance date, or material can be removed after the event has occurred.

Case Displays

Many hospital libraries own or have access to flat or upright display cases. Such cases are ideal for featuring a medical instrument or piece of equipment and corresponding literature about the instrument or equipment displayed. Old editions of medical books or a montage of nursing hats and pins are other possible displays. By adding a bibliography to the case, the librarian takes the interested viewer one step beyond the material displayed.

In arranging a display, the librarian should take care to identify all materials shown with adjacent labels. A strip of clear plastic placed near the outer edge of the pages of a book and pinned to the surface of the flat case can hold open books on display. Paper clips and rubber bands should not be used. Any book held open should be reopened periodically at another page to prevent the spine from cracking.

Book Displays and Exhibits

Many hospital libraries place new books in an identified display area so that users can quickly locate new acquisitions. A library can also arrange book displays around a theme or topic, pulling together related titles or calling attention to a part of the collection. Copies of a bibliography of the materials on exhibit, possibly including reviews, should accompany such displays.

More elaborate exhibits usually revolve around a special collection, such as historical or rare books, a unique reprint file, or a selection of medical prints or old photographs. Exhibits might use techniques of bulletin boards, case displays, and book displays to show the special collections to the fullest extent. For such exhibits the librarian should prepare a catalog or list of the items on display. Because an exhibit often features a significant collection or acquisition of some value, the librarian should make certain to provide adequate security for the items.

PERSONAL INTERACTIONS

Personal interaction between the librarian and library users is one of the most obvious, and most effective, forms of library promotion. Several of the most common opportunities for this type of promotion will be discussed here.

Figure 17-2
Orientation Master Schedule: Sample

Group	Type of Orientation	Time and Schedule	Purpose
Staff physicians	Welcome letter and packet	As appointed; notification received from medical staff secretary.	Identify library as information center Describe services Invite to library
Residents	Presentation at orientation to program	In June: call secretaries in April to get on calendar.	Identify library as information center Describe services
	Review of literature searching	One hour lecture each fall	Briefly present policies Review use of *Index Medicus* Explain Medline service
Nurses (newly hired)	Ten-minute tour as part of Nursing department orientation	Every second Monday between 1:00 p.m. and 2:00 p.m.	Identify library as information center Stress services of interest to nurses Stress access by telephone Give examples of library use by nurses
Head nurses	Presentation at head nurse meetings	Annually in Spring; call in March to get on calendar.	Highlight new services Discuss library services for managers
Department heads (newly hired)	Welcome letter and packet	As hired; notification arranged through personnel.	Identify library as information center Describe relevant services
	Follow-up personal visit to their office	Make appointment one month after starting date.	Discuss library and information needs
Administrative staff	Welcome letter and packet	As hired	Identify library as information center Describe relevant services
	Follow-up personal visit to their office	Make appointment one month after starting date.	Discuss their library and information needs
Department heads	Ten-minute presentation at department head meetings	Annually in Fall; call in Sept. to get on agenda.	Highlight a new or existing service
All new employees	New employee orientation (Five-minute presentation)	Biweekly and ongoing	Identify library as information center Describe services with examples, showing applicability to many types of jobs Review resources briefly Stress telephone access Give library facts: location, hours Invite to library for tour

Group	Type of Orientation	Time and Schedule	Purpose
Support services	Presentation at departmental meetings	At least once every two years; rotating schedule	Highlight services and sources applicable to each department Discuss information needs
Nurse refresher students	15 minute tour and orientation	In June at beginning of program; arrange in April with Nursing Education.	Describe services Describe resources Present policies and procedures for use
	One hour class	After first paper is assigned; arrange in April with Nursing Education.	Review use of card catalog and indexes
Ward clerk students	15 minute presentation during unit on communication	Varies with class schedule; notification by Education Department.	Describe relevant services Give examples
Pharmacy interns	15 minute tour	In Sept. start program; call pharmacy office in July.	Describe services Describe resources Discuss use of the library

Orientation

When an institution has a fairly constant rate of turnover of hospital staff and affiliated students, the librarian will wish to develop a systematic orientation program. This program will ensure that all user groups know how to make the best use of the library. If the librarian spends a small amount of time planning and organizing orientation sessions for various groups, presenting the actual orientations should not be overly time-consuming (6). In planning an overall orientations program, the librarian needs to make several key decisions, such as which groups to aim for, what types of orientation to use with which groups, how to schedule the orientation sessions, and what to include in the content of the sessions. This information can be summarized and recorded on a master chart like the one in Figure 17-2.

Scheduled Library Orientations

Holding orientation sessions in the library acquaints users first-hand with the facilities and allows them to see for themselves the resources available. In-depth discussions of how to use the library are most effective if the tools are readily available. Scheduled tours of the library can often be arranged, as part of the departmental orientation of nurses or other new staff members. Frequently student groups visit the library for a general overview at the beginning of their orientation programs; return visits covering specific aspects of library use can be scheduled at a later time.

Informal Library Orientations

In addition to the formal, previously arranged orientation sessions, most libraries like to conduct an informal orientation session for new physicians and hospital employees on their first visit to the library. Every member of the library staff should be alerted to identify new users and to offer them a 5- to 10-minute guided tour of the library pointing out its services and resources. The librarian will wish to conduct some training sessions of the library staff, so that all staff members communicate the same information and attitudes of service during these impromptu orientation sessions.

New Employees' Orientations

In many hospitals, all employees are eligible to use the library. If that is the case, the best time to introduce them to the library is during the hospital's orientation program for new employees. The librarian may arrange to make a short presentation at such programs, which are usually the responsibility of the personnel or education department. Even if all new employees do not actually make use of the library, the employee's orientation still provides the library with an opportunity to increase its visibility to a wide range of people.

Presentations at Meetings

Regular meetings of a specific user group, such as the medical staff, nursing staff, administrative staff, or other departments can be occasions for brief presentations about the library. The librarian may need to convince the clinical chief or department head of the relevance of library orientation to the group, but once permission is granted, scheduling can usually be accomplished with a telephone call.

Orientations by Mail

Even a well thought out series of orientation sessions may miss the one group that the library should be particularly interested in reaching: the hospital's top medical and administrative management. One method of reaching members of this group is to prepare a letter of welcome from the library and routinely send it, along with a library brochure, to newly appointed clinical chiefs, administrators, and department heads. The library can also send a "welcome packet" to physicians newly appointed to the medical staff. Some librarians follow up letters of welcome three or four weeks later with a request for an individual appointment to discuss library services.

Content of Orientation Sessions

The content of each type of orientation session will vary slightly according to the librarian's analysis of what each user group needs to know and the time available. A general outline that can be expanded or contracted to suit individual situations appears in Figure 17-3.

Orientation sessions for student groups or other groups that use the library without assistance often go into greater detail on how to use the library. Possible topics for these orientation sessions might include:

- Using the card catalog
- Understanding the classification system
- Using the indexes
- Understanding MeSH
- Locating journals
- Understanding journal citations

Orientation sessions for groups already familiar in general terms with the library might focus on a specific service or combination of services that meets the needs of that particular group. For example, a special presentation to a medical staff meeting might focus on obtaining a MEDLINE search. The librarian, in designing these presentations, might wish to think of the task as "selling" the service to potential "buyers." The "sales" presentation might follow this outline:

1. Catch and hold the audience's interest
2. Discuss a real "need" or "problem" of the specific audience

3. Demonstrate how one or all of the library's services could fill the need or solve the problem
4. Convince the audience that solving the problem by using library services is convenient, efficient, and cost-effective
5. Give details about using library services

Although designing, scheduling, and presenting a wide variety of orientation sessions might seem like a full-time job, with a little organized planning a librarian can make the orientation program fit easily into the library's routine. The use of a master chart will help to establish a schedule for each group. A "tickle" file will remind a librarian to contact the appropriate people to schedule orientations in the library or to secure a meeting place. A one-page outline kept on file for each type of orientation will reduce preparation time.

Hospital Meetings

Working with committees provides another opportunity for the librarian to promote library services. Committees such as those dealing with safety, patient education, cost containment, and quality assurance can all benefit from the library's information services. The librarian should indicate a willingness to serve on such committees by sending a letter to the hospital administrator expressing an interest and detailing potential contributions. If not appointed to a committee, the librarian might wish nevertheless to make a presentation to the committee.

If the librarian is also a department head, meetings with other department managers provide opportunities to inform them about library activities and offer library services. Often the librarian can gradually assume a role as information provider at such meetings by asking questions that clarify information needs and then offering to find the necessary answers.

One-to-One Promotion

Discussions with department heads or key administrative staff on a one-to-one basis are another form of promotion. The librarian will find such an approach

---

Figure 17-3
A General Orientation: Topical Outline

A. Brief welcome

B. Purpose of the library

C. Explanation of services relevant to each user group

D. Policies and procedures

   1. Hours

   2. Circulation policies

   3. After-hours use

E. Review of resources relevant to each user group

productive both in learning about the information needs of other departments and in communicating ways in which the library can meet those needs. Meetings with department heads often can identify topics for short programs or presentations for later meetings of that department. Informal meetings with department heads or administrators over lunch or during coffee breaks can be as successful as formal appointments. Both approaches should be utilized.

Visibility

Another way the librarian can personally promote the library is to maintain high visibility in the hospital. Serving on committees, attending meetings, and occasionally delivering library searches in person provides a chance for others to become more aware of the library staff.

The library staff can raise its own credibility in the hospital community by participating in professional library activities, particularly if such participation results in benefits to the hospital. Staff honors, such as being named to a professional committee or being elected to a regional or national office, can be publicized through the library or hospital newsletter. The publication of papers that document successful library programs or techniques can also increase the hospital's awareness of library activities.

EVENTS

Both publications and bulletin boards are essentially passive ways for the library to reach its audience. A more active approach to promotion is the staging of events, either in the library itself or elsewhere in the hospital. Library service or the library collection can be the focal point of such events.

Open Houses

Library open houses focusing on some specific activity or service can be effective promotional events. An open house might be staged to open new library facilities; to demonstrate new services, such as computer searching; to display historical materials; or to celebrate library week. Open houses must be held at convenient hours in order to draw busy staff away from work routines. Good refreshments may draw a crowd when other techniques fail. The library can serve local favorites or something less common, such as apples and cider. If library rules normally prohibit food and drink inside the library, some space can be set aside where visitors can enjoy the refreshments.

For a hospital-wide event, invitations can be issued through the hospital newsletter, the library newsletter (if one exists), table tents, fliers posted in appropriate places, or, if feasible, pay envelope stuffers. Key personnel, such as members of the library committee, clinical chiefs, department heads, and administrators might war-

rant personal invitations. If the open house is geared to a less comprehensive audience, invitations should be distributed only to the specific target group.

Detailed planning is essential to a successful event. The librarian will need to consider the probable traffic flow and to rearrange furniture if necessary. Housekeeping may need to supply extra waste cans. Good directional signs can help move guests along. Volunteers can help serve refreshments and keep the library in order during times of peak traffic.

Since only a limited amount of the information provided will be retained, handouts should be available that reinforce the message of the open house. A guest book or sign-up sheet asking for name and department will help in the follow-up evaluation of the event.

Book Fairs

Another popular library event is the book fair, when publishers' representatives or book jobbers come in to display the latest monographs and journals. Often such salespeople visit the hospital periodically and ask permission to set up displays in public areas such as a main corridor or outside the cafeteria. The library can organize a book fair simply by coordinating their visits and offering to promote them.

A book fair can be set up in the library itself or in another central spot in the hospital. If staged in another part of the hospital, the library should make certain that its sponsorship of the fair is conveyed in the publicity and announcements. Physicians, department heads, and personnel involved in education, in particular, should receive invitations, though a general invitation might be issued to all medical and hospital staff members. One way to get double benefit from such a fair is to ask staff members to indicate those materials they would like to see added to the library collection. The librarian can also make use of the opportunity to review the latest materials.

Workshops

An effective way to increase the hospital staff's awareness of the library as more than just a reading center is to prepare, market, and present workshops or programs for meetings. A wide range of topics relating to library skills and services are of potential interest to all the hospital staff. An example might be a workshop on the legislative process, which explains how bills are tracked through state and federal legislatures and emphasizes the importance of timing lobbying efforts. Other possible topics for programs or workshops are how to prepare transparencies, research and deliver speeches and presentations, write for publication, use hospital microcomputers, locate statistics, or use government documents. The librarian can present the entire program or can arrange for speakers for all or part of the program. When outside speakers from other libraries, institutions, companies, or agencies are brought in, the library staff must still be responsible for the overall planning of the workshop, including audiovisual support.

In some institutions all educational workshops are developed or coordinated by a centralized education department. The library nevertheless can offer ideas for topics and instructors and provide bibliographic support.

Effective workshops of any size depend on thorough planning. The appendix provides a checklist that can be modified to fit individual situations.

Planning Events

The more thoroughly an event is planned, the more successful and easier it will be. A librarian should develop a checklist for special events similar to the one suggested for workshops and begin to maintain it during the planning stages of any event. With both the workshop and the special events checklist, the key word is *detail.* Will guests be able to balance refreshments as they walk around, or will they require seating? Is there a mop in the back room for emergency clean-up of spills? What are the responsibilities and location of each library staff member during the event? The librarian must mentally rehearse the entire event from start to finish in order to anticipate as many contingencies as possible. Further information on planning special events is available in the *Library Promotion Handbook,* listed at the end of the chapter.

OTHER PROMOTIONAL EFFORTS

Good library service is always excellent promotion for the library, and outreach services are especially effective because they move beyond library walls, often to groups that are not normally heavy users of the library. Programs using the clinical medical librarian concept, Literature Attached to Charts (LATCH) or Literature Attached to Staff Studies (LASS) programs, library carts on the floors or wards that carry materials for the use of patients or professionals, all increase the visibility of library services.

Good directional signs to the library are another often neglected method of promoting the library. If the hospital does not already have directional signs to the library, the librarian could work with the administration and any other necessary department to see that signs are produced and hung or posted. Signs inside the library help orient new users and make them feel less dependent on library staff. Further information on directional signs appears in Chapter 16.

Another way of promoting library services and resources is to provide "drawing cards." These are devices designed to entice or "draw" users or potential users into the library for purposes that are marginally related to library services. Such drawing cards might include morning coffee, the *Wall Street Journal*, the *New York Times Book Review*, an employee book exchange, personal copying for a minimum charge, or a drawing for a free dictionary for users who visit the library during a specific month. Advantages of drawing cards are that they may make nonusers more comfortable about visiting the library, bring new patrons into the library, and change thinking patterns about the library. Disadvantages include the necessity of devoting scarce resources to support marginal activities and the disruption to library routines and services.

REFERENCES

1. Davis BB. User needs: The key to changing library services and policies. Bull Med Libr Assoc 1975 Apr;63:195-198.

2. Sherman S. ABC's of library promotion. Metuchen, NJ: Scarecrow, 1980.

3. Cooper E. A one year "promotion campaign" at St. Luke's Medical Library. Hosp Libr 1977 Sept;2:8-11.

4. Wales LH. A practical guide to newsletter editing and design. 2d ed. Ames, IA:Iowa State University Press, 1976.

5. There's nothing duller than a book display. Show-Me Libr 1980 May;31:29-34.

6. Stoffle CJ, Bonn G. An inventory of library orientation and instruction methods. RQ 1973 Winter;13:129-133.

READINGS

Bowen AM. On-line literature retrieval as a continuing medical education course. Bull Med Lib Assoc 1977 Jul;65:384-386.

Davis EB, Northup DE, Self PC, Williams M. A two phased model for library instruction. Bull Med Lib Assoc 1977 Jan;65:40-45.

Edsall MS. Library promotion handbook. Oryx Press, 1980.

Fryzel, RJ. Marketing non-profit institutions. Hosp Health Serv 1978 Winter;23:8-16.

Hall VB. A slide tape program for beginning pharmacy students: effects on learning. Bull Med Lib Assoc 1977 Oct;65:443-445.

Hicks JT. Computer assisted instruction in library orientation and services. Bull Med Lib Assoc 1976 Apr;64:238-240.

Kahn R and Tepper K. You can do it: A PR skills manual for librarians. Metuchen, NJ: Scarecrow Press, 1981.

Kotler P. Marketing for non-profit organizations 2nd ed. Englewood Cliffs, NJ: Prentice-Hall, 1982.

Levitt T. Marketing when things change. Harv Bus Rev 1977 Nov/Dec;55:107-113.

Massey ME. Market analysis and audience research for libraries. Libr Trends 1976 Jan;1982:473-481.

Messing RE. Examining marketing. Hosp Forum 1978 Jul/Aug;21:6-9.

Maina W. A class in library use for allied health personnel. Bull Med Lib Assoc 1975 Apr;63:226-228.

Nickels WG. Marketing communications and promotion. 2d ed. Columbus, OH: Grid, 1980.

Pencils with a message. Libr J 1977 Apr;102:868.

APPENDIX

Workshop and Special Events Checklist

Assigned Person	Item	Needed	Completed
	1. Planning committee		
	a) Formulation of		
	b) Determination of theme		
	c) Overview		
	d) Objectives		
	e) Set date		
	f) Choose place		
	g) Determine speakers or activities		
	h) Alternate speakers arranged.		
	i) Schedule of activities		
	2. Budget		
	a) Proposed budget		
	b) Approximate number expected to attend		
	c) Fee (a - b)		
	d) Post program (actual) budget		
	3. Apply for CEUs (2-3 mos. prior)		
	4. Flier/brochure		
	a) Designed		
	b) To print shop (5-6 wks prior)		
	(if open to outside)		
	5. Mailing list (select audience)		
	6. Mail brochure (4-5 wks prior)		
	7. Equipment and facilities		
	a) Speaker's requirements		
	b) Podium		
	c) Tables		
	d) Table covers		
	e) Seating arrangements		
	f) Microphone (stationary/portable)		
	g) Lighting		
	8. Audiovisual equipment		
	Chalkboard/chalk		
	Flipchart/pens		
	Easel		
	Overhead projector		
	Opascope		
	Screens		
	Tape player		
	Recording equipment		
	CCTV		
	DuKane		
	Slide projector		
	Movie projector		
	Other		
	9. Projectionist		

Note: Courtesy of St. Joseph Hospital, Alton, Illinois

Assigned Person	Item	Needed	Completed
	10. Speakers		
	a) Confirmed		
	b) Honorarium required		
	Honorarium prepared		
	c) Lodging		
	d) Transportation		
	e) Special meetings/meals arranged		
	11. Food		
	a) Beverages		
	b) Food		
	c) Water pitcher, glasses for speakers		
	12. Signs		
	a) Directional		
	b) Registration		
	c) Welcome		
	d) Eating facilities		
	e) No smoking		
	f) Other		
	13. Publicity		
	a) Public relations		
	b) News media		
	c) Professional organization publications		
	14. Handout preparation		
	a) Name tags		
	b) Folders (include extra paper)		
	15. Duties - day of program		
	a) Registration table		
	List of registrants		
	Name tags		
	Folders		
	Certificates		
	b) Coffee		
	c) Welcome		
	d) Message board		
	e) Audiovisual equipment		
	f) Signs		
	g) Troubleshooter		
	16. Points to check just before workshop		
	a) Seating arrangements		
	b) Personnel in place and know what to do		
	c) Signs in place		
	d) Registration ready		
	e) Audiovisual equipment in place and working		
	f) Coffee ready		
	g) Speaker's podium/table in place		
	h) Microphones in place and on		

Assigned Person	Item	Needed	Completed
	17. After the workshop		
	a) Registration materials/money in office		
	b) Audiovisual equipment returned		
	c) Evaluations collected		
	d) Evaluations compiled		
	e) Permanent folder completed		
	f) Thank you note to speakers		
	g) Thank you note to helpers		

Management Issues in Hospital Libraries

Jana Bradley
Director, Library/Media Services
Wishard Memorial Hospital
Indianapolis, Indiana

CHAPTER 18

Management Issues in Hospital Libraries

Jana Bradley
Director, Library/Media Services
Wishard Memorial Hospital
Indianapolis, Indiana

Appendixes

Figures

Previous chapters have focused on management skills important to the hospital librarian, such as planning, budgeting, and communicating. This chapter will consider management issues that frequently arise in hospital libraries. These include the library's place in the hospital's organizational structure, the role of the library committee, departmental libraries, the use of consultants, and problems of managing a small library.

Any discussion of these issues must take into consideration the great diversity that exists among hospital libraries. Not only do hospital libraries vary greatly, but their parent organizations, the hospitals themselves, differ in organizational structure and in political dynamics. Thus it is impossible to describe a single management model that will work in every situation. This chapter will analyze the issues involved and discuss common practices. The librarian can then assess his or her own environment and develop a system that will be effective in that context.

THE LIBRARY'S PLACE IN THE HOSPITAL'S ORGANIZATION

The library's position in the overall organization of the hospital may vary considerably depending on the institution. The standards for professional library service issued by the Joint Commission on Accreditation of Hospitals (JCAH) require that the library's place on the hospital's organizational chart be defined. These standards, however, do not include recommendations about what that place should be.

Organizational Models

Figure 18-1 shows three models for the placement of the library in the hospital's organizational chart. In model A, the library is an independent department. The librarian as head of the department reports to a member of the hospital's administrative staff. This person may be an assistant or associate administrator, or even the hospital administrator. The person to whom the librarian reports often has jurisdiction over other departments related to the library, such as the audiovisual department or the education department.

In model B the library is a separate section within a larger department, with the librarian reporting to the head of the department. In some cases, the library may be closely related to the larger department. In others, the library many have little functional connection with its parent department and may be placed there because of convenience, necessity, or tradition.

In model C, the library is again part of another department, but the librarian reports to a supervisor rather than to the department head. Frequently, the person in charge of the library works part-time or has other responsibilities in addition to running the library. Model C libraries are usually not well-developed and often represent the beginning stages of organized library service.

Organizational model A, with the library as an independent department reporting directly to the hospital administration, usually allows for the most effective development of library services. There are many strong arguments in favor of model A. These arguments will be discussed below.

Almost all hospital libraries serve a number of user groups. The JCAH standards require service for the medical and hospital staffs. In practice, the library's clientele almost always includes physicians and nurses, and often a wide variety of other health professionals as well. Placing the library in a department responsible for only one group, such as medical or nursing education, may create conflicts of interest and may restrict library services to other user groups.

Second, library programs usually provide information services to staff physicians and nurses, as well as services that support educational programs. Linking the library administratively to a department whose responsibility involves only educational programming may restrict the development of information services to professionals outside the educational sphere, such as attending physicians or administrators.

Providing library service for medical and hospital staff involves assessing needs, defining levels of service, and determining appropriate resources. These tasks are most effectively performed when the librarian has the authority and the access to management information that comes with the position of department head. Also, library science is a separate discipline with its own body of knowledge and accepted practices. The librarian has the appropriate education and experience in the field to make recommendations directly to the hospital administration. A person trained in an unrelated discipline is usually far less effective in making decisions regarding the administration of library services.

Finally, placing the library in an unrelated department often works to the disadvantage of both. Such an arrangement forces both departments to become familiar with unrelated disciplines so that they can work together effectively.

Although librarians may feel that these arguments are self-evident, it is often necessary to document them for the hospital administration. Departmental status should not be pursued as an end in itself, without an understanding of how it will benefit library service. The benefits may include (1) control over the administrative functions of the library, such as budget, staffing, and policies; (2) a strong line of communication to hospital management and to other departments; and (3) recognition of the library as a department that serves the entire hospital.

In many cases, departmental status also allows the librarian to participate in management activities as a peer with other department heads.

Although these benefits are usually a part of departmental status, they are not automatically conferred with it nor are they limited to department heads. The librarian can, and should, work to gain these benefits regardless of his or her position in the organization.

Figure 18-1
Place of the Library in the Hospital's Organization Chart: Three Models

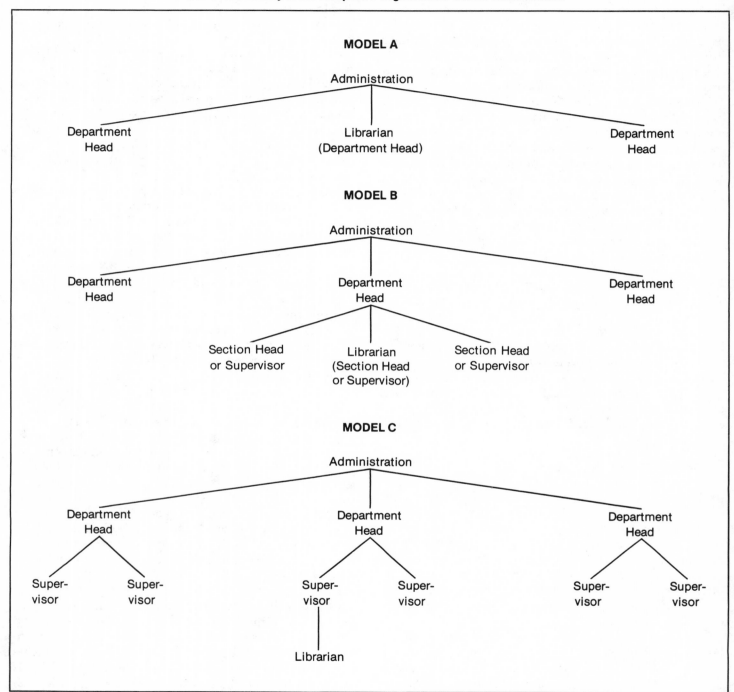

Independent status is not always feasible, necessary, or even desirable. Undeveloped or newly formed libraries are often not able to function independently and are placed under the wing of an established department. With nurturing, these libraries can grow toward independence. Well-developed libraries that have effective, supportive relationships with other departments may prefer to continue as part of the departmental team and grow within that structure.

Changing the Library's Position in the Organization

Changing the library's place on the hospital's organizational chart can be a delicate business and may result in conflict and antagonism. Before requesting a change, the librarian should carefully study the library's present situation to determine whether a change in status will result in improved library service. The librarian should also consider whether there are less drastic ways of solving the library's problems, and whether there is a strong possibility of getting the change approved. Any request for a change in supervisor is political in nature, and the implications and long-range effects should be carefully considered. Independent departmental status is not an automatic solution to all problems. In fact, it may be more difficult to demonstrate the importance of the library to a busy administrator than to the head of medical education.

Timing of the request is also important. Many hospital libraries that function as independent departments achieved that status after a long period of growth and development. Others were granted independence in conjunction with other organizational changes. The advice of local hospital librarians, the staff of the regional medical library, or the extension librarian from a local medical school may also be valuable when deciding whether to request a change.

Once the decision is made to seek a change, the strategy for doing so should be carefully planned. The librarian must thoroughly document the reasons why more effective library service would be possible under the new organization. Support for the change should be sought informally and should be fairly certain before a formal request is submitted. If possible, the support of the librarian's immediate supervisor should be gained first. Such support usually results when the supervisor understands the mutual benefits of the change. The library committee, influential users, and members of the administrative staff are also potential sources of support.

Supervisory Relationships

Whether the librarian reports to the hospital's administration or to the head of a department, success in achieving the library's goals will be affected by the librarian's relationship with his or her immediate supervisor. Supervisors have varying amounts of authority over the library depending on their own place in the organization.

However, they usually control the upward flow of information to the hospital's decision makers. Thus a supervisor's recommendations are usually very influential. Trying to work around a supervisor is extremely dangerous and seldom successful. A more effective approach is to try to create a relationship in which the supervisor, whether medical records administrator or associate administrator, works with the librarian to achieve mutually acceptable goals.

The extent to which a supervisor supports the library depends on many factors, some of which are beyond the librarian's control. Two important factors that the librarian can influence are the supervisor's understanding of the value of library service to the hospital and the supervisor's perception of the librarian's managerial competence.

Supervisor's Understanding of Library Services

A supervisor's perception of the value of library service often depends on previous experience with libraries. In many cases, the librarian must "educate" management about the benefits of library service in the hospital. This can be accomplished by regular, concise reporting on the results of the library program. Tying these results to unit costs, especially if comparisons are made with alternative costs, can further demonstrate value received for money spent. Further discussion of the role of reporting in increasing a supervisor's understanding of the library appears in Chapter 15.

Supervisors can also gain an understanding of the library's value and its potential by observing its usefulness to other departments. If library visibility is high and if services are genuinely wanted and needed by other departments, the supervisor is more likely to support the library's programs. Another way to increase the supervisor's awareness of the library's value is to provide service directly to the supervisor. A thorough analysis of the supervisor's information needs and a consistent effort to meet them can be very effective. Routine meetings with the supervisor regarding the operation of the library provide other opportunities to show what the library does and for whom.

Supervisor's Perception of Managerial Competence

The hospital's management, from the supervisor upward, often judges the librarian as much on managerial competence as on the provision of library service. Successful performance of such specific management responsibilities as budgeting, program or space planning, and personnel supervision is often essential to strong support for library development. In addition, management usually values those who show leadership qualities. Such qualities may include the ability to make appropriate decisions; a clear and concise reporting style; the ability to analyze problems, propose solutions, and implement them; and the ability to plan and operate productive, well-received programs. An understanding of the organization and its channels is also important. The librarian's place in the hospital's organization often depends on how the administration evaluates his or her effectiveness as a middle manager.

THE LIBRARY COMMITTEE

The library committee may be a useful, or even powerful, force for the development of the library. It can provide an essential base of support for library activities by providing evidence that certain library services are needed. The committee may even be able to exert pressure on the administration in support of new library services. For example, having physicians propose the addition of a MEDLINE terminal has meant the beginning of online services for many libraries.

In addition to presenting the users' needs for library services and acting as an influential advocate for these services, the library committee may function as a group of "representative users." In this role, it can give the librarian information and advice on matters of policy, selection of materials, promotional activities, and other library issues.

Although it is essential to recognize the important roles the library committee can play, an awareness of its limitations is also necessary. For each member of the library committee, the library is a secondary responsibility. In most cases, committee members' primary jobs are both demanding and time-consuming. Thus time for working on library matters will be limited, and members' primary jobs will understandably take priority.

Physicians and other members of the library committee can be influential advocates of funding for library services. However, they usually are not in direct control of approval for such funding. Even when the library is financed from medical staff funds rather than through the hospital's general fund, the library committee rarely controls the purse strings.

These limitations do not lessen the importance of developing an effective relationship with the committee and using it as a support group for the library. They do, however, make it advisable for the librarian to work toward a strong management structure within the library itself, with minimal dependence on the committee for operational decisions. The librarian should also seek support outside the committee, particularly from administrative personnel responsible for decisions that affect the library.

Not all hospital libraries have library committees. Libraries that operate successfully without a committee usually are viewed by the hospital administration as another service department and report directly to the administration. The librarian must make special efforts to assess user needs and to obtain broad-based user support, since there is no committee to assist in this effort.

Composition and Structure

The composition of the library committee will depend on the circumstances in each hospital and should be documented both in the committee's charge and in library policy documents. Colaianni recommends 5 to 15 as a workable number of members[1]. The JCAH standards state that the committee, if one exists, " . . . shall be multi-disciplinary and have representation from at least the medical staff, nursing department/service, and administration"[2].

Some committees have traditionally had a representative from every medical service. Although this arrangement does provide a subject expert for most medical fields, it can create a very unwieldy committee, particularly when other hospital user groups are included. If subject area representation is a sensitive issue, committee appointments can be rotated. The librarian may wish to seek advice on book selection from the department involved as well as from the library committee.

The committee and its chairperson may be appointed by the hospital's medical director, medical executive committee, administrator, or other person or group responsible for the appointment of committees. The librarian may be asked to recommend users interested in joining the committee.

The chairperson's role usually consists of calling meetings, determining the agenda, distributing any necessary materials, and reporting the committee's activities to the appropriate person or group. In practice, the chairperson often delegates many of these responsibilities to the librarian, committee secretary, or recorder. The librarian may also serve as chairperson or cochairperson, either on a permanent or a rotating basis.

The committee secretary or recorder is responsible for taking minutes and distributing them for approval after the meeting. This person may be asked to send materials to members before meetings and to handle other committee correspondence. The librarian may be asked to serve as secretary to the committee. However, this role may limit the librarian's participation in committee discussions.

The number of committee meetings held each year will depend at least partly on the committee's responsibilities. The JCAH standards state that " . . . the committee shall meet as often as required, but not less than twice annually"[2].

The JCAH standards also require that " . . . when a qualified medical librarian serves the hospital on a full-time or part-time basis, the individual shall be a member of the committee, with a defined role in committee functions"[2]. The librarian's role will vary and may include that of chairperson, secretary, ex officio representative, or simply committee member. Whatever the formal definition of the librarian's role, he or she is the individual with library training and experience. The librarian must play an active role on the committee, including providing agenda items, developing and recommending policies and procedures for committee approval, and providing information and recommendations on all issues. The librarian should also work to increase members' awareness and understanding of issues involved in library service.

Roles for the Library Committee

The role of the library committee may depend less on the committee's written charge than it does on other factors. These factors may include the interest of individual members; the leadership of influential administrators, physicians, or the librarian; and the committee's traditional role. The written charge is necessary both for documentation and for providing guidelines. However, the energy and resourcefulness of committee members usually determine what the committee does and how successful it is. The librarian should be the key person who provides either official or unofficial leadership and direction for the committee.

Advisory Body

The committee's most effective role is an advisory one. Committee support of policies can aid in their acceptance by the hospital. Selection is an area in which committee advice is often useful. Committee members can help to identify subject area priorities and can provide expertise in various subject areas. They can review materials and recommend titles for acquisition.

Library committees sometimes have decision-making authority for library functions. Although such authority is usually limited to selection, sometimes it may extend to other administrative functions. Such a situation may exist when a professional librarian has been employed for only a short time, or when the committee has traditionally had a dominant leadership role. From the point of view of library development, there are some disadvantages to placing decision making and leadership in the hands of a committee. Many of these disadvantages relate to the inherent strengths and weaknesses of any committee. Committee members have other responsibilities and thus do not have large amounts of time to devote to understanding library operations. Each member represents one user group or subject area and so is limited in his or her outlook. Also, members are professionals in fields other than library science and thus view the library from the users' perspective. The librarian views it from the perspective of the provider and manager of library service.

The objective of giving decision-making power to the committee is to assure that the library will meet the needs of subject experts. The assumption is that to achieve this objective, subject experts must make the decisions. When it becomes clear that the librarian can, in consultation with the subject experts, design and organize services that fully meet their needs, then the committee will usually agree to an advisory role. Such role shifts, however, often take time and are accomplished either in stages or as a result of changes in committee personnel.

Consumer's Representative

The committee can also serve as the official voice of the user and can identify problems, trends, or areas of need. It can do this by dealing with user complaints and comments as they arise or by systematically seeking user opinion. The librarian should try to be aware of the needs and opinions of all user groups. The library committee provides a core of individuals who have been specifically charged with this responsibility.

Advocate for the Library

Either as individuals or as a group, the committee can present the need for library services to the appropriate administrative or funding authority. This "proof of user need" often gives the hospital's management assurance that requests are justified. The committee's recommendations can be supported by needs analysis, whether conducted by the librarian or by the committee.

Working with the Library Committee

Skill in working with groups of people is essential when dealing with the library committee. Regardless of whether the committee makes final decisions or provides advice, its support is essential for a successful library program. Sources that discuss working with groups are listed at the end of the chapter.

Keeping the Committee Informed

Much of the librarian's work with the committee is accomplished outside of formal meetings. The librarian must keep the committee informed of library issues and operations. Well in advance of the official presentation of an issue, such as a request for a MEDLINE terminal, new space for the library, or a revised selection policy, the librarian should discuss the issue informally with individual members. The purpose of these discussions is to identify potential problem areas and to begin to educate members on the issue. Ideally, by the time the issue appears on the agenda, committee members will already be knowledgeable about it. The librarian should also feel fairly certain of members' support for the issue before it is presented.

Committee Meetings

The importance of an organized approach to library committee meetings cannot be overstated. The agenda and any background material should be distributed several weeks before the meeting, and important items should be discussed informally with individual members. At the meeting, additional summary information should be available, including the proposed text of any recommendations or motions. During the discussion, the librarian can act as a resource person, clarifying and summarizing issues under consideration. The librarian should participate in the discussion of various alternatives and yet still present the needs of the library clearly. In this way, the final decision will most likely meet the library's needs.

In addition to items that require committee action, the agenda should include items for the committee's information. The librarian's skill in choosing and presenting items can increase the committee's understanding of the factors involved in successful library service. The librarian should apply principles of good reporting when preparing such items. Information reported should relate clearly to the committee's needs and interests, and the terminology used should be understandable. The librarian should limit the number of statistics used, and try to compare them with statistics presented at earlier meetings.

Follow-up on assignments accepted or services offered in meetings is essential. The librarian should set aside time soon after the meeting for all such follow-up action and for filing any documents related to the meeting.

DEPARTMENTAL COLLECTIONS

Departmental collections of books, journals, and audiovisuals may vary from a small shelf of outdated textbooks to a large collection of books and bound journals. Many departments subscribe to journals, and some attempt to collect and bind them. Volunteer organizations or the medical staff may support collections in specific departments or on certain subjects.

The existence of these separate collections of materials can pose management problems for the hospital librarian. Even when policies on existing collections have already been set, questions still arise. Departments may wish to start new libraries of their own, or a new staff member may wish to purchase a small number of standard works for his or her office. Departments may request that the library order their materials for them. The librarian will also be concerned about the depth of the library's holdings in areas covered by departmental collections. Access to departmental collections and sources of funding for these collections may also pose problems.

Policy decisions are needed to deal with these concerns. The JCAH standards state that "It is desirable that all professional library collections be under a single library service, at least administratively when not physically possible"(1). Such centralized control may or may not be feasible in a given hospital.

In recommending policies on departmental collections, the librarian should analyze the situation realistically. He or she should seek the support of the departments involved, the library committee, user groups, and the administration. Because such decisions involve level of services, access to services, and funding, the librarian should work closely with the hospital administration in formulating policies. When discussing alternatives, it is often useful for both the librarian and the hospital administrator to consider the issue of departmental libraries in light of the following question: In what ways will the total range of books, journals, and audiovisuals needed by the medical and hospital staffs be provided?

Developing a consistent policy on departmental collections is an ongoing process and may take several years. Approaching the process from an analytical viewpoint should result in better understanding of all the factors involved, deliberate decisions about funding and the utilization of resources, and a systematic policy coordinating the hospital's information resources. When formulating a policy on departmental collections, seven areas of concern must be considered. They include (1) type of need, (2) location of materials, (3) access to materials, (4) quality of the collections, (5) relationship with the central library, (6) security, and (7) funding. In each area, the librarian, in cooperation with the administration, can determine which elements are important and at what levels they should be supported. It should be noted that the seven areas are interrelated and are separated only for purposes of discussion. The discussion below assumes the existence of a hospital library with the JCAH-mandated responsibility of serving the medical and hospital staffs.

Type of Need

Departments usually justify their collections on the basis of specific needs for particular materials. Defining these needs formally can help to identify the reasons certain departments want separate facilities. Formal definitions also tend to separate valid needs from less valid ones. Once needs have been identified, decisions can be made about their importance and about the amount of resources that will be allocated to meet them. Definitions of need should come from each individual department. Types of need that are frequently listed are discussed below.

Materials such as directories, handbooks, and standard reference works may be needed for immediate consultation at the work site. Personnel in areas like the emergency room may not be able to leave the work station and may request a greater number of reference materials. Staff members on call may also want a collection of materials close to their work stations.

Immediate access to material purchased for a specific project or course is often needed. The project or course may extend over a period of time longer than the combined checkout and renewal period. Thus the user would prefer to keep materials in the departmental collection.

Special collections of materials are often requested on the grounds that they are of interest to only one department or area. However, because disciplines overlap so much, almost all health care subjects are of interest to various user groups. The need to review literature as soon as it is published may also prompt a request for departmental journal collections.

Location of Materials

Departmental collections are sometimes justified based on convenience. Centralization of any service involves trade-offs. The benefits of centralization include better organization, access for all users, more services, and professional management and direction. Although keeping certain materials in departmental collections may be more convenient for the primary users, it should be remembered that the advantages of centralized service are lost.

Security

Lack of security is a major drawback of unsupervised collections. Materials are often taken to other areas for use and not returned, or are sometimes deliberately removed. When departments do provide security for their collections, such as housing them in an office or in a locked room, access often becomes limited. Any decision concerning security of departmental collections is best made by comparing the loss percentage over the past few years with the loss level that the hospital finds tolerable.

Access to Materials

Departmental collections are often less accessible than central collections, even for personnel within the department. The room in which materials are kept may not always be open. There may be restricted borrowing or limited facilities for use of materials, or there may be restrictions based on users' status or position. If unlimited access is provided, security becomes a problem.

In addition to the problem of physical access to materials, the problems of intellectual access, or knowing what materials are located where, must be considered. Many librarians have experienced the frustration of acquiring an expensive text only to discover that another department already owns it. One of the strongest arguments against departmental collections is that materials are not readily available, simply because their existence is not known. Documenting instances of overlapping need and unnecessary duplication is an excellent way to show that centralization of library materials can be cost-effective.

Once the hospital administration sees that lack of information about what is available can result in both underuse and duplication of expensive materials, the question of a catalog or a central list of materials arises. A list of materials by author is sometimes maintained by individual departments. However, even simplified cataloging involves more time than most departments are willing to devote to their collections. Cataloging also involves training that department staff members may not have.

The decision as to whether the library should catalog materials located throughout the hospital depends on several factors. These factors include the availability of library staff time, security of materials in departmental collections, access to these materials, and sources of funding for collections.

Advantages of cataloging include general access to all library materials in the hospital and the prevention of unnecessary duplication of resources. The librarian benefits from knowing the content of departmental collections and has the opportunity to be involved with collection development in the hospital as a whole.

Library involvement with departmental cataloging does have a number of disadvantages. It increases the library's cataloging and processing work load and thus increases library expenses for personnel and materials. Cataloging departmental materials makes collection management issues such as access, security, and inventory more important. When the library plays an active role in cataloging and managing departmental collections, additional resources and administrative support are usually needed. If such support is not available, the librarian may wish to keep a simplified list of materials in other departments. This can be done by arranging to be notified, via a copy of the purchase order, when library-type materials are ordered by other departments.

Some libraries order all the books, journals, and audiovisuals needed by all the departments in the hospital. Although this has many advantages for the library, it also involves considerable staff time and cannot be viewed as a simplified means of obtaining knowledge about hospital acquisitions.

It may not be feasible for the librarian to either catalog departmental collections or to maintain a simplified list of materials. In these cases, the librarian should try to become familiar with the acquisition patterns of departmental collections in order to provide as much coordination as possible.

Quality of the Collection

Since most collections outside the library are not professionally managed, many contain outdated editions. Selection is usually not systematic, so subject coverage is often spotty. Materials may be chosen from publishers' promotional literature rather than from more comprehensive reference sources.

Library assistance in building special subject collections helps to ensure their quality. The librarian can replace outdated editions, identify standard works in various areas, monitor new publications in a wide range of fields, and order needed materials. The librarian's knowledge of selection techniques can ensure that the collection meets the needs of users.

Relationship with the Central Library

The relationship of departmental collections to the central library may range from total separation and lack of coordination to centralized administration of all departmental collections by the hospital librarian. Centralized administration provides the most effective coordination of activities and is recommended by the JCAH standards for library service.

When centralized administration is not possible, the library may provide cataloging services or assistance with selection and ordering. Policies governing these services need to specify the kind and depth of services that will be provided. The costs, in terms of materials and staff time, should also be determined.

Decisions also need to be made regarding duplication of resources in the central library and the departmental collections. The extent to which the central library will collect in specialized areas and the procedures for keeping the library informed of various departments' acquisitions should also be specified.

The relationship between departmental collections and the central library can be very positive. Policies governing this relationship should be considered in terms of the needs of the departments, the central library, and the hospital as a whole. The librarian should work with the hospital administration, the individual departments, and the library committee to find the most cost-effective approach to meeting the total information needs of the hospital. In this way, the librarian can work toward a balance between departmental collections and the central library. Cooperation, flexibility, and a sense of perspective all help to ensure good relationships. Further information on the subject of departmental libraries can be found in the sources listed at the end of the chapter.

Funding

Money for departmental collections can come from hospital funds, grants, or gifts. The responsibility for the expenditure of these funds can rest with the library or with the department. Funding decisions are best made from the perspective of obtaining the most effective library service for the money spent.

USING CONSULTANTS

Employing a consultant is a means of securing professional expertise for a particular task, assignment, or project. Consultants are used in hospital libraries in two types of situations: 1) when the hospital does not regularly employ a qualified medical librarian, and 2) when the medical librarian employed by the hospital wishes the advice of an expert on special projects.

In the first case, the purpose of the consultant is to provide the hospital with the services of a qualified medical librarian. The JCAH standards for library service state the following:

> When employment of a full-time or part-time qualified medical librarian is not possible, the hospital shall secure the regular consultative assistance of such an individual. Consultative visits should be documented (2).

A consultant retained on a regular basis for organizing and overseeing general library operations can be involved in assessing needs, proposing and planning services, writing policies and procedures, selecting library materials, weeding the collection, and providing reference referral services.

In the second case, the hospital already employs a librarian, and that individual may wish to use a consultant for a project that involves special expertise. A consultant might be hired to review the plans for a new library or to help design a new audiovisual program. Consultants may be needed when adapting hospital computer facilities to the library or when establishing an archives service.

Consultants offer advantages besides professional expertise. In most cases, experienced consultants will have probably encountered similar situations before and thus will be aware of a variety of possible solutions. Also, they usually approach a situation with no preconceptions and therefore can provide an objective appraisal.

Consultants are usually unfamiliar with specific conditions in a particular hospital and will not be involved with daily operations. Thus they will need to acquaint themselves with the hospital and its needs for library services.

What to Look for in a Consultant

The minimal qualifications for a hospital library consultant are a matter of debate. However, a consultant who provides service to a library with no staff librarian will usually be a qualified medical librarian, as defined by the JCAH standards. He or she should be familiar with both hospital and academic medical libraries and with networking. The Medical Library Association (MLA) has endorsed a statement on hospital library consultants, which appears in Appendix A.

Choosing a consultant, whether for assistance with basic services or for expert advice on a specific project, is similar to filling any other professional position. The employer seeks, from a pool of qualified applicants, an individual whose training and experience are suited for the position. If possible, the consultant should have successful experience in solving the specific problems involved. If library service is to be initiated from the ground up, the consultant ideally would have done this before. Understanding of the particular environment in which library service is to be provided is also highly desirable. For example, if library service is being initiated for a teaching hospital affiliated with a medical school, the consultant should be familiar with the structure of medical education in a clinical environment.

Hiring a Consultant

The names of qualified persons who may meet the requirements for a particular consulting job can be obtained from a variety of sources. These sources include regional medical libraries, hospital library consortia, and state health science library associations. Local hospital libraries and medical school libraries with hospital library extension programs may also be good sources of information. One-time assessment consulting may be available in some areas through the regional medical library, extension programs offered by other library consortia or agencies, or neighboring hospital or academic medical libraries. Such one-time consultation usually serves to identify needs and does not take the place of regular consultative assistance. This type of consultation is usually not appropriate for extensive help with a specific project, such as the building of a new library.

The services of a consultant, beyond the assessment and advice offered by various extension programs and individual libraries, usually involve a fee. Fees vary depending on the project and the consultant, and obtaining job quotations from several qualified candidates is probably the best way to determine the going rate. Fees are usually based on qualifications and experience, and a more experienced consultant is likely to be more expensive than a novice.

Before interviewing candidates, the responsibilities of the consultant should be clearly defined. A formal statement of the duties of the position should include tasks to be accomplished and a tentative time schedule. It should be clearly stated if the consultant is to produce written objectives, policies, or procedures. The person to whom the consultant is responsible and the manner in which reporting is to be done should also be specified.

In most cases, an administrative representative should be actively involved in defining the consultant's role. The representative may also wish to participate in the interviewing and orienting process.

Once an agreement is reached with a consultant, it should be documented. This may be done using either a letter of agreement or a contract. The consultant's visits should also be documented, both to comply with the JCAH standards and to verify that the terms of the agreement are being fulfilled. Such documentation usually consists of the following information about each visit: date, length, purpose, proposals or reports submitted, and action taken on recommendations.

Providing Support for a Consultant

The role of the consultant is to recommend, design, organize, or oversee services or projects. He or she is hired because of specific knowledge or professional expertise. The consultant is usually not responsible for the daily operation or implementation of programs or projects, although he or she might be hired to evaluate them on a regular basis. Daily operation of library service is the responsibility of library staff members. The JCAH standards state the following:

> When the medical librarian serves only on a part-time or a consultative basis, a suitably trained employee shall be designated and available to provide basic library services. The individual should have basic library skills and, wherever possible, should be at least the equivalent of a library technician or library assistant (2).

The exact nature of the support provided for the consultant should be specified in the initial agreement.

The consultant is employed as an objective third party. The value of the consultant lies in this objectivity. Thus it is best, if at all possible, to avoid situations in which the consultant must take sides on partisan issues.

MANAGING A SMALL LIBRARY

When applied to a hospital library, the term "small" is of course relative and may be based on several criteria. These criteria include space, collection, budget, services, and staff. From an administrative viewpoint, staff is a key indicator of size, simply because the number of available working hours limits what can be accomplished. However, the term "small staff" is also relative. For example, a staff that may be considered large by hospital library standards may be too small to meet users' needs in a particular hospital.

A great many hospital libraries, probably the majority, are small in the sense that they are staffed by one person. Operating a full-service library with one person presents very real management difficulties. The librarian must not only perform the duties of the library director, but also those of the public services staff and the technical services staff. In addition to delivering services, the librarian must also plan and administer these services. Although a small library may not be able to provide all services, the librarian can choose the services that best meet the needs of the hospital. A list of basic manuals for small hospital libraries appears in Appendix B at the end of the chapter.

The discussion that follows will focus on the problem of too much to do in too little time. For many librarians, the time dilemma becomes a vicious circle. Library duties related to technical and public services pile up, leaving little time for administrative tasks such as analysis, planning, and report writing. Suggestions on ways to achieve a workable balance between what has to be done and the amount of time available are discussed below.

Assigning Priorities for Services

With the approval of the hospital administration, priorities can be set regarding certain services and requests. For example, all reference questions relating to patient care may be given first priority. Priority can also be given to certain services or projects. For example, attention may be focused on providing services for attending staff or on developing a reprint file for floor nurses. Although concentration on one service or on the needs of one user group means less attention to others, this may sometimes be necessary. Similarly, services that are seldom used might be discontinued until there is time to develop and promote them.

Quotas can also be used. For example, each department can be limited to a certain number of searches or loans. However, outright refusal of services in the face of legitimate need may undermine support for the library. Quotas that are part of approved policy may discourage chronic overusers, but unless quotas are so high as to be meaningless, they can interfere with the needs of special projects. Also, overusers can usually be dealt with on a case-by-case basis, especially if library policy states that services are subject to the availability of staff time.

When demand for service is so high that there is no alternative other than to limit or cut service, the administration should be involved in formulating policy on cutbacks. Such involvement allows the administration to see the effects of inadequate staffing in the library.

Using Time Effectively

Time management experts believe that most people do not use time as effectively as possible. The best way for an individual to determine patterns of time usage is to analyze exactly how he or she spends time. Although filling in a time analysis chart for a week can be tedious, it can give an accurate picture of how time is spent.

There are many methods of time analysis. One method uses a chart divided into 15-minute blocks of time. A timer or similar device is necessary to ensure regular recording of activities. All activities in each time block should be listed honestly and should include an estimate of time spent on each activity. Once the chart is completed, it can be analyzed to determine how time is being spent and whether more efficient methods could be employed for certain activities.

Techniques and systems for making efficient use of time abound. Several are listed at the end of the chapter. Lois Ann Colaianni discusses many of these techniques as they apply to hospital libraries (1).

Some suggestions for efficient time management are listed below.

- Assign specific times for accomplishing routine tasks.
- Make notes of points to cover in telephone calls before calling.
- Use lists to keep track of tasks and to organize the work day.
- Arrange for at least some uninterrupted work time.
- Learn your personal work rhythms and plan to do routine tasks at the time of day when you are least effective.
- Break large tasks into smaller ones.
- Assign priorities and do important tasks first.
- Don't let others waste your time.

Improving Library Operations

Efficient operation of library services is essential in a one-person library. The librarian may wish to evaluate routine procedures to determine whether they are efficient and necessary. Questions to consider might include the following.

- What is the purpose of the routine?
- How much staff time does it take?
- What materials are needed?
- Can the routine be simplified?
- What compromises does a simplified routine involve, and what are the implications?
- How valuable is the routine, especially when considered in light of the time and materials it involves?
- What alternatives might accomplish the same or similar purposes?

Evaluations of routines can be performed on a continuing basis by allotting some time each week to the activity. Procedures may also be evaluated when a change in the library is being considered, such as the addition of a new staff member or a computer terminal; when a problem in the system becomes obvious; or when a particular task is not being done on a timely basis.

When major library functions like cataloging are being examined, the possibilities for automation or for contracting with a commercial service should not be overlooked. Network participation may also be possible. Some hospital libraries have developed automated operations in conjunction with computer systems already available in the hospital.

Improving Staffing Levels

Although adding a new staff position is often thought of as a remedy for time shortages, staffing level increases in most institutions are related to increases in services provided, particularly to new services or new user groups. To justify a request for a new position, the librarian usually must document an increase in work load.

Volunteers can be useful in the library, although the time involved in supervision must be balanced against the assistance they provide. Determining staffing levels and using volunteers effectively are discussed further in Chapter 14.

Exploring Cooperative Relationships

Cooperation with other libraries is an excellent way to increase access to materials and to expand services. However, it rarely results in a saving of time. Cooperative efforts may have the effect of shifting the amount of time spent on various activities. But cooperation is primarily a way of sharing resources, not of saving time.

REFERENCES

1. Colaianni LA, Lyon FI. Hospital library management. Chicago: Medical Library Association, 1981. (MLA courses for continuing education, CE-129)

2. Joint Commission on Accreditation of Hospitals. Accreditation manual for hospitals. 1983 ed. Chicago: Joint Commission on Accreditation of Hospitals, 1982:147-149.

READINGS

Bormann EG, Bormann NC. Effective small group communication. II 2d ed. Minneapolis: Burgess Publishing, 1976.

Bradford LP. Making meetings work: A guide for leaders and group members. La Jolla: University Associates, 1976.

Cressaty M. The library committee in the medical school. Bull Med Libr Assoc 1969 Oct;57:352-361.

Douglass ME, Goodwin PH. Successful time management for hospital administrators. New York: AMACOM, 1980.

Dyer SR. Decentralized, departmental library collections in health care systems. Hosp Top 1980 Sep-Oct;58:19-22.

Edson JB. How to survive on a committee. Soc Work 1977 May; 224-226.

Fanning T. Get it all done and still be human: A personal time-management workshop. Radnor, PA: Chilton, 1979.

Howard E, Kharibian G. Mechanization of library procedures in the medium-sized medical library: XIII. Computer applications in hospital departmental libraries. Bull Med Libr Assoc 1972 Jul;60:445-466.

Jay A. How to run a meeting. Harv Bus Rev 1976 Mar-Apr;54:43-57.

Kasses CD, Taylor SD, Jones CL. Departmental libraries: curse or blessing? Bull Med Libr Assoc 1978 Apr;66:77-84.

Pletzke CJ. On the road to effective hospital library committees. Hosp Libr 1976 Jul 15;1:4-5; Aug 1;1:6-7.

Stefanacci MA, Wood MS, Huff LA. Departmental libraries: why do they exist? Bull Med Libr Assoc 1977 Oct;65:433-437.

Wheeler DD, Janis IL. A practical guide for making decisions. New York: Free Press, 1980.

APPENDIX A
Hospital Library Consultants

Role Statement for Hospital Library Consultants

The hospital library consultant serves as advisor to the hospital administration, medical staff, library staff, and/or library committee in defining and designing hospital library services and/or facilities to meet the informational, educational, research, and patient care-related needs of the entire hospital community including, where appropriate, the instructional needs of patients.

Consultation is provided on a contractual basis.

Hiring a hospital library consultant is not a substitute for the employment of permanent library personnel.

Qualifications for Hospital Library Consultants

A hospital library consultant should have a master's degree in library/information science from a program which is accredited by the American Library Association, should be certified as a medical librarian by the Medical Library Association, and should have at least three years of administrative hospital library experience. If the consultant does not have all of the above qualifications, he/she should have an equivalent combination of training and experience, such as eight years of progressively responsible health science library experience including at least five years of hospital library management, administration of a medical center library, or working with hospital libraries in a consultative capacity.

The consultant should have supervisory and administrative experience with ability to provide assistance on personnel and fiscal issues. The hospital library consultant must show evidence of regular participation in continuing education courses in consulting, management, health sciences, and/or hospital librarianship such as those sponsored by the Medical Library Association.

The consultant must be familiar with existing national, state, and local library networks, and have a working knowledge of the National Library of Medicine's Regional Medical Library Program. The consultant should also have a thorough working knowledge of the Joint Commission on Accreditation of Hospital's (JCAH) standards and other hospital library standards.

Membership in the Medical Library Association and its Hospital Library Section is preferred. Membership in other local, state, regional, and national professional library associations is desirable.

Note: Hospital library consultants for certain types of facilities such as federal or psychiatric hospitals may require additional qualifications.

Functions/Process for Hospital Library Consultants

A. Identify objectives with the hospital administrator, library staff and/or library committee, and other appropriate hospital personnel.

B. Negotiate a contractual agreement with the hospital administrator which would include:

- Consultant and client responsibilities
- Purpose of consultation
- Period of contract
- Number and frequency of visits or amount of time to be spent by a consultant during the contractual period
- Verbal and written reporting mechanisms
- Fee for service
- Terms of termination by either party

C. Conduct a needs assessment for library services profiling all disciplines in the total hospital environment. Functional elements identified might include:

- Placement of library staff within the hospital organizational structure
- Job descriptions for library staff
- Library staff recruitment, training, and development
- Budget
- Facility planning and/or space allocation
- Policies and procedures
- Availability of current materials for each discipline at the hospital
- Acquiring, cataloging, arranging, organizing, and evaluating library materials
- Answering questions and providing other information
- Circulation or control of materials
- Notifying hospital staff of new information in their area of interest
- Audiovisual services
- Patient education
- Promoting library services
- Cooperation with other libraries

D. Provide specific written recommendations for administrator, library manager, and/or library committee.

E. Develop a methodology for implementation of recommendations by hospital employee(s) assigned to the library.

F. Evaluate and assess progress regularly during the contractual period.

Recommendations for the Documentation of Consultative Visits

The hospital library consultant shall document each visit. At minimum, such documentation should include:

- A record of the date and length of each visit
- An account of the consultant's activities during each visit
- Recommendations for action based on the needs assessment
- Progress reports
- Suggestions for follow-up

A record of documented visits shall be maintained on file for review by the appropriate reviewing or surveying agencies and for continued reference by the administration, library staff, and/or library committee. Meetings with the administrator, library manager and library committee to discuss recommendations, questions, or concerns should be held as needed and followed by a formal written report.

Endorsed by the Medical Library Association

APPENDIX B
Basic Library Manuals for
Small Hospital Libraries

Bloomquist HJ, Rees AM, Stearns NS, Yast H, eds. Library practice in hospitals: a basic guide. Cleveland: Case Western Reserve University Press, 1972.

Colaianni LA, Lyon FI. Hospital library management. Chicago: Medical Library Association, 1981. (MLA courses for continuing education, CE-129)

Colaianni LA, Mirsky PS. Manual for librarians in small hospitals. 4th ed. Los Angeles: Biomedical Library, University of California, Los Angeles, 1978.

Gadzikowski C. Hospital library operations: an overview of technical and public services. Omaha: Midcontinental Regional Medical Library Program, 1980.

Library Services Committee, Ohio Hospital Association. Hospital library services manual. 1980.

Midwest Health Science Library Network. Basic library management for health science librarians. 2d ed. Chicago: Midwest Health Science Library Network, 1982.

Wender RW, ed. Organizing and administering the small hospital library. Dallas: TALON Regional Medical Library Program, 1979.

Cooperation Among Libraries

Sandra Clevesy
Director of Library Services
Cesare G. Tedeschi Library
Framingham Union Hospital
Framingham, Massachusetts

CHAPTER 19

Cooperation Among Libraries

Sandra Clevesy
Director of Library Services
Cesare G. Tedeschi Library
Framingham Union Hospital
Framingham, Massachusetts

Figures

Although cooperation is well established in the library field, it is relatively new in hospital libraries. Before 1970, many hospital libraries with small collections and limited staffing had few cooperative connections and operated in relative isolation. In teaching hospitals or in hospitals with nursing schools, libraries were generally more developed and more likely to be staffed by a professional librarian. In these libraries cooperation, usually in the form of interlibrary loan, resulted from personal contact between librarians.

In the last decade, the need for formal cooperation has grown rapidly. Hospital and medical staff need timely materials to solve clinical problems, to keep up-to-date in their fields, and to meet continuing education requirements. As bibliographic searching services become more available in libraries, the variety of materials needed to meet user needs expands. As the teaching and research responsibilities of hospitals increase, the pool of materials needed to support these programs grows. The need to meet a wide variety of requests for informational services and materials has encouraged cooperative activity in general and resource sharing in particular.

Today the central role of library cooperation is well established. A significant responsibility of hospital librarians is participation in cooperative arrangements. Because even simple cooperative tasks involve complex processes, functioning effectively as a group member requires knowledge and skills. To provide a basic understanding of hospital library cooperation, this chapter examines types of cooperation, the range of possible activities, and some fundamental principles.

Traditional cooperation is generally based on personal contact between librarians rather than on formal agreements between libraries. As Felter describes it, traditional cooperation is perceived as a moral rather than a contractual obligation, with the larger library serving as a patron to the smaller one principally by providing free interlibrary loans(1). Such one-to-one cooperation has considerably aided the development of hospital libraries and can provide a valuable extension of services for small libraries that are unable to take part in more formal programs. Traditional cooperation can also provide a foundation on which to build more extensive and formal cooperative arrangements. A number of types of formal structures have evolved during recent years.

THE REGIONAL MEDICAL LIBRARY PROGRAM

In 1965 Congress passed the Medical Library Assistance Act, which held the National Library of Medicine (NLM) responsible for improving information transfer to support health services delivery, education, and research. A major result of this charge has been the development of the Regional Medical Library Program (RMLP).

The Regional Medical Library Network

One purpose of the RMLP is extending cooperation between existing libraries. The network consists of a four-tiered pyramid, with institutions at each level serving as backup resources for the level below.

Level I—Basic Health Science Libraries

Basic health science libraries, primarily located at hospitals, are the first places where many clinicians and other health professionals seek biomedical information. If the information is not available at the primary library or a nearby cooperating library, the request is referred to the next level of the network. By providing physicians with access to the network, the library is a principal agent in providing health professionals the biomedical information they need.

Level II—Resource Libraries

Libraries with major health science collections comprise the next level of the network. Most are affiliated with medical schools or medical centers. They supply materials and programs not available from the basic health science library.

Level III—Regional Medical Libraries

Regional Medical Libraries (RMLs) serve not only as backup for resource libraries in providing interlibrary loans but also as a source of programs designed to promote and improve medical library services. Supported by the NLM under contract, each RML provides services that meet the needs of its particular region. These typically include reference services, consultation by extension librarians, newsletters, and training of library personnel. In 1983 the regional structure was reconfigured from eleven to seven regions. A list of the Regional Medical Libraries and their addresses can be found in a current volume of *Index Medicus*.

Level IV—The National Library of Medicine

At the top of the pyramid, the National Library of Medicine represents a comprehensive national resource. Its responsibility is providing materials not available from other libraries.

Effects of the Regional Medical Library Program

The dramatic success of the RMLP has significantly altered the traditional role of the hospital library. Whatever their geographical location, health care practitioners are able to get needed information from medical collections throughout the United States without leaving their hospital. Clinicians have been so receptive to network services and have used them so extensively that the demand has exceeded the funds allocated for its support at all levels. A variety of strategies including quotas, fees, and restricted lists of available titles have been implemented to encourage local self-sufficiency and to stretch available support funds.

Hospital libraries have increased their efforts to cooperate among themselves, an action influenced by the NLM Policy Statement of 1972. That statement outlined expectations of more self-sufficiency at each level of the network than had been required during earlier stages of the RMLP (2). Thus the Regional Medical Library Program has been instrumental in stimulating a growing grass roots movement: the development of formalized local networks of basic units, called consortia.

CONSORTIA

A library consortium is an organized group of at least two autonomous libraries. Consortia vary in membership, purpose, organizational structure, resources, and activities, but each represents a voluntarily organized formal group that pursues activities of mutual benefit to members. The formal organization and reciprocal sharing of services differentiates the consortium from more traditional forms of cooperation.

Types of Consortia by Function

In her classic work on consortium planning, Patrick identifies four general types of consortia(3):

- Large consortia concerned primarily with computerized, large-scale technical processing
- Small consortia concerned primarily with user services and everyday routine
- Limited-purpose consortia cooperating with respect to limited special subject areas
- Limited-purpose consortia concerned primarily with interlibrary loan or reference network operation

The first category, large consortia, includes national or regional networks such as OCLC, Inc., and New England Library Network (NELINET). As products and services of these large-scale cooperatives expand, the advantages of membership become more evident. Many librarians are investigating the feasibility of participating through direct membership, through regional or state groups, or through commercial vendors. Further discussion of these networks can be found in the readings listed at the end of this chapter.

The second category includes consortia of basic health science libraries, which have recently emerged in conjunction with the RMLP. Most of these consortia consist of libraries located close enough together to allow daily interaction by telephone and occasionally by personal visits. This kind of grass roots consortium frequently develops from formalizing traditional cooperation already existing between librarians. The development of this type of consortium has been widely reported in the literature.

The third category includes limited-purpose consortia concentrating on special subject areas. Consortia of this type are concerned with coordinating and sharing materials usually of interest to a particular user group, such as nurses.

The fourth grouping consists of consortia limited to interlibrary loan or reference network operations. The distinction between limited-purpose consortia and all-purpose consortia is blurred because many emerging consortia focus on interlibrary loan and the development of union lists. When operations are functioning smoothly, such consortia often expand their activities to other areas of cooperation.

Types of Consortia by Membership

Consortia can be divided into two types according to membership: (1) a single-type library cooperative composed of similar libraries and (2) a multitype library cooperative. The latter type consists of two or more types of libraries, such as academic, public, school, or special libraries. Because similar libraries serve similar users, operate within similar institutional environments, and face similar problems, single-type cooperatives generally provide closer interaction among members than multitype cooperatives. Single-type cooperatives, however, lack the diversity of collections offered by multitype cooperatives. As hospital libraries receive requests for a broader scope of materials to meet the needs of an increasingly diversified clientele, access to information from public, academic, or special libraries becomes highly desirable.

The multitype cooperative can be both all-purpose, such as state library groups, or limited-purpose, such as online bibliographic searching networks. The diversity of libraries found in a multitype consortium represents its biggest advantage.

Structural Documents

A major difference between traditional cooperation and a consortium is the consortium's formal structure, usually defined in one or more organizational documents. These documents establish the conditions of cooperation, provide guidelines for daily operation, and serve to maintain the consortium's structure. Although the documents for each consortium are different, some basic categories are discussed below.

Cooperative Agreement (Contract)

This document defines the conditions of cooperation. Usually it is an agreement between institutions rather than librarians. It is signed by the administrator and kept on file as documentation of cooperative arrangements for the Joint Commission on Accreditation of Hospitals (JCAH.)

Usually, the document states the goal of the cooperative group. This goal may be given a broad definition such as "to facilitate the sharing of resources and services," or a narrow one such as "to provide centralized bibliographic retrieval services." The contract also describes the group's organizational structure. It enumerates the responsibilities of the members, including staff time, costs, and other commitments. Finally, it states the duration of the agreement and conditions for both joining and withdrawing.

Some documents of agreement are detailed and formal and may be reviewed by the hospital's lawyer. Others are more generally phrased, expressing an intent to cooperate and leaving the details to be worked out in other documents or informal agreements.

Bylaws

Some consortia follow the example of professional organizations and have bylaws, either in addition to or in place of a cooperative agreement. When bylaws stand as the sole agreement of cooperation, they contain all the elements discussed above.

Policies and Procedures

Each activity the group undertakes should be guided by written policies and procedures. This standardizes practices and ensures continuity.

Funding

Most consortia depend heavily on trading and donating labor. Many consortia projects are completed through the cooperative efforts of members with costs covered indirectly by individual library budgets. Still, a consortium's progress is often determined by the level of additional funding the group is able to obtain. Several funding alternatives used to support consortia operations are examined below.

Grant Support

Agency or foundation funding is often a way to begin highly visible projects. Many health science consortia have benefited from grant funds such as the National Library of Medicine's Resource Improvement Grants. Generally, the terms of the grant require supplemental support from participating institutions. Almost all grants are for limited periods to allow planning and resource improvement. After this period, support of the entire program falls to the member institutions.

Fees

Collecting fees is another way to increase funds. Membership fees may be levied at a flat rate per institution or on a sliding scale based on such variables as size of institution, rate of use of services, or number of services used. Another method for determining membership fees is to divide the projected budget for the year's operation by the number of members.

If a consortium provides several cooperative programs, such as audiovisual sharing, online services, and cooperative cataloging, another alternative is for member libraries to pay only for the services they use. Users of individual libraries may also be asked to pay for services provided through cooperative arrangements. In this way, the consortium avoids soliciting institutional support for cooperative services. Each library decides whether to charge users or to absorb the cost in the library budget.

Revenues

Fundraising activities have not been widely used by consortia. Some groups, however, have charged fees for workshops, publications, or services provided to users outside their organization.

Activities

The cooperative activities of a consortium reflect the goals and objectives of the group. The single-purpose consortium, such as one made up of several institutions that agree to share MEDLINE costs, readily demonstrates this concept. In a consortium with the broad purpose of "sharing resources to avoid unnecessary duplication and improve service," cooperative activity tends to expand as the consortium develops. A group may elect to concentrate exclusively on one project at a time or undertake several activities simultaneously. Most initial consortium activities produce quick and tangible benefits but require low levels of compromise and low costs. The primary example is the basic cooperative activity—interlibrary loan.

Interlibrary Loan

In health science consortia, books constitute only a small portion of the materals that are loaned. The major items loaned are journal articles. Providing journal articles, both originals and photocopies, is often called document delivery. It is the basic activity of most networks. Through it, each library has access to materials in the collections of the other libraries. The effectiveness of this access depends on the efficiency of the consortium's procedures and the speed with which the materials are sent. In some consortia, requests are made by telephone, and the lending library processes the material for mailing within 24 hours. Some librarians have obtained permission to use the hospital's courier service for picking up interlibrary loans. When requests are mailed and materials returned the same way, turnaround time is extended to allow for the vagaries of the postal service. To expedite delivery, larger libraries have used TWX for many years to communicate requests. Some librarians now use the interlibrary loan subsystems of bibliographic utilities such as OCLC, Inc.

Union Lists and Catalogs

Locating libraries that own a needed journal is the essential first step in an efficient interlibrary loan transaction. Therefore the development of a union list of journals is often one of the first cooperative activities of any group. Union lists are produced either manually or by computer and vary considerably in detail and sophistication.

Several guides for the development of union lists for serials have been published(4,5). The NLM is developing its National Biomedical Serials Base, which it intends to use to aid regions and subregions in producing union lists. Some major utilities, such as OCLC, Inc., have also implemented union list services. Whatever the format or source, the development of a union list must be combined with a formal structure for sharing the materials.

Cooperative Cataloging

The dramatic success of OCLC, Inc., demonstrates the potential of cooperative cataloging. For hospital libraries, the necessary duplication of a large percentage of core materials makes cooperative cataloging a logical consortium activity. Cooperative cataloging, however, requires standardized policies and procedures that involve more compromise, cost, and structure than other consortium activities. Further details on cooperative cataloging alternatives may be found in Chapter 5. As more libraries participate in networks such as OCLC, the incidence of cooperative cataloging should increase.

Computerized Bibliographic Services

Sharing the costs of MEDLINE access is widely practiced. A terminal and searcher at one institution may serve several other institutions on a regular basis. Perhaps the terminal and the searcher may rotate regularly among member institutions. A third alternative uses technology to transfer information from one terminal to another. First the searcher and the user discuss the question over the telephone. Then the search is performed at the primary terminal, and the results are printed out at both terminals. Thus one searcher can serve many locations, provided each has a terminal(6).

Duplicate Exchange

Exchanging of surplus materials among members of local consortia is another activity that produces large benefits at low cost. Through such an exchange, libraries can replace missing issues and complete journal volumes. Lists of surplus materials are compiled and circulated among members before being offered to other exchange programs. Or one library serves as a clearing house for requests, providing a centralized "matching service."

Cooperative Acquisitions and Holdings

Promoting the development of complementary collections has resurfaced as an important reason for cooper-

ation. One way to coordinate resources is to develop union lists. Another way is to share acquisitions by pooling funds for the joint purchase of an expensive journal or reference book. A more frequently used alternative is for one library to buy or maintain an item on behalf of the group. Such a system of "serials rationalization" is described by Jones(7).

A similar method of coordinating resources is for each hospital to develop collections in subject areas that reflect the services of the hospital. For example, a library in a hospital with a CT scanner would buy materials on computerized tomography. In a hospital with a psychiatric department, the library would agree to expand its collection of psychiatric literature. This method eliminates any pooling of funds, which is often cumbersome and difficult to accomplish. Conversely, assigning subject specialties is generally difficult in a single-type library consortium where all hospitals offer similar services. While cooperative acquisition is frequently set as a goal, achievement is often very slow.

Inter-institutional Delivery Service

Some cooperating libraries located near one another share the costs of an inter-institutional delivery service. Such a service greatly reduces the turnaround time for interlibrary loan transactions. When delivery services already exist among hospitals, perhaps in relation to other shared activities or among other libraries in the area, affiliation is often possible.

Reference Referral

As Patrick states, "Not only can the library collection be considered as a resource of the whole consortium, but the combined library staffs may also be considered a consortium resource" (3:130). Reference referral among consortium members makes use of the combined knowledge of the group and the expertise of individual members. It also provides backup during vacations. Reference referral is often the only way to extend services into peripheral subject areas. The library that routinely serves administrators, managers, and support services staff almost certainly needs channels for referring questions to libraries with broader collections. Many hospital librarians have found cooperative reference referral arrangements with public and academic libraries extremely beneficial.

Continuing Education of Members

Continuing education is another basic component of consortium activities. Consortium meetings provide regular opportunity for discussing problems; the exchange of ideas can be both educational and therapeutic. Since recertification requires documented participation in MLA-accredited continuing education programs, many consortia sponsor workshops for members and outside groups. For the same reason, consortia may subsidize the costs of members' attendance at national meetings and training sessions.

Setting Up and Operating a Consortium

The above discussion describes the basic organization and possible activities of consortia. Guidelines for establishing a consortium and developing specific activities can be found in the readings listed at the end of this chapter. Especially useful are the following: *Guidelines for Library Cooperation, Getting Into Networking: Guidelines for Special Libraries, Dynamics of Hospital Library Consortia,* and *The Development and Operation of Health Science Library Consortia* (3,8,9,10).

PRINCIPLES OF COOPERATION

Although the details of cooperation may vary, certain principles are common to all successful cooperatives. The road to cooperative activity is not always smooth, but an understanding of these principles and the issues surrounding them will provide insight and perspective when problems occur.

Necessity

It is well recognized that no one library can independently provide all the materials required by its users. Resource sharing has long been essential to libraries of all types. The necessity for broad cooperative action by hospital libraries has never been more apparent. JCAH standards reflect the validity of cooperation among libraries. The structure of the RMLP illustrates the interdependence of all medical libraries and the basic "first line" position of the hospital library in the information transfer process. This structure encourages libraries to build their collections in the context of resources available locally, regionally, and nationally.

As more library operations are computerized, libraries that fail to participate in networks are likely to become further isolated, restricting access and limiting use of new technologies. This prospect represents a grave danger for small libraries that already tend to be isolated. Librarians should stress that cooperation is fundamental to effective library service. They should vigorously pursue existing potential for cooperative action and actively participate in ongoing cooperative programs. However limited these programs may be initially, they provide a foundation upon which to build.

Support

All cooperative activities should reflect written library policy and procedures approved by the administration. This includes informal arrangements of traditional cooperation, which have been largely interpersonal relationships. It is essential that the administration of each institution makes a philosophical commitment to the program. If financial commitment is required, the necessity of administrative approval of the project is obvious.

As in other aspects of library operation, gaining hospital support for cooperative programs constitutes one of the largest challenges confronting many librarians. Building a supportive environment takes effort and energy, but it is essential to the success of the consortium.

Support for cooperation should be sought from those affected by proposed cooperative arrangements as well as those responsible for their implementation. The librarian should make users aware of existing networks and their essential role in the delivery of information. One common method for increasing awareness of cooperation is marking each cooperative item with a stamp, bookmark, or form identifying the consortium or the source: for example, "This material has been provided to you by the cooperative activity of _____ Consortium."

Library committee members can serve as a sounding board for new ideas and can promote support throughout the institution. Although the role of the library committee should always be advisory, the librarian should solicit committee approval of any proposal to be presented to the administration. This technique of raising the expectations of library supporters can have a subtle but positive effect on cooperative progress.

Even with enthusiastic support from users and the library committee, administrators' awareness and approval of all cooperative programs is vital. The approach to administration must be thoroughly professional. The librarian should begin by telling administrators about the role of health information networks. Needs for cooperation should be documented, and the costs of the program and alternatives, including no cooperation, must be projected. The librarian should also define the roles and responsibilities of the hospital within the group structure. Letters of support from as many groups as relevant should be solicited. A literature search may locate pertinent articles documenting the success of similar projects and data should be professionally presented. Finally, approval should be enthusiastically and confidently expected.

A strategy that has been used successfully is soliciting consortium endorsement from administrators as a group. For example, the geographic region for a consortium may coincide with that of an existing body of hospitals or administrators. Then the consortium can request formal approval from that body or even organize under its auspices. Perhaps several institutions have already established shared services and could provide support for a cooperative library program. State or local hospital associations might provide support or endorsement for cooperative efforts.

Finally, librarians should be diligent and patient in seeking and maintaining administrative support. If a proposal is rejected, the librarian should learn the reasons so that the problem can be eliminated or the proposal can be modified and resubmitted. Often cooperation is initiated on a very limited basis, so a librarian may have to accept a small beginning and then persistently seek support for expanded objecties. Visible participation in a successful cooperative program, however narrow, frequently enhances the status of the librarian and generates additional support. Bolef notes that "as services improve, the ability to attract money and qualified staff increases, which in turn further improves services"(11).

Every hospital library situation is unique. If the librarian, however, identifies true needs within the institution, works out cooperative programs to meet those needs, and then finds creative ways to demonstrate to administrators the value of participating in the program, support will in all likelihood be won eventually.

Costs

While lower cost is powerful motivation for sharing resources, cooperative programs cannot be developed and administered without investing staff, time, and money. Librarians should not assume that cooperation cuts costs. It often adds costs, directly in the form of dues and indirectly in the form of staff time. Because the cost of self-sufficiency is higher than the cost of cooperation, cooperative programs that expand resources and increase the quality of services are desirable and justifiable. The concept is one of cost-effectiveness, or providing the best service for the money spent.

When considering costs, it is important to note that traditional types of cooperation, while not involving fees, are not free. Often related expenses are simply not identified as costs. If requests are few, the effect on the lending library is negligible. As the volume increases, however, costs may rise, possibly straining the cooperative spirit of the lending library. The requesting library also sustains the indirect cost of the time needed to process and arrange for requests. Traditional nonreciprocal cooperation may also have the hidden effect of inhibiting the borrowing library's development. As Felter points out:

> . . . librarians in small libraries . . . overlooked opportunities to help each other and thus become more self-sufficient. On the other hand, institutional administrators, especially in hospitals, took free assistance for granted, and tended to value the librarian according to his ability to provide library service at little or no cost(1:2).

Typically, when a group first begins to organize, consortium activities tend to involve low costs and broadly-distributed tasks. While this practice is more equitable than traditional cooperation, it disperses costs to the degree that the real expense of an activity is once more not recognized. Because consortia exist for the mutual benefit of the participants, each member library should pay for itself either in currency or services. For example, a consortium may find that for some libraries the interlibrary loan traffic is all in one direction: a particular

library may either lend more than it borrows or borrow more than it lends. The consortium should decide what levels are tolerable and work out ways of equalizing demands beyond those levels. Some consortia have resolved this problem by designating one library as the holder of record for each title and requiring borrowers to call that library first. Other solutions are imposing quotas or fees after traffic reaches a specified level, trading services, or providing searches or other services in exchange for loans. The group benefits by developing a logical cost-sharing system that reimburses any library giving considerably more than it receives. This is important because any significant imbalance jeopardizes the cooperative effort. As suggested by Kent, resource sharing can be beneficial if it is understood that the motivation is not to salvage one library at the expense of another(12).

Cost analysis can contribute significantly to the planning, implementation, and evaluation of cooperative programs. Isolating the hidden costs of traditional cooperation (or lack of cooperation) could prove that maintaining the status quo is expensive and perhaps not the most effective method. Chapter 13 discusses ways of reflecting costs of cooperative activity in budget reports. Demonstrating that resources and service capabilities increase as costs are stabilized will promote support and maintain interest among cooperative members.

Leadership and Structure

Enthusiastic, strong leadership is a key element to successful cooperation. The early leadership role is that of initiator. Attributes required of an initiator have been described by Topper:

> The individual must have energy, determination, and the ability to generate enthusiasm and a spirit of cooperation where previously there may have been indifference and competitiveness. It is a task requiring a broad spectrum of skills and the time to exercise them(13).

Strong communication skills are especially important for the individual charged with guiding the members toward group goals. As the cooperative structure develops, committees are established and tasks assigned, and the role of initiator usually evolves to that of coordinator.

Getchell has identified two types of leadership required for successful cooperation. First, administrative leadership is needed to direct activities such as planning, budgeting, and evaluating cooperative projects. A second type, operational leadership, is the leadership and expertise of members needed to execute consortium activities (14). In planning cooperative programs, the requirement for both types of leadership should be addressed. Leadership, or at least advice, may also be sought from groups representing each institution.

A mechanism for providing leadership must be in-

Figure 19-1
Consortium Organizational Chart: Full-time Staff

```
                        ┌─────────────────────┐
                        │ Board of Directors  │
                        └─────────────────────┘
                                   │
                        ┌─────────────────────┐
                        │ Full-time Coordinator│
                        └─────────────────────┘
                                   │
        ┌──────────────────────────┴──────────────────────────┐
 Working Committees                                  ┌──────────────────┐
                                                     │ Library          │
                                                     │ Consortium       │
                                                     │ Staff            │
                                                     └──────────────────┘
```

Cooperative Cataloging	Online Services	Special Collection Development		Library Consortium Staff			
Continuing Education	Policies and Procedures		Union List	Evaluation Specialist	MEDLINE Search Analyst	Secretary	Cataloger

Note: An independent full-time coordinator directs all activities and supervises a central consortium staff, providing service to all members. Librarians participate in working committees that are responsible for each cooperative activity.

cluded in the organization's structure, usually through adopted bylaws. A variety of structures are possible. Leadership may be centralized, as illustrated in Figure 19-1. Under this arrangement leadership responsibilities are concentrated in the role of full-time coordinator. Another type of structure is based on a committee and a chairperson (Figure 19-2). Under this structure, responsibility for consortium activities is distributed among members.

Sometimes a unique aspect of the consortium determines its organizational structure. For example, the composition of the membership may suggest the most effective structure. Organizational structure may be influenced by the goals and objectives of the group. The availability of funds may determine whether an independent coordinator is appointed.

Whatever the organizational structure, librarians must remember that cooperation is a dynamic process. As members come and go and group activities shift or ex-

pand, reorganizing the consortium structure may be required. Generally, a structure that distributes responsibilities broadly will prove most durable. Because it does not depend solely on one individual, the structure will absorb leadership shifts with less disruption to the group. When major responsibilities are placed under a single leader, the danger of "burnout" is very real. Members can guard the leader against this threat by accepting delegated responsibilities and by enthusiastically contributing their time and skills to cooperative activities. A clearly defined set of responsibilities must be provided so that each participant's place within the structure is clearly visible. Because the organizational structure delegates authority and responsibility, selecting a structure that will be responsive to a consortium's needs is vital.

Standardization

Standards are the foundation upon which cooperative activities are built. Establishing standards will be one of

Figure 19-2
Consortium Organization Chart: No Full-time Director

```
                    ┌─────────────┐
                    │ Chairperson,│
                    │  Executive  │
                    │  Committee  │
                    └──────┬──────┘
                           │
                    ┌──────┴──────┐
                    │  Executive  │
                    │  Committee  │
                    └──────┬──────┘
                           │
                  Working Committees
                           │
   ┌───────────┬───────────┼───────────┬───────────┐
┌──┴───┐   ┌───┴───┐   ┌───┴───┐   ┌───┴───┐   ┌───┴────┐
│Coop. │   │Inter- │   │Online │   │Policies│  │Continu-│
│Cata- │   │library│   │Ser-   │   │and    │   │ing     │
│loging│   │Loans  │   │vices  │   │Proce- │   │Educa-  │
│      │   │and    │   │       │   │dures  │   │tion    │
│      │   │Union  │   │       │   │       │   │        │
│      │   │Lists  │   │       │   │       │   │        │
└──────┘   └───────┘   └───────┘   └───────┘   └────────┘
```

Note: This decentralized library consortium (without full-time director) uses a committee structure. An executive committee composed of the chairperson of each working committee is responsible for the administrative activities such as planning, budget, and evaluation. If a coordinator is not elected, the chairperson of the executive committee serves as coordinator. Working committees direct the cooperative activities of the group.

the objectives of any resource-sharing network. Indeed, the concept of creating a network implies the acceptance of standardization. Without standardization, policies and procedures of individual libraries may produce incompatibilities that hamper communication. Standards of cataloging, collection, and methods of operation help facilitate cooperation.

Reaching agreement on standard policies and procedures frequently is a significant challenge to the group, because unfortunately, long-standing local traditions and practices seem to abound. Standardization that requires substantial compromise is likely to encounter resistance and may threaten the group's stability. Dougherty noted that libraries that have consistently adhered to one policy over the years may reject innovative proposals because the value of change is not worth either the cost or the headaches. Dougherty's first law of cooperation is, "The more a cooperative affects a library's local policies and procedures, the less the likelihood that the cooperative will be viewed with enthusiasm"(15:1769). Many consortia therefore find it best to start with activities such as interlibrary loan that typically require little compromise. Cooperative activities that demand considerable standardization and extensive alteration of local practices, such as cooperative cataloging and joint collection development, are usually best undertaken by older groups whose structures are firmly established.

Commitment

Cooperation requires a cohesive group of committed participants. To assure progress, the group must be composed of individuals who realize the opportunities of participation and hold reasonable expectations of the program. Participants must commit themselves with the full awareness that they will be expected to serve the consortium in addition to the parent institution. This dual role may involve some conflicts of interest, some rearrangement of priorities, and a measure of compromise. If the librarian is not convinced of the merit of joining a consortium, commitment will be marginal and can hamper the progress of the project. If lack of commitment stems from the reluctance of the institution, a group effort may be necessary to define roles and secure institutional commitment.

Cooperation implies that all decisions will be achieved democratically. If the program is to succeed, the decisions establishing it and guiding its operation must reflect the consensus of the membership. Active participation in the decision-making process strengthens the commitment to make the activity a success. Effective communication is critical to any network because participation in decision making requires the communication of ideas. Transforming the abstract notion of cooperation into active channels of communication is a constant and complex task. Although leadership is the key element in initiating communication links, every participant must assume a share of responsibility for the process.

Brong warns, "Cooperation is a fragile way to accomplish tasks, a cooperative chain being only as strong as its weakest link" (16:273). Ultimately the success of any cooperative effort depends on the performance of the participants. Cooperative goals cannot be attained without shared efforts. Each consortium member brings a unique set of professional skills and personal characteristics to the group. Sensitivity is needed to assure that each member's strengths are identified and can be used for the group's benefit. Basic differences between individuals are invitable and must be accommodated in a supportive environment. Functioning in an inter-institutional group requires flexibility and tolerance.

Rewards

Reports of cooperative experience stress the complexity of cooperation and the rigorous demands on time and energy required for even basic interlibrary activities. In a checklist of recommendations and advice to other librarians entering consortium arrangements, one consortium gives as both its first and final statement, "Realize that belonging to a consortium will take a lot of time and energy"(17). The democratic process may not always be the most efficient method of accomplishing tasks, yet the overall effectiveness of group decision making is well proven.

However demanding collective action may be, working with colleagues as a cooperative team is usually professionally rewarding and brings satisfaction and strength that may justify cooperative systems. Particularly for the librarian who previously operated in relative isolation, participation presents a stimulating challenge. The pooling of experience and expertise that occurs not only increases the competence of members but also subtly raises the expectations of individual librarians, contributing to professional growth and maintaining a positive influence on performance. The increased job confidence fostered by sharing of ideas and problems within a supportive group has always been a strong testimony to the benefits of joining a consortium. In addition, as a result of the visibility of successful cooperation, librarians almost invariably report that their professional status and the status of the library within the hospital is raised.

THE FUTURE OF LIBRARY COOPERATION

With rapid developments in technology and the ongoing standardization of bibliographic format, the linking of the nation's libraries in a comprehensive national network appears possible. OCLC, Inc., Research Library Group's Research Library Information Network (RLIN), and the Washington Library Network (WLN) represent key components in the developing framework for nationwide cooperation and are investigating the feasibility of linking databases. Several other organizations are attempting to coordinate the fragmented network explosion. L. C.'s Network Development Office, the Network Advisory Committee, and the Council on Library Resources Bibliographic Services Development Program are addressing the complex political, economic, and technical issues involved in the linkage and coordination of existing databases and their products.

To say that advances in technology will continue to alter library operations dramatically is now a cliche. In the pivotal study sponsored by the Association of American Medical Colleges, *Academic Information in the Academic Health Sciences Center: Roles for the Library in Information Management*, Matheson details the evolution of the health sciences library from a collection of books and resources to an electronics-dominated academic information management services center(18). An increase in cooperative activity seems assured as faster and cheaper communication facilitates resource-sharing among libraries. Cooperation will be extended at and across all levels—local, regional, national, and international.

The trend toward multitype cooperatives will undoubtedly increase as computer applications force the standardization of procedures. Libraries will place greater reliance on network communication rather than on paper communication, and networks will be expected to provide a broad range of services and products to members. Online searching and online interlibrary loan systems can accelerate interlibrary lending and dramatically alter exchange patterns enabling even small libraries to carry their share of the interlibrary loan workload.

To take full advantage of emerging bibliographic capabilities, libraries must internally develop a capacity for change and growth. The librarian must view each library as a component of an undefined whole, as part of a "process" that contributes to both local and national information objectives.

REFERENCES

1. Felter JW. Library cooperation: wave of the future or ripple? Bull Med Libr Assoc 1975 Jan;63:1-6.

2. National Library of Medicine Regional Medical Library Program policy statement. Bull Med Libr Assoc 1972 Apr;60:271-273.

3. Patrick RJ. Guidelines for library cooperation:development of academic library consortia. Santa Monica, CA: System Development Corporation, 1972.

4. Morris RT, ed. Union Lists of serials: guidelines. Chicago: Locator/Union List Committee, Midwest Health Science Library Network, 1981.

5. Bell CL. A SERLINE-based union list of serials for basic health sciences libraries: a detailed protocol. Bull Med Libr Assoc 1982 Oct;70:380-388.

6. Graham DL. Simultaneous remote search: a technique of providing MEDLARS services to remote locations. Bull Med Libr Assoc 1980 Oct;68:370-371.

7. Jones CL. A cooperative serial acquisition program: thoughts on a response to mounting fiscal pressures. Bull Med Libr Assoc 1974 Apr;62:120-123.

8. Special Libraries Association. Networking Committee. Getting into networking: guidelines for special libraries. New York: Special Libraries Association, 1977.

9. Fink WR, Getchell ME, Hughes CW, Moulton BL, eds. Dynamics of hospital library consortia. Waltham, MA: West Suburban Hospital Research and Education Association, Inc., 1975.

10. Medical Library Association. Continuing Education Committee. The development and operation of health science library consortia. Chicago: Medical Library Association, 1977. (MLA courses for continuing education; CE 37).

11. Bolef D, Fisher JS. A health sciences libraries consortium in a rural setting. Bull Med Libr Assoc 1978 Apr;66:185-189.

12. Kent A, ed. Resource sharing in libraries: why, how, when, next action steps. New York: Marcel Dekker, 1974. (Books in library and information science: vol. 8).

13. Topper J. Grants for hospital library consortia. In: Supplemental material; Hospital librarians conference, January 30-31, 1978. Bethesda, MD: National Library of Medicine, 1978.

14. Getchell ME, Moulton BL. Principles of cooperation. In: Fink WR et al, eds. Dynamics of hospital library consortia. Waltham, MA: West Suburban Hospital Research and Education Association, Inc. 1975:12-29.

15. Dougherty RM. The paradoxes of library cooperation. Libr J 1972 May 15;97:1767-1770.

16. Brong GR. The state of Washington's search for intrastate cooperation. Libr Trends 1975 Oct;24:257-275.

17. Fink WR, Getchell ME. West Suburban Hospital Association. Consortium for Information Resources. Continuation Report, January 1, 1975-April 30, 1976. Waltham, MA: West Suburban Hospital Research and Education Association, 1976.

18. Matheson NW, Cooper JA. Academic information in the academic health sciences center: roles for the library in information management. J Med Educ 1982 Oct;57:pt2:1-93.

READINGS

Bailey AS, Tibbetts P. The Twin Cities Biomedical Consortium. Bull Med Libr Assoc 1975 Jul;63:252-258.

Bury B. The Coastal Bend Consortium: an overview. Bull Med Libr Assoc 1978 Jul;66:350-352.

Byrd GD, Smith MK, McDonald N. MINET in K. C.: a report on the Kansas City Libraries Metropolitan Online Bibliographic Network. Libr J 1979 Nov 15;104:2405-2407.

De Gennaro R. Resource sharing in a network environment. Libr J 1980 Feb 1;105:353-355.

DeGennaro R. Resource sharing in a network environment. Libr J 1980 Feb 1;105:353-5.

Drake MA, Olsen HA. The economics of library innovation. Libr Trends 1979 Summer;28:89-105.

Fink WR, Bloomquist H, Allen RG. The place of the hospital library consortium in the national Biomedical Communications Network. Bull Med Libr Assoc 1974 Jul;62:258-265.

Gartenfeld E. The Community Health Information Network: a model for hospital and public library cooperation. Libr J 1978 Oct 1;103: 1911-1914.

Giuliano VE. A manifesto for librarians. Libr J 1979 Sep 15;104: 1837-1842.

Huston MM. Fee or free: the effect of charging on information demand. Libr J 1979 Sept 15;104:1811-1814.

Martin SK. Library networks, 1981-82. White Plains, NY: Knowledge Industry Publications, Inc., 1981.

Millard SK, Andriate GS. MEDCORE: commitment to cooperation. Bull Med Libr Assoc 1978 Jan;66:57-58.

Moulton B, Fink WR. Components for consideration by emerging consortia. Bull Med Libr Assoc 1975 Jan;63:23-28.

Rochell C. Library development and legislation: a call for unity. Libr J 1979 Sep 15;104:1856-1862.

Sekerak RJ. Cooperation strengthens small hospital libraries in a rural area of New England: a five year experience. Bull Med Libr Assoc 1979 Jul;67:322-329.

Swartz RG. The need for cooperation among libraries in the United States. Libr Trends 1979 Oct;24:215-227.

Professional Development

E. Jean Antes
Medical Librarian
Robert Packer Hospital
Sayre, Pennsylvania

and

Jane Lambremont
*Medical Librarian
Earl K. Long Medical Library
Baton Rouge, Louisiana

*Currently:
Reference Librarian/AHEC Liaison
Health Sciences Library
University of North Carolina
  at Chapel Hill
Chapel Hill, North Carolina

CHAPTER 20
Professional Development

E. Jean Antes
Medical Librarian
Robert Packer Hospital
Sayre, Pennsylvania
and
Jane Lambremont
Medical Librarian
Earl K. Long Medical Library
Baton Rouge, Louisiana

Today conditions are changing and information is increasing so rapidly that no matter how much formal education we have, we must continue to add to that knowledge merely to keep current. Changing conditions and the "information explosion" are nowhere more challenging than in the fields of science, technology, and medicine. In order to provide information effectively in these areas, librarians, like the health care professionals they serve, must stay abreast of change.

The field of librarianship is itself changing. Technology is introducing new methods of handling information. The medical librarian needs to be aware of new ideas in the management of circulation, reference requests, budgets, and personnel, regardless of the size of the library or the hospital. Only through a continual process of self-development can the hospital librarian maintain professional competence and meet the challenge of change. This chapter discusses some of the opportunities for self-development that are available to the medical librarian, including informal and formal programs of education, certification requirements, and the resources of professional associations.

CONTINUING EDUCATION

Continuing education, or ongoing education designed to update the professional's knowledge and skills, has been a part of the health care scene for many years. The medical and nursing professions early on identified the need for continuing education. Hospital librarians also must recognize that, as part of the health care team, they too must continue to learn in order to be competent in their work.

Informal Continuing Education

Hospital librarians have many informal ways to expand their knowledge and awareness. Scanning the contents of major library and health science journals increases an awareness of current trends and issues. When a new concept is encountered, whether in the areas of medicine, management or librarianship, further reading can be undertaken.

In addition to having an overview of trends and issues in the health professions and an in-depth knowledge of developments in librarianship, the librarian also must have a thorough understanding of the organization, operation, and current issues in hospitals. Moving from the library out into the hospital proper; becoming acquainted with physicians and nurses; visiting the laboratory, pharmacy, and other departments of the hospital; and having coffee or lunch with hospital personnel are all important. They help the librarian find out what is going on in the health care professions. The librarian needs to know what kinds of programs are in operation in the hospital and what kinds of information hospital staff members require in order to carry out their work.

Conferences and annual meetings of professional associations are also valuable opportunities for continuing education, both through formal, planned activities and through exchanges of information and ideas with colleagues. Such occasions for informal continuing education not only increase the librarian's ability to provide effective services but also prevent stagnation, or becoming bogged down by the daily routines of the library.

Formal Continuing Education

Formal continuing education involves programs designed to assist persons with professional training to keep abreast of new developments in their fields. Such programs can be used, under certain conditions, to meet recertification requirements. These programs are usually provided under the auspices of an institution of higher learning or a professional organization. Frequently the sponsoring institution or association awards credit on completion of the course; this credit is usually expressed in terms of continuing education units (CEUs). This way of measuring continuing education activity was formulated by the Council on the Continuing Education Unit in an effort to establish uniform recognition of nondegree education. The council, made up of more than 260 individual organizations concerned with education and training, defines one CEU as "ten contact hours of participation in an organized continuing education experience, under responsible sponsorship, capable direction, and qualified instruction"(1). The Council encourages the use of this unit by groups sponsoring educational programs but does not itself provide certification for CEUs for specific programs. The Council has, however, published guidelines concerning the awarding of CEUs, and member institutions agree to comply with these guidelines(1).

Continuing education courses are usually described by sponsors in terms of content, sponsoring agency, contact hours, and credit (usually CEUs) awarded. When CEUs are required in fulfillment of recertification requirements, it is the certifying body's prerogative to define the conditions under which CEUs will be accepted.

The Medical Library Association (MLA) has since 1964 operated a program of formal continuing education (CE) courses. These now include more than 30 offerings, which range from the literature of various health sciences to courses in various aspects of library management. Thus many courses needed by hospital librarians can be obtained through MLA itself. The courses are presented to annual and regional meetings of the MLA, or to any group that wishes to organize a course and that can guarantee 12 or more participants. One-day courses consist of 8 contact hours and provide 0.8 CEUs; two-day courses provide 1.6 CEUs. Descriptions of courses offered for the following year are published in the *MLA News*, usually in the September issue, and announcements appear regularly in the *MLA News*. A list of MLA courses offered in any one year can be obtained by writing to MLA headquarters.

Syllabi used in the CE courses offered by the MLA are available for purchase from the association, but because a syllabus is only one part of an integrated educational package, CEUs are currently not awarded for independent study. The MLA is exploring alternate forms of continuing education for credit, and some may be available in the future.

Fees for MLA courses are set by the board of directors. Rates, which are higher for nonmembers than for members, are listed in the *MLA News*.

Other associations such as the Special Libraries Association (SLA) also offer formal educational programs in specific subject areas. The SLA's offerings focus on management, technology, and communications. Information about current course offerings can be obtained from SLA's headquarters.

Self-study or independent study programs are ideal for the hospital librarian who may find it difficult to attend courses outside a local area. In independent study the opportunity for exchange of ideas with other participants and the instructor is of course lost, but such courses can provide stimulating educational opportunities. Self-study courses may be found on television or through colleges and universities. Some self-study audiovisual courses have been developed commercially for or by professional associations.

Workshops, which are short courses usually given without credit, are another widely available source of continuing education. The Regional Medical Libraries (RMLs) throughout the country sponsor workshops on such topics as cataloging, document delivery (interlibrary loan services), and audiovisual services. To find out about workshop activities in a particular region, librarians should contact their RML. Local, state, and regional library associations and networks also often present workshops. Finally, many hospital library consortia are defining continuing education as a priority and are offering workshops on topics of local need.

In pursuing opportunities for continuing education, hospital librarians should not overlook the possibility of sponsoring, through a local cooperative group or association, a particular course they feel is needed. Expertise to develop courses or workshops may be found within the group, or outside instructors may be located—from other libraries, from nearby library schools or other educational institutions, or from library associations such as the MLA. Such instructors are usually paid an honorarium plus travel expenses, so a fee for participation in the workshop will usually be required. As mentioned earlier, the MLA will work with local groups in presenting CE courses and will provide the instructors, materials, and certificates. Local groups need to guarantee a registration of 12 people. For further information, librarians can

write to the Education Department, Medical Library Association.

The Continuing Library Education Network and Exchange (CLENE, Inc.) is a national organization that has as its chief mission the advancement of continuing education for all information, library, and media personnel. One function of CLENE of particular interest to hospital librarians is the provision of a mechanism for recognizing educational attainment and for building a system that encourages better quality continuing education activities.

CLENE's program includes five components:
They are:

- Criteria for quality continuing education
- A system for the approval of providers of continuing education who effectively apply the criteria
- A national mechanism for keeping records of an individual's participation in continuing education activities
- A statement of acknowledgment of participation in continuing education at a specified level expressed in number of contact hours
- Support services for the individual participant and for the providers of continuing education

Further information can be obtained from CLENE.

Participation in Continuing Education

A primary problem for many librarians in pursuing continuing education is getting away from the library for any period of time. This can be particularly difficult if the library is staffed by only one person. Nevertheless, librarians should attempt to work out temporary arrangements that will allow them to leave while ensuring that users have access to the library. Involving the administration in the arrangements to provide temporary coverage in the librarian's absence can increase the administration's awareness of the importance of education to the librarian and of the importance of library service to the librarian of the importance of library service to the hospital. Using volunteers or part-time, temporary staff or locking the library and providing access with a key are all arrangements that allow the librarian to be away for a continuing education program. If the library has more than one staff member, the librarian should carefully train the staff so that service can continue unhampered when the librarian is away. Often local hospital librarians can agree in advance to provide backup service for one another via the telephone.

Even though the hospital administration may recognize in general the need for continuing education for hospital personnel, the librarian may need to show how a specific course will benefit both the library and the hospital. In such a case, the librarian may wish to relate courses to current projects, problems, or plans in such areas as budgeting, space planning, or patient education services. Many librarians write a brief report after they have completed a course, either summarizing relevant information or applying it to the local situation. Standards for library services issued by the Joint Commission on Accreditation of Hospitals (JCAH) offer a further argument for supporting a librarian's participation in continuing education (2).

A librarian who expects to participate in some continuing education activity may wish to put together an annual continuing education budget, even if presentation of such a budget is not normally required. Identifying educational needs, locating appropriate courses, and determining related expenses demonstrate the librarian's willingness to plan systematically for educational opportunities. The librarian may wish to make some inquiries about the continuing education practices and policies followed in other departments of the hospital. Some hospitals will grant time off with pay but will not pay registration fees or travel expenses. By demonstrating the relevance of desired courses to hospital responsibilities, the librarian may eventually receive both time off and paid expenses. When continuing education is funded, it is up to the librarian to show how the hospital benefits from the expenditure.

CERTIFICATION

Certification is necessary for many positions in the health sciences and is available for medical librarians through the MLA. The requirements for MLA certification are:

1. Graduation from an American Library Association (ALA) accredited library program
2. A passing grade on the certification examination administered by the MLA
3. Two years of postgraduate experience as a health sciences librarian at the professional level or the equivalent, within ten years of having received a library degree

The MLA certification examination, following recent trends in professional certification, tests for competency in on-the-job performance rather than for recall of details and historical knowledge. The competencies tested for were defined by practicing medical library professionals. They appear in the booklet *Certification Examination for Health Sciences Librarians* available from the MLA(3). Librarians who do not have two years' postgraduate experience may obtain provisional certification.

Recertification is required of all certified medical librarians every five years. This can be accomplished in either of two ways:

- Participating in at least 35 contact hours of continuing education activity (either 3.5 CEUs or the approved equivalent of 35 contact hours), or
- Passing the current certification examination

According to the MLA's definitions, continuing education activities include approved courses and approved individual accomplishments. Lists of approved activities appear in *MLA Requirements for Recertification of Health Sciences Librarians*, available from the MLA(4).

PARTICIPATION IN PROFESSIONAL ASSOCIATIONS

A professional organization is made up of individuals who have in common their dedication to and respect for the contributions to society made by their profession. Such organizations support the development of the profession and of individual professionals in a variety of ways:

- By providing educational programs
- By working via committees on problems of concern to the profession
- By speaking in a unified voice for the profession
- By striving to improve its status
- By promulgating standards and guidelines concerning professional practice
- By participating in the definition of educational requirements
- By providing certification
- By encouraging research

Professional associations also offer opportunities for contacts with colleagues in other parts of the country.

Hospital librarians have a special need to participate in professional library associations because they frequently work in settings isolated from other librarians and the library community. The meetings, conferences, and other activities provided by professional library organizations offer hospital librarians a vital opportunity to exchange ideas with other librarians in similar institutional settings. Participation in professional meetings also provides opportunities to learn about the broader issues of the profession and the newest techniques for improved library service.

The hospital librarian can benefit also from publications sponsored by professional organizations. Through these publications the librarian can share in the research and experience of other librarians who work in different settings but who have similar interests. Through meetings and publications, professional organizations provide forums by means of which hospital librarians can contribute to the body of knowledge of their profession and exchange ideas with other librarians. Many improvements in hospital service have emerged through the formal and informal presentation of new projects and through new interpretations of methods of service discussed under the aegis of professional meetings, conferences, and publications.

To attend professional meetings, as to participate in continuing education programs, the librarian must first solve the problem of getting away from the library. Many of the suggestions discussed earlier for securing administrative approval to attend continuing education sessions apply as well to attending professional meetings. Generally a hospital will encourage the staff to participate in professional organizations. The recognition gained by the hospital as a result of staff participation is a favorable argument that can be used. The librarian may find the library committee a useful ally in such matters. Whenever submitting a request to attend a professional meeting, the librarian should always present a plan detailing how library service will be provided during the librarian's absence.

The hospital librarian will find many potentially beneficial organizations on local, state, regional, and national levels. The remainder of this chapter details the activities, publications, and membership benefits of the professional associations most often joined by hospital librarians.

Medical Library Association (MLA)

The most prominent organization made up of medical librarians and the primary national forum for progress and activities in the field of professional health sciences librarianship is the MLA. Founded in 1898 by four physicians and four medical librarians from the United States and Canada, the MLA now has over 5,000 members.

Since 1961 the headquarters of the MLA has been located in Chicago, Illinois.* Information concerning membership, publications, scholarships, placement, and committee services can be obtained from its executive director. The headquarters' staff also includes a director of education, a publications manager, a meetings manager, a business manager and support staff members. The headquarters' staff handles the operational aspects of the MLA's diverse programs and assists the elected officers and committees with their responsibilities. Headquarters also serves as a focal point in the dissemination of information about issues of interest to librarians working in health sciences libraries. The association urges its members to contact the MLA staff members with questions or concerns about the association. Full information about the association can be found in the introductory pages of the *Directory of the Medical Library Association*.

Organizational Structure

The organizational structure of the MLA includes elected and appointed officials, headquarters' staff, association committees, regional chapters (formerly called regional groups) and sections (formerly called special interest groups). The board of directors of the MLA is the planning and policy-making body of the association. It consists of the president, the immediate past president, the president-elect, and six board members, all elected by the membership. The chairmen of the chapter and section councils serve as ex officio, voting board members, while the executive director of the association is an ex officio, non-voting member of the board. Appointed officials of the association include the trustee, editors of the *Bulletin of the Medical Library Association* and the *MLA News*, and the archivists. The names and institutional affiliations of the current officials appear in the latest edition of the MLA *Directory*. Applications for committee appointment appear annually in the *MLA News*. Criteria for appointment include a written statement of a member's willingness to serve; the individual's professional contributions and experience; and the individual's record of service to the association. Appointments are recommended by the Committee on Committees and made by the president.

MLA committees provide opportunities for active participation by members; some committees that may be of particular interest to hospital librarians include:

- Continuing Education Committee
- Health Sciences Library Technicians Committee
- Hospital Library Standards and Practices Committee
- Audiovisual Standards and Practices Committee

The MLA *Directory* publishes information concerning the charges of all MLA committees, their membership, and their activities and publications. The January issue of the *Bulletin* contains reports of committee activities and the proceedings of the previous annual meeting.

The MLA recently undertook an intensive examination of its organizational structure and implemented some changes referred to as the new MLA group structure. The new structure created sections to take the place of the former special interest groups. Each section has its own bylaws, officers, and committees. The section elects a representative to the Section Council, which meets once a year at the annual meeting. The chairman of the Section Council serves as an ex officio voting member of the board of directors.

The Hospital Library Section, formerly called the Hospital Library Interest Group, grew out of a discussion held at the 1974 annual meeting. It has now become an integral part of the association and promotes the special interests of hospital librarians. Members of the Hospital Library Section must be members of MLA; as one benefit of membership, they receive the *Hospital Library Section Newsletter*, which publishes news and articles of interest to hospital librarians. Many of the other sections, such as those concerned with nursing libraries or audiovisuals, are also of interest to hospital librarians; a current list may be found in the most recent MLA *Directory*.

The MLA has also sponsored the growth and development of regional chapters, which meet annually, usually in the fall or spring. The regional chapters provide information programs and continuing education opportunities

---

* The addresses for the MLA and other organizations mentioned in this chapter appear in the Appendix.

for their members. Under the new group structure, the regional chapters elect a representative to a chapter council. The chairman of the chapter council is also an ex officio voting member of the MLA board. The regional chapter structure provides for association activities to be organized in a relatively small geographical area, thus allowing greater participation and with less of an outlay of travel time and money. The *MLA News* regularly reports regional chapter activities, and the MLA *Directory* lists chapter officers.

Publications

Publications of the MLA include the *Bulletin of the Medical Library Association*, which began in 1911 and continues to be the journal most widely read by medical librarians. The *Bulletin* publishes articles concerning health science librarianship in a variety of settings, including academic, hospital, industrial, and specialized subject libraries. The proceedings of MLA's annual meeting and the annual reports of committees are printed in the *Bulletin*. Other features include letters to the editor, notes on journal articles of interest to MLA members, book reviews, and notices of new books of interest. The *Bulletin* subscription is included in MLA dues; the publication can be ordered separately.

The MLA also publishes a monthly newsletter, the *MLA News*; a subscription to the *News* is also included in the MLA annual dues. The *MLA News* contains items of current interest to health science librarians, information about the activities of the association and its committees, and regular features such as "Capital Notes," "International Notes," and "Media Notes." The newsletter also regularly lists continuing education courses and employment opportunities.

In addition to the *Bulletin* and the *MLA News*, MLA also publishes a number of other serials and monographs. A current listing can be obtained from the association.

Health Sciences Communication Association (HESCA)

The Health Sciences Communication Association (HESCA) is an organization concerned with the coordination of educational programs in the health sciences, especially the promotion of communication technology for continuing education. HESCA considers all forms of media in studying resources for these educational programs. Of special interest to hospital librarians is the association's biomedical libraries section. Publications include the *Journal of Biocommunication and Feedback*.

Special Libraries Association (SLA)

The Special Libraries Association is an international organization composed of 11,000 professional librarians and other information scientists. Its objective is to provide an association of individuals and organizations having a professional, scientific, or technical interest in library or information service. The SLA provides continuing education courses, consultation services, and employment information. Publications include a quarterly journal called *Special Libraries* and a monthly newsletter, *The Specialist*, as well as bibliographies and monographs. Its organization encompasses 53 regional groups and 29 special interest divisions.

American Library Association (ALA)

The 30,000 members of the American Library Association represent the entire range of library interests. One of ALA's many divisions is the Association of Specialized and Cooperative Library Agencies, which deals with health care library services to professionals working in institutions and to handicapped and institutional library patrons. Hospital librarians who offer patient education or consumer health information as part of their library service will find this division of ALA especially valuable.

American Society for Information Sciences (ASIS)

The American Society for Information Sciences (ASIS) seeks to improve the information transfer process through research, development, application, and education. The ASIS has 22 special interest groups, including one for special librarians and other information scientists.

American Hospital Association (AHA)

The American Hospital Association (AHA) was founded in 1898 and currently has over 31,000 members. The stated purpose of the organization is to promote the public welfare through the development of better hospital care for all people. Since its establishment, the AHA has been concerned with libraries in hospitals and their contributions to optimal patient care through the provision of information to health professionals. This encouragement of hospital libraries is reflected in the publication *Health Science Libraries in Hospitals*(5). The AHA also publishes a bimonthly periodical entitled *Hospitals* and the annual *AHA Guide to the Health Care Field*. Information concerning library-related activities of the AHA may be obtained from the director of the library of the American Hospital Association.

Regional, State, and Local Library Associations

Many hospital librarians also value participation in regional, state, and local library associations. Hospital and other health science libraries often form consortia to share resources and cooperate in other ways. In many communities, librarians from different types of institutions organize as local groups. Belonging to these organizations increases the hospital librarian's knowledge of and access to local library resources.

Another way hospital librarians can participate in cooperative activity is through the programs of the RML. This network is described more fully in Chapter 19. Further information about it and other National Library of Medicine (NML) programs is available from the Extramural Programs Office of the Division of the Biomedical Information Support, National Library of Medicine.

Professional Health Organizations

Regional, state, and local organizations of other health care professionals may be other valuable sources of information to hospital librarians. As with the professional organizations of librarians, the educational interests of the health care personnel served by hospital libraries are reflected in the programs and activities of their professional organizations. Local health educators, nurses, in-service training groups, and coordinators of continuing education for all allied health workers can offer materials and suggestions for collection development of the library. The local or regional Health Systems Agency (HSA) often can supply data on health personnel, certification procedures, and supply and distribution of personnel. These and other organizations often reflect new directions taken in the field of patient care, and the hospital librarian will usually benefit from such associations.

David Bishop, in an address to the MLA on June 15, 1976, characterized the hospital librarian as "an unsung hero or heroine, manning these (library) outposts, meeting those needs that can be met from limited resources, sending for reinforcements when necessary—and, as a group, forestalling an invasion by information-hungry hordes before whom the larger centers would quickly crumble." The solitude of the hospital librarian can be greatly reduced through participation in professional organizations that supply reinforcements, both professional and personal.

REFERENCES

1. Council on the Continuing Education Unit. Criteria and guidelines. Silver Spring, MD: Council on the Continuing Education Unit, 1979.

2. Joint Commission on Accreditation of Hospitals. Accreditation manual for hospitals. 1983 ed. Chicago: Joint Commission on Accreditation of Hospitals, 1982:147-149.

3. Medical Library Association. MLA certification examination for health sciences librarians. Chicago: Medical Library Association, 1981.

4. Medical Library Association. MLA requirements for recertification for health sciences librarians. Chicago: Medical Library Association, 1979.

5. American Hospital Association. Health science libraries in hospitals. Chicago: American Hospital Association, 1975.

READINGS

Colaianni LA. Librarians in the hospital: you and the MLA. Bull Med Libr Assoc 1977 Jan;65:67-68.

How to be appointed to an MLA committee. MLA News 1979 Aug; 116.

Lentz RT. Professional associations. In Annan GL and Felter JW, eds. Handbook of medical library practice, 3d ed. Chicago: Medical Library Association, 1970: 368-380.

Love E. The evolutionary process of organizational development. Bull Med Libr Assoc 1978 Oct;68:468-470.

Perl ML. Professionals: their problems, their fears, and their social responsibilities. Bull Med Libr Assoc 1973;61:15-20.

Procedure for MLA Group Structure. MLA News 1979 Aug;116.

Yast H. The program of the American Hospital Association. Bull Med Libr Assoc 1969 Apr;57:177-182.

APPENDIX
Organizations and Associations of
Interest to Hospital Librarians

American Hospital Association (AHA)
840 N. Lake Shore Drive
Chicago, Illinois 60611

American Library Association (ALA)
50 E. Huron Street
Chicago, Illinois 60611

American Society for Information Science (ASIS)
1155 16th Street, N.W.
Washington, D.C. 20036

CLENE, Inc.
620 Michigan Avenue, N.E.
Washington, D.C. 20064

Health Sciences Communication Association (HESCA)
P.O. Box 79
Millbrae, California 94030

Medical Library Association (MLA)
919 North Michigan
Chicago, Illinois 60611

National Library of Medicine (NLM)
Extramural Program Office
Division of Biomedical Information Support
Bethesda, Maryland 20209

Special Libraries Association (SLA)
235 Park Avenue
New York, New York 10003

SECTION IV:

Providing Special Services

Library and Health Information Services for Patients

Rebecca R. Martin
Chief, Library Service
Veterans Administration
Medical Center
San Francisco, California

*Currently:
Head, Biology Library
University of California
Berkeley, California

CHAPTER 21

Library and Health Information Services for Patients

Rebecca R. Martin
Chief, Library Service
Veterans Administration
Medical Center
San Francisco, California

Hospital librarians serve patients in a fundamental way by providing support for their medical care. By furnishing information services to health care providers, librarians have an indirect effect of the quality of patient care. Some librarians also contribute directly to patients' welfare by providing them with library services.

Patients have a basic need for library services that goes beyond the information needs they experience as healthy members of their communities. They need information on how to interact with the health care system, on their specific conditions and how to deal with them, and on community resources they might use after leaving the hospital. They also need recreational materials to relieve the fatigue of hospitalization, to provide a therapeutic means of dealing with their conditions, and to assist them in the rehabilitation process. In long-term care institutions, patients often need vocational guidance and training in daily living skills to assure a successful return to community life. The American Library Association (ALA) standards for library services in health care institutions summarize these needs well when they state, "The Patients' Library...provides and makes accessible adequate library materials and services to patients of all ages which will assist in their rehabilitation or adjustment to their illness and/or handicapping conditions" (1:12).

These standards imply the necessity for an established patients' library as a basis for service to patients. Full-scale patients' library programs, with staffing and budgetary support, do exist in many hospitals. The absence of such a program, however, should not preclude the provision of library services to patients. Effective programs for meeting the information needs of patients are present in many hospitals that have only limited resources designated for this purpose. Outreach services to patients' rooms and waiting areas utilizing small collections of recreational materials can provide reading material for patients, especially those in acute care facilities. Health information services at several levels of development are often based in the medical library with great success. Patients' services can become a valid component of the hospital library program in a variety of settings, given the basic recognition of the patient as a legitimate recipient of library services. This chapter discusses both recreational and health information library services to patients. Health information services for the community are considered in Chapter 22.

HEALTH INFORMATION FOR PATIENTS

The growth of the consumer movement in health information over the last decade has had a significant impact on the interaction of health care providers with their patients. Individuals receiving medical care are becoming active participants in this process and are asking for information about their treatment. The response of the health professional to these demands is now addressed by both public law and professional code(2). Perhaps the most compelling statement for hospitals comes from *A Patients' Bill of Rights*, published by the American Hospital Association (AHA) in 1975. This document states, "The patient has the right to obtain from his physician complete current information concerning his diagnosis, treatment, and prognosis in terms the patient can reasonably be expected to understand"(3). Furthermore, the Joint Commission on Accreditation of Hospitals (JCAH) now requires patient education in a number of clinical areas as well as documentation that such teaching is taking place(4).

The Joint Committee on Health Education of the AHA has defined the health information process in this way:

"Health education is an integral part of high-quality patient care.... The major emphasis...is health promotion, which includes health maintenance, disease and trauma management, and the improvement of the health care system and its utilization"(5). For patients receiving information in the hospital setting, a distinction should be made between health information and health or patient education. Health information refers to communication with the patient regarding basic procedures for dealing with the health care system, general facts about diseases or conditions, and information on different forms of therapy. This interaction is very often initiated by the patient. Patient education is a more structured program of teaching that is related to an individual patient. It includes assessment of patient needs, development of motivation, attempt at behavior change, and evaluation. Patient education is usually provided by a physician, nurse, or other health care provider in a one-to-one situation or a formal group class.

Roles for the Library: An Overview

The library can offer much in the field of health education and information for patients, both to the professional conducting patient education and to the patient seeking information. The library's role as already defined in the hospital environment can be a starting point in these efforts(6). Support services similar to those routinely provided to staff educators might include the provision of information from the health care literature to patient education planners; the assessment of existing health information resources in the hospital and community; the procurement of teaching materials; and the storage, classification, and organization of these materials. A less familiar but equally important area for library involvement is the provision of health information directly to the patient. Here the librarian's reference skills and expertise in matching available materials with individual information needs can be an important resource.

Libraries can provide various levels of support for health information and patient education programs in the hospital. The library's space and funding and especially its staffing will have a direct impact on the support it can provide. Many of the services discussed in this chapter could be incorporated into an existing hospital library program, but the effect on the library when the services are fully utilized and the possible need for additional resources should be carefully considered in the planning stages.

Another factor influencing library involvement is the degree of development of patient education in the hospital(7). Many institutions have active patient education programs, but others have been reluctant to support organized efforts in this area. While the library can in some ways become a focal point for patient health information and education services, the hospital staff and administration must participate in the development of the program and support it with appropriate resources.

Finally, the staff's acceptance of the librarian as a team member in patient education activities is crucial to the success of the library's involvement. The library's role in the patient education process raises many questions for both the librarian and the health practitioner. This is particularly true when considering the provision of information directly to the patient relating to the patient's own health care. Many of these ambiguities are resolved once the librarian becomes involved in actual patient education activities and the library's role is clearly defined.

Services to Staff

As with any new library service, one of the most difficult steps is the first: to make users aware of the resources that the library can offer. If the hospital does not have an organized patient education program, then a good starting point is a study or survey to identify existing patient teaching programs and the key personnel participating in them. In-depth interviews with these people probably will have a number of positive outcomes. First, this process will demonstrate to those involved in patient teaching both the interest of the library and the potential support the library can provide them. Second, considering the fragmented state of many hospitals' patient education programs, the survey might bring together health professionals teaching in similar areas who might benefit from cooperative efforts. Perhaps most important, the survey will enable the librarian to assess whether library involvement in patient education would be accepted. In conducting such a survey, it is important not to overlook any segment of the health care team. The librarian should remember to consult not only physicians and nurses, but also dieticians, social workers, pharmacists, physical and occupational therapists, and psychologists, all of whom may be teaching patients in some way.

The librarian should try to become involved in the planning stages of formal patient education programs from the outset. As a resource person, the librarian should be an active member of the patient education committee as well as an advisor to informal groups who

may be planning programs on specific topics. When used effectively, the material already available in the hospital library can yield much valuable information for planning patient education programs.

Literature Searches

Providing traditional literature searches to support patient education planning is a preliminary way of establishing the librarian as a member of the patient education team. This service is actually no different from that already provided by the hospital library to other clinical programs. Published information on patient education has expanded rapidly over the past several years as formal programs have been developed and described in the literature. A comprehensive search of this literature can yield practical information on model programs, guidelines and protocols for program development, teaching techniques, and assessment and evaluation tools. Especially in hospitals with limited staff resources devoted to health education, building on the experience of others can save a great deal of time and energy.

Materials on Patient Teaching

Continuing education for patient educators is another area in which libraries can be involved. In-service training for staff members who are identified as potential patient teachers is usually an integral part of a growing health education program. Patient teaching is a new field for many health practitioners, and the level of formal preparation in this field varies widely within each discipline and from one discipline to another. Patient education is now being included in the curricula of many health care training programs, but this has not always been the case. Studies indicate that often the health professional does not feel sufficiently informed about teaching techniques to provide patient education(8).

The growing body of educational material for staff members on patient teaching is a resource that should not be overlooked. Current awareness services should also be provided to educators to keep them abreast of new trends and developments in such areas as program innovations, record-keeping requirements, evaluation techniques, and quality assurance. All of these services can be easily incorporated into the existing hospital library program, enabling even a small library to be involved in patient education.

Identification of Existing Resources

Patient education has been an integral, although not necessarily formalized, part of hospital services for years (9). In all probability, informal teaching programs have gathered their own resources, such as pamphlets, charts, filmstrips, and other teaching materials. When developing an organized patient education program, a survey should be made to assess the availability of existing resources in the hospital. If possible, these materials should be assembled in one location to form the basis of a centralized collection of patient education materials. Centralization of these materials in the library, media center, or other information center provides many benefits to the health care provider and the patient education program as a whole. It provides a focus for patient education activity within the hospital, bringing together at one point both the diversity of teaching activities and the resources that support them. The need for duplication of expensive materials is frequently eliminated, and a single access point to all patient education information in the hospital for both staff and patients will ensure wider utilization of available materials. Once this collection is developed, it will provide the librarian with a base of health information materials with which to respond to patients' questions.

Resources within the community should also be investigated. Using contacts developed in hospital networks, the librarian can often identify programs in other hospitals that might serve as models and possibilities for resource sharing. Some public libraries have, or are developing, programs and collections in health information, and this avenue should be explored.

The librarian must approach with caution the use of professional information in the medical library as a resource for patients. In most hospitals, the medical library is the most well-developed source of health information in the hospital and may be looked upon by some as a resource for patients as well as staff. Sometimes the librarian can locate appropriate information for the lay person in the medical library collection. Generally, however, this material is widely scattered and once located, is not always suitable for patients. A librarian who is willing to conduct such a search must spend a great deal of time gathering the materials and then condensing and simplifying the information before effective communication with the patient can begin(10).

Though the medical library collection can occasionally be used to answer patient questions, it is a limited source at best and one that will not support a full-scale health information and education program. This is not to say that a patient information service cannot be effectively based in the medical library. With a collection of health materials designed for the lay person, the medical library can be a good location for these programs. The differences in the health education materials and the rest of the collection, and in the primary users of each, must, however, be recognized.

Selection of Health Information Resources

Financial support for patient education programs is likely to be as limited as other education funding in the hospital setting, and will probably not cover the costs of all desired materials. While patient education has been developing into an integral part of many health care delivery programs, publishers and producers have quickly identified this field as a new market for their products. The amount of material in this area has mushroomed in recent years. The quality and cost of these materials varies widely, and thus choosing appropriate teaching aids and other informational sources for patients can be a difficult task. The role of the librarian in selecting patient education materials is an important one, for the librarian can contribute both formal training and extensive experience in the many facets of the selection process.

The first step in building a collection of resource materials in patient education that will be useful both to the patient seeking information and to the practitioner providing information is to define the specific needs of both groups. In the initial stages of collection development, this process can begin with one or two areas where active teaching is already taking place. Good candidates are common chronic conditions that require training for continued self-care, such as diabetes, hypertension, and heart disease. Those selecting the materials should review any existing plans for specific health teaching programs to identify topics requiring resource support and the type of support desired. The planners should decide how resource materials will be used—to instruct, to illustrate, reinforce, or elaborate. They should consider the educational setting, because a different program might be selected for group versus individual use. They should identify the preferred format of the materials—print or nonprint, pamphlet, model, book, or audiovisual program. The selectors should consider the characteristics of the intended audience and pay particular attention to the educational level, age, perception or language problems, and anticipated level of patient motivation. They should also consider subjects not included in teaching programs but likely to be the basis of patients' questions, again taking into account the factors listed above.

Health information resource materials come in a wide variety of formats, including pamphlets, books, models, charts, slides, audiocassettes, and videocassettes. The specific attributes of these different types of media are addressed in Chapter 10. The way the material will be used and the subject presented should determine the format selected. A collection that is made up of a combination of these formats rather than a concentration on one type of media is inherently more flexible and will better accommodate the varying needs of individual patients and teachers who use the materials(11).

The sources of patient education materials are as diverse as their types and purposes. Roughly speaking, they can be divided into five main groups: (1) commercial publishers and producers, (2) voluntary health organizations, (3) pharmaceutical companies, (4) professional health organizations, and (5) individual health care delivery programs. These materials are elusive and difficult to identify because bibliographic control in this field is virtually nonexistent. A good starting point is getting on as many mailing lists as possible to accumulate a good collection of catalogs. A method for indexing these catalogs for easy access is described in Chapter 10. A number of source lists have been developed by individuals and organizations involved in health education. In addition, various agencies have developed clearinghouses for information on specific health problems, such as the Cancer Information Clearinghouse. A listing of clearinghouses can be found in Chapter 8.

The selection process for patient education materials contains many elements that are familiar to the librarian and some that may be new. With a good knowledge of the hospital's programs, the librarian can select books in all but the most controversial areas, based on reviews. Journals that regularly publish reviews of health information materials include:

- *American Journal of Nursing*
- *Health Care Education*
- *Health Values*
- *Journal of Nutrition Education*
- *Library Journal*
- *Medical Self-Care*
- *Rehabilitation Literature*

Once the books arrive, the librarian may wish to have staff members review those on topics such as nutrition or weight control that might be subject to fads. Such reviews should be the exception, however, for as the librarian develops a familiarity with the program philosophies of the health care team, the librarian will wish to make most book selections based on his or her own judgment. Although the librarian should retain selection responsibility, the librarian should encourage participation by the staff involved in patient education.

Transient materials such as pamphlets and booklets can provide an important resource for health information. In selecting these, the librarian should consider carefully the costs involved. What may at first seem to be a low-cost or free resource can turn out to be a considerable investment, because this type of material is usually given to the patient and therefore must be continually restocked. Pamphlets used in patient teaching programs should be selected with the assistance of the educator; those in general information areas generally can be chosen by the librarian.

Audiovisuals pose a different set of problems, and their careful evaluation for content and quality is imperative (12). As the investment can be quite large, the librarian needs to exercise prudence in their purchase. Moreover, philosophies and modes of treatment vary in many fields, so that it is essential that local practices be reflected in programs selected. If practitioners do not agree with the information presented in a piece, they will not use it, nor will they wish their patients to have access to it.

Many producers of audiovisual programs make the programs available for preview to the prospective buyer, either free of charge or for a rental fee. Previewing, even when a charge is involved, should be part of the selection process for every audiovisual purchase. The librarian and media staff should review the programs for technical quality, and the subject specialists who will be ultimately responsible for teaching patients in the particular area should review them for content. Potential reviewers could include but should not be limited to physicians, nurses, dieticians, instructional designers, and others involved in teaching the patient. Some librarians like to have patients preview programs under consideration in order to obtain a user-oriented response to the material (13). The use of subject specialists for previewing is preferable to having a preview committee with fixed membership. Using the individuals directly involved in a teaching program as reviewers results in the selection of the most relevant materials for that area and helps to stimulate patient referrals and the use of the resource materials once the program is underway.

The desire for hospital-produced materials tailored to specific programs is likely to be encountered repeatedly in the development of resource support for patient teaching programs. The librarian should critically evaluate any proposal for such a venture in terms of time, cost, and facilities required for a production of quality. A complete search of materials available from other sources should be made before giving serious consideration to producing the materials locally. Many times such a review will turn up suitable commercially produced items at a much lower overall cost to the institution. Whenever the decision is made to develop an item locally—whether it be an instruction sheet, a pamphlet, or an audiovisual program—the librarian should be a member of the multidisciplinary committee planning the production. The librarian, having a familiarity with a range of patient education materials in many areas of health care, can offer advice on the most effective format, level of presentation, and informational approach to use.

Organization of Patient Information Materials

The storage and organization of educational materials falls within the purview of the traditional function of the librarian, and patient education resource materials should be no exception. Centralization of these materials under the control of the library will enhance both their use and their availability to the hospital at large.

In organizing a health information collection, the librarian should consider who the primary users of the materials will be. The answer to this question will influence the choice of classification scheme and cataloging procedures. If patients are to gain access to the collection through the librarian or other health professional, a more sophisticated system may be appropriate than if patients are to use the catalog and the materials directly.

Alternatives for classification are limited to the Dewey, Library of Congress (LC), and National Library of Medicine (NLM) schemes. Although the first is probably most familiar to the public, it does not offer enough detail for most collections of health materials. LC and NLM classifications provide for a more complete organization of the subject, and in small collections are manageable for both patients and staff. Selection of subject headings poses much the same problem of specificity versus familiarity to the patient. The conventional lay tool, *Sears' Subject Headings*, will not provide the comprehensive coverage of the LC system or the NLM *Medical Subject Headings* (*MeSH*). An alternative designed for this field is the *HEIRS Thesaurus* (Health Education Information Retrieval System) that was developed by the Public Health Service and is now located at Johns Hopkins University, School of Hygiene and Public Health. This thesaurus uses over 900 health education topics to categorize the information(13).

Documentation of Use

The librarian, acting as an intermediary between patients and health information materials, can furnish evaluators of patient teaching programs information on the use of educational materials. For some special studies, the librarian can gather initial reactions from patients using specific items. The JCAH now requires patient education in a number of clinical areas, so documentation that such teaching is taking place has become necessary(4). In a number of programs, such documentation is initiated by the librarian for inclusion in the medical record. Methods vary from placing a library-issued consultation report in the chart to actual recording in the nursing notes information on material provided to the patient(14,6). The librarian can also assist with informal documentation, using lists and sign-up sheets that can be forwarded to the appropriate educator.

Services to Patients

The librarian can also support patient education efforts by providing information directly to patients. Such activity may range from distributing pamphlets and other materials prescribed by a health care provider to dealing directly with the patient to determine the best method to meet the patient's information needs. Physician resistance to active participation of the librarian in the patient education process may be encountered. However, if the role of the librarian is well defined as one of resource provider rather than teacher, such resistance can be mitigated. The importance of a formal policy delineating the librarian's role cannot be overemphasized and will be discussed in detail later in this chapter.

Patients as Library Users

Patients bring to the library a set of needs that make them very different users from medical or hospital staff members. The stress of hospitalization can have an important effect on a patient's approach to the librarian, especially in the area of health information. Age should also be considered when dealing with patients, for the librarian is often faced with providing service to the very young or the very old. Handicaps such as blindness, hearing disorders, and emotional problems also have an impact upon the communication process. In addition, the educational background of patients varies widely, demanding a broad range of materials and services. These aspects of the interaction between patient and librarian call for a special set of skills on the part of the librarian and can make provision of information services to patients a difficult but rewarding challenge.

At some point in a librarian's involvement in patient education, the librarian in all probability will be approached by a patient seeking health information. It is important for a number of reasons that the response to such an inquiry be positive and that the patient not be turned away. Most patients come to the hospital because they have been made aware of symptoms that indicate physical or mental problems. Many factors can cause anxiety, fear, and doubt in a patient who is entering the hospital. For some patients, the loss of self-identity has been characterized as one of the most difficult aspects of hospitalization(15). Often the library will provide a more comfortable or familiar setting for the patient within the larger hospital environment. The librarian may be one of the few staff members the patient will see who does not wear a uniform. In addition, many patients may feel that the library is the most accessible source for health information, since the health care providers may often seem too busy to be approached with questions. The positive response that patients may have to the library may encourage them to seek out health information, and thus can become an important factor in the patient education process.

Because the majority of patients encountered in this setting will be adults, it is important to recognize the differences between teaching adults and teaching children. Adults are nearly always voluntary participants in learning experiences, and they do not continue to learn in situations that do not satisfy them. Although the adult who is a hospitalized patient may be a captive audience in a learning environment, the teaching will have little effect if the patient does not wish to participate. The implications for the librarian concern motivation and the importance of responding to the inquiring patient when the patient is receptive. As Bille points out, if the patient "recognizes a need to learn, and asks a librarian to help him meet that need, he must be helped at that time—the teachable moment; otherwise, the need will dissipate and not come back"(16:7). Or in Elsesser's words, "it is important to recognize the patients' curiosity and self-directed inquiry as positive and necessary components in the health education process"(13:24).

Librarian's Role

To meet patients' needs for health information competently, the resources of the library must be well developed in several areas. As previously indicated, a collection of health information materials designed for the lay person and coordinated with the hospital's programs is of primary importance. Next in importance is recognition of the librarian as a working member of the health care team, with the clearly defined role of providing information to patients. The librarian is not a substitute for the health professional and should not diagnose conditions or interpret information(17).

Perhaps the most important resource the librarian has to offer the patient is the professional ability to match the information needs of the patient with the appropriate available materials. The training that librarians receive in reference skills—to first define what information the user actually needs and then identify resources at hand that will meet that need—is unique in the hospital setting. In health information, the problem of specifically identifying the exact question is complicated by the unfamiliarity of medical terminology to most patients. Furthermore, the anxiety and tension that often surround key topics related to an individual's health can make posing direct questions difficult. Reference work with patients will continue to be one of the most challenging areas in the provision of patient health information services, but many feel it is also the most rewarding.

Family members should also be considered appropriate recipients of health information, and in many cases it is they who will best use the resources of the library. Information on dietary modification, exercises, and aids for the handicapped are especially useful when family members will be providing specialized home care. Referrals to associations, groups, or publications that provide support for the relatives may also be helpful.

It should again be emphasized that in all of these activities the librarian acts as a member of the health care team. Communication with the health care provider following contact with a patient is an important element in this process. The patient who has further questions regarding a particular medical situation should always be referred back to the health care professional. The resources and services of the patient education library cannot stand alone in the patient teaching process.

Policy for Patients' Services

Before a hospital librarian embarks on the development of patients' library services, such services must be recognized as an activity or responsibility of the hospital library, and the role of the hospital librarian in providing health information to patients must be reflected in formal hospital policy. The review, approval, and support of such policy by the administration and by the medical departments, nursing staff, and education committees involved is essential for the success of the program. Formal acknowledgment of these services as the patients' rights and the hospital library's responsibility will be the key to both policy and program.

A policy for health information programs should include at least the following four elements:

• The purpose or goal of providing health information materials to patients
• Definition of the patient population eligible to use

health information materials, whether all patients or only those with referrals or prescriptions from health professionals
• A statement of the responsibility for selection of materials, whether it rests with the librarian, the health professional, or a combination of the two
• Descriptions of the services that will be provided to patients

An example of such a policy, which also covers recreational reading services, may be found at the end of this chapter. This policy has been adapted from one in use for a patients' library that is separate from the health sciences library for professional staff. However, similar elements would be required in a patient-use policy for a library that combined professional and patient services.

RECREATIONAL AND OTHER LIBRARY SERVICES

Patients also have needs for library services that may not be specifically related to information on their health problems. For many years, libraries have been providing traditional services to patients for the purpose of diversion and rehabilitation. These programs, which largely emphasize recreational reading, range in scope from book cart services to fully developed and staffed libraries with extensive collections, large reading areas, and group activities. Such programs are based on the premise that reading promotes recovery by helping the patient adjust psychologically to illness and by relieving the fatigue of hospitalization.

Patients' library programs vary widely among institutions, and responsibility for services to patients may or may not reside with the librarian. Recreational programs in particular are often organized by hospital auxiliaries or volunteer groups. In institutions with recreation departments, the patients' library may fall under this jurisdiction. Many hospitals, however, do not have patients' library services of any kind, and they would welcome program development by the librarian in this area.

Services

The services that a hospital library offers patients will depend on the type of institution the library serves, as well as the budget and staff time available for such services. In acute care facilities, book cart service with magazines and paperbacks may suffice. In a long-term care setting, educational and rehabilitative materials as well as programming may be required. These materials may be housed in a patients' library or in browsing collections in patient-care areas. Therapeutically oriented library programs can be important in psychiatric hospitals.

The Library

An active patients' library is similar in many ways to a

small branch of a public library. A collection of fiction and nonfiction books comprises the basis for the library and is augmented by a selection of current popular magazines and newspapers. A reading area and perhaps facilities for listening to music and other recordings can also be provided. Ambulatory patients and their families will be the primary users of the library, although services are sometimes also extended to staff members. The patients' library should be located in an area convenient to the patient floors and should be attractively decorated to create a warm, inviting atmosphere. In addition to providing assistance to library users in locating and selecting materials, the librarian may be involved in such activities as storytelling, showing movies, and organizing reading discussion groups.

Book Carts

Any patients' library program must provide service to patients unable to leave their rooms or floors. Such service is usually provided through rounds with a book cart stocked with library materials. Individualized service is provided at the bedside. In the absence of a patients' library, this type of program may serve all patients, both bedridden and ambulatory. The librarian should select the materials for the cart with ease of use in mind. Paperback books and current magazines are especially popular. The librarian should see that materials on the cart are changed regularly and displayed attractively. A consistent schedule of visits should be maintained and coordinated with the unit staff to ensure that most patients will be present and unoccupied when the librarian arrives. Cooperation between the librarian and hospital staff members is always important in providing library services to patients and is essential in intensive care units, isolation rooms, psychiatric units and detention areas.

Browsing Area

Another way of providing patients with recreational library service is to maintain deposit collections, or browsing shelves, in patient-care areas throughout the hospital. Although deposit collections may meet patients' needs somewhat less effectively than libraries or book carts, they require less library staff time. The deposit collections may be located in patients' lounges, in waiting areas, and on units to which the librarian may not have access. The loss rate in this type of collection can be quite high, and the librarian can never be certain that the patients are the recipients of the materials. However, this method of providing recreational reading material to patients should be considered if the situation warrants it.

Bibliotherapy

Another area of interest for the patients' librarian, which has been a recognized library activity for many years, is bibliotherapy. The official ALA definition of bibliotherapy, taken from *Webster's Third New Interna-*

tional Dictionary, describes it as "the use of selected reading materials as therapeutic adjuvants in medicine and in psychiatry; also: guidance in the solution of personal problems through directed reading"(18:242). Monroe, in her book *Reading Guidance and Bibliotherapy in Public, Hospital, and Institutional Libraries*, views bibliotherapy as part of a continuum of library services, closely related in function to reference and reading guidance(19). While reference services are objective, reading guidance is subjective. Librarians see bibliotherapy as a long-term approach to library services for therapeutic purposes. In the hospital setting, bibliotherapy is usually conducted under the direction of a physician, psychologist, or social worker. It is used primarily when psychopathology is present but can also be effective with the physically disabled or ill patient. Detailed discussions on the methods and materials of this complex topic are listed in the suggestions for further reading at the conclusion of this chapter.

Collection Development

Selection criteria and procedures for the patients' library should incorporate the basic tenets of selection as expressed in the ALA's *"Library Bill of Rights."* This topic should be covered in the written policy on library services to patients. The scope, size, and character of the collection will depend on many of the same factors that govern the development of the patients' library program. These factors include the size and type of institution, whether it is a short-term or long-term facility, and the emphasis made in its care and rehabilitation program. Other factors are the characteristics of its patients: their age range, nature of illness or handicap or both, and how many are readers and nonreaders(15).

Most of the materials in the patient's library will be books. These should include both current, popular titles and standards of fiction and nonfiction. The reading interests and age of the patient population should be primary factors in selection. Materials in languages other than English should be included as appropriate. The value of paperback books has been discussed and should be reemphasized here; not only are they convenient for many patients, they stretch limited budgets as well. Rental services that provide a rotating collection of best-sellers should also be considered, if funds permit. A small general reference collection is often appropriate. Collections to support the institution's vocational rehabilitation and bibliotherapy programs should be provided. Books on health information should also be included; selection of these has been discussed in detail earlier in this chapter.

The collection of current subscriptions to popular magazines should be as comprehensive as funding allows. Guides to selection of magazines for small public libraries are useful in identifying possible titles for consideration. Multiple copies of several standard titles should be provided for book cart service. Local daily newspapers should also be available. Normally, long back runs will not be required, since interest will be primarily in current materials. Donations of out-of-date magazines will be frequently offered, but because they are usually of little interest to patients, they should be avoided if possible.

Audiovisual materials are sometimes included in the patients' library collections. These usually include audio-cassettes or records of music and other entertainment, and talking books. Films for recreational programs may also be present. Audiovisual materials used to support patient teaching programs should be placed in the library, as indicated earlier.

Special Services for the Handicapped

Some of the patients who will use the patients' library will be handicapped, and provisions should be made for them when designing space, selecting materials, and developing programs. Accessibility to both the library and its materials is the right of all patients, and it is especially important that handicaps are not barriers to receiving library services in the hospital. A wealth of information and materials for the handicapped is available from the Division for the Blind and Physically Handicapped of the Library of Congress. Individual patients may be eligible to receive talking books and specially designed equipment directly. Anyone unable to read or use standard printed materials as a result of visual or physical limitations may receive special services free of charge, usually through the local public library(15). Hospital libraries serving such patients also qualify for receipt of talking books and accompanying equipment. These should be considered for use not only with the blind but also with patients who have difficulty holding books and other printed material. Large-print books and magazines form a useful component of the library collection. Reading aides such as book stands, page turners, and optical aids or magnifiers should also be provided. Any library area to be used by patients should be designed with wheelchairs in mind.

Children's Services

The presence of a large pediatric program in the hospital will necessitate the development of special library programming for children. A collection of children's books and magazines should be provided. In addition, story hours, film programs, and other special activities may be beneficial. Cooperative programs with public libraries may be useful in this area.

Volunteers

If well chosen and carefully trained, volunteers can provide a valuable resource for the patients' library. It is essential, however, that both the library staff and the administration understand that volunteers should never substitute for professional or clerical staff. Trained volunteers can be effective at such tasks as staffing the circulation desk, making deliveries of special requests, processing books, and in some cases providing supplemental book cart service. Because of the problems with scheduling, seasonal fluctuation, and dependability inherent in the use of volunteers, great care should be taken to avoid developing basic library services that are completely dependent upon volunteer assistance. In addition, the librarian should be aware of the large investment of time required to operate an effective volunteer program. Training and supervision are essential but time-consuming elements of this process and should be carefully weighed against the benefits received. The use of volunteers in hospital libraries is discussed more thoroughly in Chapter 14.

Resources Outside the Hospital

In some areas, the services of local public libraries can augment library services to patients. The most substantial type of support usually offered is a deposit collection program. Typically, each participating hospital receives a deposit collection of several hundred books, which is changed on a regular basis. The selections most frequently consist of titles and subjects of general and popular interest aimed at the patient who is looking for recreational reading. Contractual agreements between the hospital and the library are important in this type of program. Usually the hospital agrees to provide the space and equipment required for storage and distribution of materials, while the public library agrees to provide books and staff. Other services that may be provided include interlibrary loan of films and books, selection assistance, and special programming. These programs vary considerably from one area to the next and are a resource that should be investigated. State libraries may also provide support to patients' libraries in funding and consultant services.

In providing library services to patients, hospital librarians make a major contribution to the quality of care these patients receive. For some, recreational reading programs improve the experience of hospitalization. For others, health information promotes understanding and acceptance of medical treatment. In even the smallest hospital library, patients' services should be considered as a fertile area for program responsibility and development.

REFERENCES

1. American Library Association. Association of Hospital and Institution Libraries. Hospital Library Standards Committee. Standards for library services in health care institutions. Chicago: American Library Association, 1970.

2. Somers AR. Promoting health; consumer education and national policy. Germantown, MD: Aspen, 1976.

3. American Hospital Association. A patient's bill of rights. Chicago: American Hospital Association, 1975.

4. Joint Commission on Accreditation of Hospitals. Accreditation manual for hospitals. 1983 ed. Chicago: Joint Commission on Accreditation of Hospitals, 1982:147-149.

5. American Hospital Association. Statement on the role and responsibilities of hospitals and other health institutions in personal and community health education. Chicago: American Hospital Association, 1974.

6. Harris CL. Hospital-based patient education programs and the role of the hospital librarian. Bull Med Libr Assoc 1978 Apr;66: 210-217.

7. Eakin D, Jackson SJ, Hannigan GG. Consumer health information: libraries as partners. Bull Med Libr Assoc 1980 Apr;68: 220-229.

8. Wise PS. Barriers (or enhancers) to adult patient education. J Contin Educ Nurs 1979 Nov/Dec;10:11-16.

9. American Hospital Association. Hospital inpatient education survey findings and analyses, 1978. Chicago: American Hospital Association, 1980.

10. Kelly, M. The consumer and health information. M.L.S. thesis, University of California, Berkeley, 1977.

11. Kucha DH. Guidelines for implementing an ambulatory consumer health information system. Fort Sam Houston, TX: Army-Baylor University, 1973.

12. Stein D. Selecting and evaluating media for patient education. J Biocommun 1979 Nov;6:22-26.

13. Elsesser L. Patient education. Chicago: Medical Library Association, 1978. (MLA courses for continuing education: CE 36).

14. Collen FB, Soghikian K. A health education library for patients: Kaiser-Permanente Health Education Research Center. Health Serv Rep 1974 May/June;89:236-243.

15. Phinney E, ed. The librarian and the patient. Chicago: American Library Association, 1977.

16. Bille DA. The librarian as facilitator of patient education. Hosp Libr 1976 Oct 15;1:6-7.

17. Quay C. Role of the librarian in patient education efforts. Paper presented before the Second Annual National Symposium on Patient Education, San Francisco, California, October 21, 1978.

18. Rubin RJ. Uses of bibliotherapy in response to the 1970s. Libr Trends 1979 Fall;28:239-252.

19. Monroe ME. Reading guidance and bibliotherapy in public, hospital and institutional libraries. Madison: University of Wisconsin Library School, 1971.

READINGS

Alock D. Books can help. Can Nurse 1979 Jan;75:52-54.

Cahn H. A library service to patients in hospitals and health institutions. NZ Nurs Forum 1979 Jun/Jul;7:11-12.

Chabon SS, Chabon RS. Annotated bibliography of health care books for children. Am J Dis Child 1979 Feb;133:184-186.

Charney N. Ethical and legal questions in providing health information. Calif Librarian 1978 Jan;39:25-33.

Conaway MC. Patient/family education: reaching out to wellness. Cath Libr World 1977 Mar;48:328-331.

Coomaraswamy SD. Therapeutic aspects of a library service to hospital patients. Health Welf Libr Q 1979 June/Dec;2:29-32.

Dunkel LM. Library to patient: new role for the patients' librarian. Bull Med Libr Assoc 1976 Oct;64:418-419.

Franzblau S, Wesley W, Horton L, Johnson FE, Hight WC. Library resources for patient education. Assoc of Hosp Inst Lib 1971 Winter; 11:11-15.

Green LW. Health information and health education: there's a big difference between them. Bull Amer Soc Info Sci 1978 Apr;4:15-16.

LaMonte SJ. What a patient education center can do for you. Group Pract 1978 Sept/Oct;27:19-21,32.

Lunin LF. Information for health is an issue: opportunities for information scientists in health care information. Bull Amer Soc Info Sci 1978 Apr;4:11-12.

McClaskey HC. Health education. Health Rehab Libr Serv 1975 Mar; 1:3-7, 10-12.

Monroe ME, Rubin RJ. Bibliotherapy: trends in the United States. Health Rehab Libr Serv 1975 Oct;1:15-17.

Pritchett S. Patient, family and community health education: design and management of hospital based programs. Atlanta: Pritchett and Hull Associates, 1977.

Rickards DJ. Providing health care information to patients in a small hospital. Bull Med Libr Assoc 1978 July;66:342-345.

Rienzo BA, Vitello EM. Development of patient education resource materials; a planned strategy. J Am Coll Health Assoc 1979 Feb;27: 224-225.

Romani D. Reading interests and needs of older people. Libr Trends 1973 Jan;21:390-403.

Roth BG. Health information for patients: the hospital library's role. Bull Med Libr Assoc 1978 Jan;66:14-18.

Rubin RJ. Bibliotherapy sourcebook. Phoenix : Oryx Press, 1978.

Rubin RJ. Using bibliotherapy: a guide to theory and practice. Phoenix: Oryx Press, 1978.

Shuler C. Documenting patient teaching. Superv Nurse 1979 June; 10:43-49.

Sorrentino S, Fierberg J, Goodchild EY. CATLINE as an acquisitions tool for health and patient education materials. Bull Med Libr Assoc 1978 Oct;66:458-460.

Swezey AM, Kaufman A. Library cart service provides information for clinic patients. Hospitals 1977 Sept;51:65-67.

Topper JM. Hospitals as centers for consumer health information. Bull Amer Soc Info Sci 1978 Apr;4:13-14.

Vaillancourt PM. The librarian and patient's information. Cath Libr World 1979 Apr;50:393-396.

APPENDIX A
Sources for Patient Education Materials

SELECTED RESOURCE LISTS

Audiovisuals: patient education. Duke P. J Biocommun 1978 Mar;5: 18-23.

> *An annotated list of sources of media for purchase or rental.*

Directory of health education sources. Medical Library Group of Southern California and Arizona, 1978.

> *An alphabetical listing of agencies primarily located in Southern California and Arizona that offer health education materials free of charge or under $25.*

Guide to medical media producers and distributors. Baltimore: Welch Medical Library, Johns Hopkins University, 1977.

> *An alphabetical listing of over 500 names and addresses of media producers and distributors of patient and health science education materials.*

Health: A multimedia source guide. Ash J, Stevenson M. New York: Bowker, 1976.

> *An annotated alphabetical guide to publishers, audiovisual producers and distributors, libraries, government agencies, societies, pharmaceutical companies, and research institutions that deal with health education materials.*

Health education materials and the organizations which offer them. Health Insurance Institute, 1968.

> *A subject listing of insurance companies, health organizations, medical associations, health-related businesses, private publishers, and government agencies that produce free or low-cost publications on health.*

Medical media directory: programs and producers. Biomed Commun 1981 Mar;9:1-56.

> *An extensive annual compilation of audiovisual programs and producers arranged in alphabetical order by medical specialty.*

Patient education: A list of societies, companies, and institutions with audiovisuals for sale, rent, or loan. Yakote G, Homan M. Los Angeles: Biomedical Library, University of California, Los Angeles, 1976.

> *A guide to sources of audiovisuals including types of media offered, costs, and subjects covered.*

Patient education resource list. Sources of patient education videotape programs. Chicago: American Hospital Association, 1976.

> *Two listings of patient education materials suppliers and the types of resources that they provide.*

Source list for patient education materials. Martyn DE, Spencer DA, Duke P. Milledgeville, GA: Health Sciences Communications Association, 1978.

> *An alphabetical directory with subject index of associations, government organizations, commercial sources, and some pharmaceutical companies, for both print and nonprint materials.*

Sources of health information for public libraries. Chicago: Library of the Health Sciences, University of Illinois at the Medical Center, 1976.

> *A selective list of health related agencies and private companies.*

APPENDIX B
Patients' Library: Sample Policy*

I. *Purpose:* To outline procedures and practices of the general library

II. *Explanatory Remarks:* The general library has been established to provide centralized facilities for the location, organization, and distribution of print and audiovisual materials for patients. Use of the general library (including materials, information, and reference help) is the right of every patient. The use of health materials for independent study or within a patient education program is encouraged to enable patients to assist in their treatment, and to allow patients to make informed decisions regarding health habits, type of treatment, and medication use. Recreational reading is encouraged to reduce the fatigue of hospitalization and to speed recovery.

III. *Responsibilities*

A. The general library houses a permanent collection of print and audiovisual materials; rents materials for patient education and other medical center programs; loans materials to patients and staff members; provides them reference service and bibliographic help (including manual searches and computerized bibliographic retrieval). Access to the collections and information in the health sciences library is provided through the general librarian, who uses these resources whenever necessary to answer health-related questions.

   1. These services are available to patients, out-patients, family members (or others who are concerned with the patient's care), staff members, and volunteers. Requests for extensive reference or bibliographic assistance (such as provided by a research assistant), extended loan privileges, or requests for rental or purchase of items are all subject to the needs of other users and the library's resources, as determined by library staff. Services are also available to other libraries and the community, subject to these constraints.

   2. Services to staff members are limited to use of materials and reference or bibliographic work in support of patient education programs. Recreational reference or interlibrary loan services unrelated to work are not provided for staff. Materials are selected, policies are decided, and services are organized to meet the needs of the patient population.

B. The collection includes recreational reading, print and audiovisual materials in health, large print and recorded materials, reading aids, teaching carts that travel to clinics or the bedside with programs, audiovisual equipment, anatomy models, resource catalogs, and material on health education and on hospital-based patient education.

C. All items purchased through the general library budget become part of the permanent collection. Items are housed, cataloged, and made accessible to the entire medical center. No materials are purchased for administrative collections. Selection decisions rest with the general librarian. Suggestions for purchase are welcome and should be forwarded to the librarian.

D. Requests for patient interlibrary loans or for rental or previewing of audiovisual programs for use with patients should come to the general library. Staff interlibrary loans are offered through the health sciences library; requests to rent or preview for staff training are also handled by the health sciences library.

IV. *Procedures:* (If desired, the policy can specify specific procedures for the use of services.)

*This sample policy has been adapted, with permission, from the general library policy of the Veterans Administration Medical Center, Palo Alto, California.

Community Access to Health Information

Ellen Gartenfeld
Network Coordinator
Community Health Information
    Network
Mount Auburn Hospital
Cambridge, Massachusetts

CHAPTER 22

Community Access to Health Information

Ellen Gartenfeld
Network Coordinator
Community Health Information Network
Mount Auburn Hospital
Cambridge, Massachusetts

HEALTH EDUCATION FOR PATIENTS AND CONSUMERS
    The Development of Consumer Health Education
    Professional and Governmental Support of Health Education

THE HOSPITAL'S ROLE IN COMMUNITY HEALTH EDUCATION

THE LIBRARY'S ROLE IN COMMUNITY HEALTH EDUCATION
    Gathering Support for the Library's Role
    Resistance from Health Care Providers
    The Role of Hospital Personnel in Community Health Information Programs
    The Librarian's Contact With Patients and Consumers
    The Librarian's Reluctance to Serve Consumers
    Policy Statements
    Selection, Organization, and Dissemination of Health Information
    Information Services
    Publicity
    Program Costs and Sources of Funding
    Interlibrary Cooperation
    Specific Programs

THE HOSPITAL LIBRARIAN'S CONTRIBUTION TO IMPROVED HEALTH STATUS

Since 1970 the public's perceptions of health and disease have changed steadily. One result of this change is an increased interest in health care delivery, disease prevention, and health maintenance. Since hospitals form such a large part of this sytem, it was inevitable that this new attitude would affect hospitals and the services they provide. It was also inevitable that this change would affect the hospital library. Demands for new services by traditional users have intensified. New users with different needs and expectations have appeared. The previous chapter considered the needs for library services to patients. This chapter will discuss the sources of pressure on hospital libraries to serve the community and some ways in which these services can best be provided.

HEALTH EDUCATION FOR PATIENTS AND CONSUMERS

To understand why hospital libraries are under increased pressure from the community for health information, librarians must be aware of the changes in attitudes and services that are taking place within health care institutions. One of the most important new services is hospital-based educational programming aimed at consumers rather than providers of health care. In contrast to informal education of patients, which has long been a part of hospital care, these formal programs include diagnosis of individual patients, written educational plans, and evaluation of the program based upon the patient's progress(1). The practice of educating patients has contributed to the growth of a new professional group: the hospital-based health educator. It has also led to increased participation by other health professionals, specifically nurses, in these educational programs. Another related development in hospital-based education is the hospital's growing involvement in health promotion programs for the community.

The Development of Consumer Health Education

The emergence of a consumer health education movement emphasizing personal responsibility for health maintenance is the result of a number of recent social and historical developments. Most important of these developments is the growing realization that sophisticated technology and numerous medical personnel have not brought about a significant improvement in the health of the population(2). Infectious diseases, which previously claimed the most lives, have been replaced by chronic conditions such as heart disease, stroke, and cancer. These conditions, together with motor vehicle accidents, are now the major causes of death in the United States and Canada. As Somers says, "The common denomina-

tor in most of this preventable morbidity and premature mortality is individual behavior or lifestyle"(3:52). No longer can poor health and premature death be blamed solely on the health care delivery system. Rather, emphasis is being placed on the relationship between the causes of illness and death and such factors as obesity, stress, lack of exercise, smoking, and alcoholism.

Economic factors have also played an important role in the development of consumer health education. If the health of the population is not improving, obviously the enormous sums of money being spent on medical care are not bringing about the expected results. A role that has been challenged, says Foster, is "the traditional paternalistic and authoritarian relationship between the professional and the client" that does not encourage "public accountability, participation, or control"(4:74). Many customers become increasingly impatient with the overemphasis on technology and the neglect of patients as responsible agents in the treatment of disease and the maintenance of health(5). Anger about the increasing cost of care, disillusionment with providers, and recognition of the system's limitations has had a variety of results. Certainly, however, the rising number of malpractice claims and the demands for informed consent and patients' rights are part of this. Also included are the growth of self-care, the success of community health programs, and the continuing interest in exercise, diet, stress management, and cessation of smoking.

Professional and Governmental Support of Health Education

The consumer movement is probably the most important factor in the public's demand for new hospital services. A growing body of health care consumers has been crucial in the development of patient and community health education programs. To encourage and assist hospitals in providing these services, the American Hospital Association (AHA) has developed two important policy statements and created the Center for Health Promotion.

The first of the policy statements was the 1973 Patient's Bill of Rights. It specifically states that "the patient has the right to obtain from his physician complete current information concerning his diagnosis, treatment, and prognosis in terms the patient can be reasonably expected to understand"(6). Other sections of this document uphold the patient's right to know information of a preventive as well as a curative nature.

In the second policy, issued in 1975, the AHA dealt directly with consumer health education. The association urged hospitals and other health care institutions to recognize the opportunity to take a leading role in health education. Three specific audiences were outlined: the patient and the family; personnel, including employees, medical staff, volunteers, and trustees; and the community at large(7). In defining key issues for hospitals in the eighties, the AHA's Council on Research and Development noted that hospitals will continue to be faced with increasing demands for consumer involvement. Consequently, this will lead to more active involvement in health education programs.

Government participation in health education has resulted in the passage of legislation and the creation of many bureaus, departments, and agencies. The first important development was the appointment of the President's Committee on Health Education in 1971. In 1973 this group issued a report that led to two significant developments: the establishment of the Bureau of Health Education at the Center for Disease Control in Atlanta, and the creation of the privately financed National Center for Health Education in San Francisco.

In 1974 the National Health Planning and Resources Development Act (Public Law 93-641) was passed, which for the first time included public health education as one of ten national health priorities. Another federal law, the National Consumer Health Information and Health Promotion Act (Public Law 94-317), enacted in 1976, called for the establishment of the Office of Health Information and Health Promotion (OHIHP) in the Department of Health, Education and Welfare. One of the major tasks undertaken by OHIHP is the creation of a national health information clearinghouse whose goal is to identify health information resources and to ensure that knowledge of such resources is widely disseminated. In addition, during the past decade, the government has created more than 20 federal clearinghouses in areas such as cancer information, arthritis, high blood pressure, and smoking. All are responsible to a greater or lesser degree for informing the public about health and disease.

THE HOSPITAL'S ROLE
IN COMMUNITY HEALTH EDUCATION

The existence of a growing body of consumers interested in assuming responsibility for their health, together with governmental and professional support for health promotion, has caused many hospitals to become more aware of their role in community health education. Although participation in community health education may seem unusual for hospitals, it is in fact a logical extension of their educational functions. Many institutions have long provided continuing medical and nursing education, in addition to training programs for housestaff. Once the need for formal programs of patient education became clear, hospital personnel obviously had a crucial role to play in providing these services. Extension of such educational services to the community has understandably progressed more slowly. Until hospitals came to accept

that their function included the promotion of health as well as the treatment of disease, they could see no rationale for involvement in such programs.

In most hospitals this involvement has begun with small-scale programs that aim to inform the community about hospital services. Such programs may include school tours, a community open house, and health career days for young people(8). Some hospitals also provide cardiopulmonary resuscitation courses and screening clinics for a variety of easily diagnosable conditions.

For an increasing number of hospitals, participation in community education has been much more extensive. Lectures, workshops, and seminars are presented both in the hospital and at sites in the community. The purpose of these programs is to present information about many health concerns and to help consumers make changes in their behavior, such as exercising more or controlling stress. In some hospitals the commitment to educate the public about health has resulted in the creation of departments specifically devoted to community health education. Such departments not only present the kinds of programs noted above but also develop needed resource materials and attempt to evaluate the impact of educational programs on the population served by the hospital (9).

THE LIBRARY'S ROLE IN
COMMUNITY HEALTH EDUCATION

Whether the participation of the hospital in community health education is minimal or extensive, it should involve the library at some level. At the very least, providers of these new services require support in selecting and acquiring quality materials. Even with the most limited community health education programs, many hospital librarians are reporting increased pressure from consumers who want to use the hospital's collections.

Gathering Support for the Library's Role

The librarian's role in serving the community should be supported by hospital staff members, administrators, and trustees. In most hospitals, doctors and nurses are already involved in patient or community health education. In seeking support, the librarian should approach this group first. The librarian can also ask the support of health educators, psychologists, nutritionists, pharmacists, and social workers.

The patient education committee or coordinator, if one exists, is another source of support for the librarian in providing information services to the public. Often the curriculum developed to teach patients can be easily adapted for the community. Nurses and health educators involved in patient education are most aware of the public's need for accurate, useful health information.

Clearly, the support of the administration must be enlisted. The development of community services cannot proceed without the approval of hospital management. In some institutions the impetus for community programs may originate from an administrator. More often, however, the librarian must convince administrators of the value of providing such services(10). A number of strategies are successful in gaining this support. The most important way is for the librarian to tell the administrators about other successful programs. Another effective strategy is to stress the role of library services in improving the hospital's community image. Van Gieson says, "As the hospital emerges as the center of health care and community health in general, a library can fill a major public relations role, showing the hospital's constituency again that the hospital and its staff care"(11:67).

Of all the departments in the hospital, public relations will probably be quickest to see the benefits of library services for the community. "The benefits to the hospital of the public relations potential of community health education programs cannot be overlooked. These programs represent the most positive image building activity that a hospital can employ to gain the confidence and respect of the community that it serves"(9:97). The public relations staff always wishes to publicize hospital programs that illustrate the hospital's commitment to the community. Given the regard in which libraries are held and the standard of quality they represent, library-based public information services are perfect for such image building. Time spent in developing close contact with public relations means that the librarian will have access to the publicity needed to inform the hospital staff and the community of new library services.

It should be noted that community access to the hospital library and information services to the public are closely related to the larger field of community health education. If the hospital has such a department, its programs and services will inevitably have an impact on the library. One of the purposes of community outreach is to build up a group of users for the hospital's services. The shift in emphasis from disease to health means that a growing group of healthy nonpatients will look to the hospital for education and information on maintaining health. The need for the hospital librarian to cooperate with community health educators in developing and implementing programs cannot be overstated.

Gathering support from the board of trustees is a slightly different matter than dealing with hospital staff members. The business executives and community leaders who generally sit on such boards are, in fact, consumers of health care, even though they have a special relationship with the hospital. One of the most effective ways of securing their support is to provide trustees with health promotion materials on topics of personal interest. Stress management and exercise are two topics that often concern individuals(9).

Resistance from Health Care Providers

No hospital librarian planning to develop services for the community can afford to ignore or overlook resistance to these programs. Most librarians expect opposition from physicians on the staff and in the community. In many parts of the country, health education has always been the province of the medical profession. Although this situation is changing, many physicians are slow to accept community programs that are not directed by physicians. Mathes warns, "The medical librarian who argues for freedom of medical information may well find herself taking a professional stand against a much more powerful professional group who find an informed public a threat to their authority and autonomy"(12:909). Public access to quality health information, however, has found strong advocates in the medical community(13). While librarians must look for ways to deal with opposition, they should by no means approach physicians with the expectation that they all will be uncooperative. Librarians should also seek support from physicians who recognize the value of such efforts.

Probably the best way for the librarian to handle objections is to present a program for the staff about the new services. The program should stress the involvement of medical personnel in selecting and evaluating materials. Many physicians resist the dissemination of health information because they are unaware of the exact nature of the services and materials provided. Often, the librarian can overcome resistance by simply inviting a physician to examine the types of books and pamphlets that will be available for public use. The librarian can also ask supportive physicians to talk to resisting staff members. Members of the library committee can be especially valuable in gaining support for services to the public. If the committee has been included in planning and developing programs, it will be familiar with the content and parameters of the services.

Librarians may find that opposition stems from the fear of disrupting traditional services. Some hospital staff members fear that new users will crowd the library, remove materials, or occupy too much of the librarian's time. The hospital librarians must plan programs in which this will not happen. Librarians may also want to spend some time allaying the fears of concerned individuals.

The Role of Hospital Personnel in Community Health Information Programs

In addition to enlisting the support of administrators and staff in developing library services for the community, the librarian must understand clearly the part these groups can play in providing such services. Probably the most important way for health care providers to participate in consumer information programs is assisting in the selection and evaluation of materials for the hospital library. This assistance includes informing the librarian about new materials and sources, as well as sharing perceptions of the information needs of the community.

Hospital staff members are best able to evaluate materials for the accuracy of their content. They are also most knowledgeable about the types of materials that will be acceptable to the community. If the hospital library becomes involved with other libraries who provide consumer health information, hospital staff members may be asked for help in building these collections. The librarian can also ask them to speak at programs on health resources sponsored by the hospital library. In-service training programs for hospital and public librarians are other places where members of the hospital's professional staff can make important contributions. Given the enormous amount of questionable and controversial information about topics such as nutrition, stress, physical fitness, and environmental pollution, it is especially important that librarians be well-informed.

The Librarian's Contact with Patients and Consumers

In some hospitals, librarians participate as members of the health care team and have closer contact with patients. Initially, the library's role in patient education was a traditional one of helping develop new programs through the creation of a collection of books and journals to meet professional educational and informational needs of the staff. It soon became apparent that, in addition to professional materials, patient educators needed help in finding materials suitable for their clients. In most situations, this information flows from the library to the patient via a staff member. In some cases, however, the development of larger collections, including audiovisuals, has meant that patients and their families now come to the library(14).

To an even greater degree, clinical librarianship has involved librarians in direct patient care. Being present on the hospital floor as part of the health care team has made librarians more aware of the patients' need to know and has also made them more accessible to patients and their families. Today an increasing number of librarians answer patients' questions. They identify the patients' request, locate appropriate materials, have them reviewed by other members of the health care team, and then supply them to the patient. In some cases the librarians make follow-up visits to patients, refer them to other staff members if the information needs clarifying, and, if necessary, supply them with additional resources(15). It is important to understand how the librarian's participation in patient education and clinical librarianship has legitimized the library's role in providing services to consumers.

The Librarian's Reluctance to Serve Consumers

Some librarians may feel reluctant to serve the general public. The librarian's unwillingness may arise from a variety of assumptions. One is the librarian's belief that the hospital staff, particularly doctors and nurses, will view such services as an interference in their relationship with patients. If hospital staff members take a stand against providing library services to the public, the librarian should meet with them to find out the reasons for their opposition.

Related to this assumption of staff opposition is the unfortunate attitude of elitism. Sometimes both librarians and health care providers have a tendency toward this attitude. They consider themselves custodians of information that is too dangerous or too difficult for consumers to understand. There may be valid, practical reasons why the hospital library cannot be open to the public, but the belief that free access to information is harmful is not one of them. Often, librarians seem to consider information harmful to readers because some readers become upset by learning particular information, usually related to specific disease prognosis. Hospital librarians need to learn how to deal with incidents involving an emotionally upset consumer and should not use such incidents as a justification for denying access to the library's collection.

Some librarians have also expressed considerable concern about the legal liability for providing medical information to consumers. Lawyers agree that as long as librarians clearly give information and not advice, they are in no danger of being sued. Although it is possible that the distinction between these two actions may not be clear, guidelines can assist the librarian in separating one from the other. Any of the following actions almost always indicate that advice, not information, is being provided(16).

- Recommendation of a method or procedure of treatment
- Recommendation of a drug under any circumstances
- Assisting a user who is known to be attempting a sel-diagnosis
- Interpreting medical or health information for the user.

Two additional situations may have some legal implications, although to date no information exists of librarians being taken to court over either. The first involves accusations of fraud or misrepresentation if the user is injured as a result of misunderstanding information. The second and perhaps more likely situation is an accusation of defamation if the librarian gives an opinion of the qualifications of a particular practitioner(17).

For most hospital librarians the practical considerations of collection size, library location, and limited staff and budget are the reasons for reluctance. The most important resource, however, in developing services for consumers is the skill and experience of the librarian. This is available no matter how limited other resources may be. Even if the hospital librarian only establishes contact with the public library, the result will be an improvement in access to information for the public. Consumer health information programs do not have to be large to be effective but they do have to be well-conceived, well-planned and well-executed.

Policy Statements

An essential part of creating new programs is developing a policy that details specific services. Such a policy is especially important when the program is new to a hospital library and there are few models to follow. Policy statements are guidelines that help the librarian answer requests for information. They also limit variations in service(18). Any policy developed by the library should directly reflect the hospital's philosophy, plans, and overall policy related to community service. It should state specifically the services that will be provided by the library and the people eligible to use them. A policy should also allow room for new developments. It should reflect knowledge of locally available resources and the health information needs of the community.

The detail of the policy statement will be determined by the library's needs. In one medical school, the library staff thoroughly reviewed the existing public services statement to determine the services that would be available to consumers(19). It is especially important to distinguish clearly between services provided to patients and services available to the community. If the librarian plans to share service programs with other hospital libraries, public libraries, or school libraries, the details of such agreements should be included in the policy. Although listing specific subjects is probably unnecessary, changes in collection development policies to include health promotion materials should be outlined. A policy on community access is not only the base upon which services are built, it is also the library's statement of its commitment to these services. Of course, administrators, doctors, nurses, the patient education committee, and the library committee will all be involved in the formulation and adoption of the policy statement. The policy, however, should be written by the hospital librarian.

Selection, Organization, and Dissemination of Health Information

Of all the members of the hospital staff, the librarian is the most competent in the selection, evaluation, organization, storage, and dissemination of information. This is true whether the librarian is selecting materials for the provider of health education or for the community. The following discussion will describe a variety of ways to create and administer a health information collection. It will include methods for use by libraries with very limited

resources as well as methods for use by libraries that plan a broader involvement.

Assessment of Need

In setting up a procedure for selecting materials, it is essential that librarians become familiar with the health information needs of the community. Librarians should be aware of the discharge diagnosis of the hospital, major health care trends, and health care topics receiving media coverage. If the hospital has a department of community health education, the department probably already assessed the needs of the community. Useful information about questions the public asks can also be obtained from the reference librarian at the public library. The hospital librarian can also analyze consumer requests that come to the hospital library. Above all, the librarian should contact all health care providers on the staff and in the community who are involved in health promotion programs for the public. The librarian will be able to use this information to select a limited number of topics of most interest to the community. Such decisions should be made early in the planning process, for without them the library will lack the necessary guidelines to prevent being flooded by the quantity of health information materials produced today.

Sources of Selection Information

The lack of bibliographic control or comprehensive selection tools means that the librarian will have to use a number of sources in selecting materials. The best of these is *Medical Self Care*, a quarterly publication that reviews a wide variety of health books, pamphlets, and other resources. In addition, *Library Journal, American Journal of Nursing, Nursing Outlook, Journal of Nutrition Education*, and other professional journals can all be used to find information and reviews of new books for the community. Valuable information on health promotion can be found in pamphlets and brochures published by the government and other organizations. The *Consumer Information Catalog* and *Selected U.S. Government Publications* can be of some assistance. Other sources include clearinghouses such as the National Diabetes Information Clearinghouse, professional organizations such as the American Hospital Association, and national voluntary agencies such as the American Cancer Society. Resources for audiovisuals are scattered, although some useful information is available in the *Boston University Film Catalog* and the *National Audiovisual Catalog*.

Selection of Materials

The quantity of materials, the variation in their quality, and the library's limited budget force the librarian to be highly selective in choosing materials. Purchased materials should be the best available to meet the widest variety of needs. The librarian should develop guidelines for evaluating books, pamphlets, and audiovisuals. Guidelines for print materials should include such factors as accuracy, currency, point of view, audience level, scope, organization, style, and physical format. In addition, guidelines for evaluating audiovisuals must include technical quality and the appropriateness of the format for the type of information being presented.

All audiovisuals being considered for purchase must be previewed by the librarian and appropriate members of the professional staff. When no money is available to pay for previewing, the librarian should ask other organizations involved in community programs and voluntary health agencies if they will lend copies for previews. If the hospital librarian is willing to gather together a group of librarians and other potential purchasers, it is sometimes possible to persuade film distributors to loan films free of charge.

The help of interested staff members in reviewing and evaluating materials should be a well-developed part of the library's selection procedure. Physicians, nurses, psychologists, dietitians, pharmacists, social workers, and other health personnel can all participate in the program. This will not only involve all of these individuals in a new library activity, it will also provide a group of supporters for the new services and mitigate criticism on the part of providers who question the librarian's ability to judge medical accuracy. The membership of such a review panel will vary with each hospital. As a minimum, however, it should include members of the library committee, patient educators, a representative from ambulatory care services, and individuals already involved in community health education. Whether this group will simply review specific pieces or whether their responsibilities will also include the development of review criteria should be determined by the needs of the hospital librarian. Final selection decisions should rest with the librarian as the person best able to create a collection responsive to user needs.

Organization of Materials

An important issue that must be addressed in planning library services for the community is organizing the materials for use. If services are to be provided in the library, should the books, journals, and pamphlets be integrated or shelved in a separate location? Since many consumers are interested in professional materials, it is probably most efficient to house the two types of materials together. Space limitations and the opposition of the hospital staff to such an arrangement will also have to be taken into consideration. If all materials are integrated, they should be cataloged and classified in the same way as the rest of the collection. In one hospital library, cataloging information for about 60 percent of the consumer book collection was found using CATLINE and the National Library of Medicine *Current Catalog* (20). For the rest of the collection, original cataloging may have to be done. Libraries with access to a general

bibliographic utility such as OCLC, Inc., will find much of the information they need on that database. The decisions made for housing the book collection should also be followed for shelving journal subscriptions.

When the two types of materials are shelved together and receive the same cataloging and classification, it is obvious that they should also share the same subject headings. While MeSH subject headings are too technical for the general public, no better listing exists at present. This difficulty can be partly solved through the use of liberal cross-references that include popular, local, and foreign language terms. The librarian should create and maintain the cross-reference list. If consumer materials are to be housed in a separate location, the librarian is free to use less technical subject headings, such as the Library of Congress. In this case, information about these books and other resources should be included in the hospital's professional library catalog to inform staff members of the existence of the collection. Cataloging for the professional library can be brief, using locational information in place of a classification number. Still, these materials should be given MeSH subject headings so that the cards can be filed together with those for books in the library's regular collection.

One of the most difficult problems for the librarian who wants to become involved in community health information services is the heavy reliance on pamphlets, brochures, booklets, and other ephemeral materials. These materials have no centralized acquisition source. The amount of material can be overwhelming, and very little exists that will help the librarian organize a useful file. Another problem is determining whether the library will act as a distributor of the pamphlets in addition to collecting them. The amount of space, money, and time required to distribute these materials puts such a service outside the capabilities of most hospital libraries. Possibly the best solution to this problem is for the library to limit itself to a small number of defined topics and to provide detailed acquisition information for those who need it. Such pamphlet information can probably be best organized using the traditional library vertical file.

Information Services

Once the librarian makes decisions about the size, scope, and organization of the community collection, attention must be given to the kinds of reference and bibliographic services that will be provided. Providing answers to the public's questions is the core of a community information program. It is also the service that presents the greatest challenge to hospital librarians. Fear of misinterpreting the user's request, providing incorrect or misleading information, or upsetting the user's physician all contribute to the difficulties involved in providing reference services. Often, however, problems can be avoided if all involved parties have a clear understanding of the information the library will provide. More important, everyone involved must understand what information the library will not provide. To further this understanding, the librarian should include guidelines for information services in the library's policy statement. These guidelines should also appear in hospital and community publicity items about the program.

When formulating a reference policy, the librarian may find the following points helpful:

• The librarian should provide information from printed sources. The user should also be told the name of the source.
• The librarian should remind users to check with a qualified health provider in the event that the information is unclear or alarming.
• The privacy of the user must be respected during and after the request.
• The librarian must take special care in using the telephone to give information. Users should be encouraged to visit the library to read the sources. It is all too easy for information transmitted over the telephone to become "the hospital said." The librarian should determine the type of information to be given over the telephone. In many hospitals, for example, information on drugs and medication is not given over the telephone.
• Above all, the librarian must make it clear that information—not advice or opinion—is being provided.

Once guidelines have been developed, the librarian can decide the extent of services. Many libraries already provide answers to short reference questions such as doctors' names and addresses, location of health services, and bibliographic citations. When an information service for the public is available, new users will make more detailed and extensive reference requests. Consequently, the librarian must establish limits on answering research questions and compiling bibliographies. If the library has access to computerized bibliographic search services, the librarian must decide whether to open these services to the public. Will the library provide interlibrary loans or should the librarian refer users to their public library for this service? Often questions from the public can best be answered by referral to the appropriate community service agency. Will the library provide information on such services or is this a function better performed by other departments within the hospital? Librarians will have to answer these questions on the basis of their own perceptions of their appropriateness and the capability of the library to answer them well.

Librarians can play an important role in two other areas of consumer health information services. The first is providing in-service training to public librarians and health educators about how health sciences information is organized and accessed. Whether or not the library provides direct services to community members, their need for information still exists. In many communities, consumers ask for information at the public library. Hospital librarians can help their public library colleagues by presenting workshops on using medical information sources and compiling core lists of reference titles for public libraries to purchase. Programs about specific resources available for educating the public about health may also be useful for health educators, nurses, physicians, and other health care providers.

The second area involves the hospital library in presenting programs to the public, either on specific health topics or on sources of health information and health services. For programs on health topics, the librarian might simply compile bibliographies and resource lists and help identify useful pamphlets. Programs on sources of information would most likely involve the librarian as one of the program presenters.

Publicity

All well-planned programs must include methods for disseminating information about the services to its users and other interested individuals. This publicity is especially important for services that are new or unusual or could affect other hospital departments. Hospital library services to the community are still rather rare, so it is very important for the librarian to give close attention to publicity and public relations. If the hospital has a public relations department, it can be asked to help develop a publicity campaign, brochures, flyers, and press releases. If such a department does not exist, the librarian can still conduct a successful program. Information about the new community services should be submitted to all in-house publications. The librarian should use every opportunity to inform the staff. No one among the hospital personnel should have to learn about the program from outside the hospital.

To inform the community of the new services, the librarian should make use of the local newspaper. These publications are always looking for stories with high reader interest and are often willing to send a reporter to interview the librarian. Information should also be sent to the newsletters of human service agencies, councils on aging and children, neighborhood health centers, and even churches and fraternal organizations. The hospital librarian should also be willing to speak to interested community groups.

Program Costs and Sources of Funding

No program for community access to health information should be undertaken without first acquiring adequate information on its costs and sources of funding. If possible, the program should be included in the regular hospital library budget. In determining costs the librarian must consider the following factors:

• *Space*. Does the library have enough space? Does any other department have space that can be used?
• *Facilities*. Will any remodeling or reorganization of the library be necessary? How will this affect services already being provided?
• *Equipment*. Will new equipment be necessary, such as files, audiovisual hardware, and shelving?

• *Materials*. What types are needed? How much money is available for their purchase?
• *Staff*. Who will provide the services? Can volunteers be used?
• *Cost effectiveness*. To determine this, the librarian must have a clear understanding of the goals and objectives of the program. Will the program be likely to meet its goals? Will those goals affect the community in a meaningful way?

Once cost factors have been established, the librarian can determine the feasibility of the program. New services require money for personnel and materials. These costs must be balanced against the library's other responsibilities. If hospital funds are unavailable, efforts can be made to secure support from outside agencies.

When approaching outside funding sources, librarians should remember that few potential funders are interested in underwriting on-going operating expenses. They are interested in helping libraries to develop programs, but they do not wish to be asked to support these services for an unlimited period of time. The librarian should plan for the program's maintenance when external support is no longer available.

Approaches to federal and state agencies should include both the library services and consumer information aspects of community health information programs. Although the National Library of Medicine (NLM) will not fund programs directly for consumers, it is interested in programs that improve services to direct care providers and which result in better use of existing resources. Library Services and Construction Act funds administered through state library agencies are already being used to support existing community health information programs(10,21). To gain access to these funds, hospital libraries must participate in cooperative programs with other types of libraries. Both the Bureau of Health Education and the Office of Health Information and Health Promotion are becoming increasingly aware of the role that libraries can play in the field of health promotion. Although neither agency has a great deal of money to distribute at present, the national emphasis on promotion may change this situation in the near future. Librarians seeking federal support for health information programs will need to review the *Federal Register* regularly. They should make sure that they are on the mailing lists for requests for proposals and announcements of the appropriate agencies. Librarians should also be willing to put in the amount of time and effort necessary to submit a government grant application.

For most hospital libraries, attempts to find local support will be much more successful. The request procedures of such groups are generally much simpler. Smaller sums of money are often available to underwrite specific programs.

The librarian can approach commercial organizations such as insurance companies, banks, and the local offices of national companies. Today many large companies have community relations departments that fund programs aimed at improving the company's image locally. Service societies such as the Junior Chamber of Commerce, the Lions Club, and the Rotary Club may also be interested in supporting community health programs. Local family foundations are another source that the librarian should investigate. If the hospital has a fund-raising or development office, attempts to find local support should be jointly coordinated.

Once outside sources of support have been identified, the librarian should write a brief letter to the organization outlining the reasons behind the request and the amount that will be needed. If a positive reply is received, it will be necessary for the librarian to write a proposal that explains the rationale for such a program. The librarian should also write about the program's goals, objectives, and activities; the budget and personnel requirements; and the support planned after initial funding runs out. Help in writing grant proposals can be sought from regional medical libraries, cooperative foundation agencies, and professional library organizations. More information on writing proposals can be found in Chapter 15.

Interlibrary Cooperation

Many successful community health information programs involve cooperative services between health sciences libraries and other types of libraries. Such cooperation is usually based on an understanding that the public uses the library that it feels is most appropriate to meet its needs, not the one that is necessarily equipped to meet these needs. Larson says, "To a patient, or to a member of a family acting as a surrogate for a patient, the hospital library may be seen as a natural place to turn for clarification of a medical diagnosis. On the other hand, a layman in good health, or with only suspected health problems, may view the public library as the place where he can best increase his understanding and, in the process, becomes a better guardian of his health"(22:xii). The public library is still the place where the largest number of consumers take their questions. The increasing sophistication of requests, however, has led to greater involvement of hospital libraries in meeting these needs. In many cases the hospital library has not indicated a willingness to answer such questions, but it may be the only resource available after the user contacts the public library. In areas with medical schools, the public often turns to the schools' libraries rather than to the local hospital(16,18). This happens not because these libraries provide services but because the public knows that a medical school will have a sizable library. Given the variety of the public's need for health information, each type of library has a role to play in providing these services.

To date, the most common form of interlibrary cooperation has been between the hospital library and the public libraries in its area(10,21). Often these programs are the result of long-standing informal cooperation. The increased pressure on public libraries for more extensive health information and a growing interest on the part of hospitals in community service led to more formal shared services. The success of these programs is largely the result of the equal participation of each member. Participants see the programs as a better way of meeting their users' needs, not as a way of shifting responsibility to the other institution. Given a large and varied public, cooperation between hospital libraries and public libraries may be the most efficient way of meeting the public's needs.

It is true that public libraries can handle large groups of users and are the most frequently used source of information. Public libraries, however, lack skill in developing medical collections, knowledge of recent developments in health care, and access to professional books and journals. Conversely, hospital libraries usually have small collections, limited staff, and inconvenient locations. Their services can include in-service training of public librarians, reference backup for questions that cannot be answered in the public library, assistance in developing collections and preparing bibliographies, and contacts with health care providers willing to participate in public health education programs. To successfully share services, hospital libraries and public libraries must recognize the need for consumer health information. Then both parties must strive to fill the need in a way that accounts for the strengths and weaknesses of each library.

Other forms of multitype library cooperation exist, although some have not been tested to any great extent. One example is cooperation between hospital libraries and school libraries. Health care experts agree that health education must begin as early as possible. Many states now require extensive health education courses for which neither the school library nor the school health department is prepared. Information services to the parents of school-aged children are also seriously lacking. Cooperation with the schools probably benefits the hospital library by improving public relations.

Another type of cooperative program is that between hospitals and health maintenance organizations (HMOs). HMOs are required by federal law to provide health education. A few have their own extensive information services, but most use hospital libraries that serve their patients(23). By the very nature of their function, HMOs often have the largest pool of providers interested and involved in community health education.

An increasing number of hospital library consortia are helping the public as part of their services. Consortia eliminate duplication of materials and services and heighten the ability to cover a wider variety of topics. One of the best examples of this type of cooperation is the patient education network of the Veterans' Admsinistration. hospitals. Although created to serve the needs of patients and their families, many of these libraries have expanded their user population to include the general public.

Specific Programs

Once the hospital librarian has decided to play a role in providing the community with health information, specific services must be planned so that they will neither interfere with on-going services nor overburden the facilities, budget, and staff. Most libraries begin with relatively small limited programs whose effectiveness can easily be measured. In some communities the librarian can make a good start by meeting with public librarians to inform them that the hospital library is willing to serve as a backup in responding to users' requests. Policies and procedures for reference referral and interlibrary loans can then be drawn up and agreed to by all participants. Other examples of limited involvement for the hospital librarian include helping the public library select medical and nursing books for its reference collection. The hospital librarian could also help the public library to develop bibliographies for use during the various national health weeks. The hospital librarian might also create small collections of pamphlets on a few topics of interest to the community. Another valuable service the hospital librarian can perform is to serve as a liaison between the public library and health providers willing to review materials.

Even a hospital library capable of providing direct service to the public must pay attention to the exact nature and depth of these services. Again it is best to start on a limited basis and extend services as money and staff become available. Attempts to develop collections should focus on topics of known interest to both the public and the hospital staff. An example of a much-needed program is assistance in locating good audiovisuals for use in health education programs presented by members of the hospital staff or community. Other valuable projects might include developing cross-references from popular terms for the subject catalog, compiling bibliographies from the professional literature on medical topics of interest to lay people, or providing informational materials at hospital-sponsored screening clinics in the community. Workshops on medical bibliography and medical library services have already been mentioned as programs hospital librarians can provide for their colleagues.

Providing identical services to both the general public and the staff is probably not possible for most hospital libraries. The librarian should examine each type of service to determine whether it can be extended to the community. Providing computer-produced bibliographies is one service in which a relatively small investment in time will benefit both the community and the library. The public will have access to such capabilities and the library can increase its revenue through fees for the service.

THE HOSPITAL LIBRARIAN'S CONTRIBUTION TO IMPROVED HEALTH STATUS

The skills hospital librarians have in selecting, organizing, and disseminating information, combined with their relationship to health care providers, can make them a vital part of the consumers' health education movement. Education—behavior change as a result of something learned—is not the same as information dissemination. However, it is important to note the vital role played by information in decision making. Recent reports on adults who have stopped smoking highlight the crucial role played by public information programs in this change in behavior.

In addition to the more passive roles of information providers, hospital librarians have educational functions within consumer health information services. The first of these is the responsibility to educate health care providers about resources that exist to support them in presenting health education programs.

Second is the role librarians can play in teaching their colleagues in other types of libraries how to find health and medical information and how to develop services that will meet users' information needs. If at all possible,

these services should also be provided directly to members of the public seeking information from the hospital library. Not only should librarians be knowledgeable about print and other materials, they should also be able to refer consumers to available human and organizational resources.

All of these programs depend on active participation by the hospital librarian. Librarians cannot simply wait for people to visit the library. Hospital librarians must recognize that they have a role, however indirect, to play in consumer health education. It is unlikely that the present emphasis on health promotion and maintenance will diminish in the future. This emphasis will result in increased consumer needs for accurate, timely, relevant information. If hospital librarians do not provide such information or help other librarians to do so, they will miss the opportunity to make themselves more visible and to communicate the important role a library can play in maintaining the public's health.

Possibly, involvement of hospital librarians in community health programs will lead to new responsibilities in librarianship. For example, librarians may work with consumers to make the public's information requirements known to providers. Hospital librarians may also be called upon to play the profession's traditional role of advocates for the individual's right to information. If librarians keep in mind that the goal of health care is the promotion and maintenance of well-being, and that their function is to assist both providers and consumers, then their participation in community information programs will benefit all concerned.

REFERENCES

1. Harris CL. Hospital-based patient education programs and the role of the hospital librarian. Bull Med Libr Assoc 1978 Apr;66: 210-217.

2. Lalonde M. A new perspective on the health of Canadians: a working document. Ottawa: Information Canada, 1975.

3. Somers AR. Consumer health education; to know or to die. Hospitals 1976 May 1;50:52-56.

4. Foster L, Self PC. Legal and medical reference: a dilemma for public libraries. Ill Libr 1978 Mar;60:243-248.

5. Somers AR. Consumer health education; a new challenge to the medical profession. J Med Assoc Ga 1976 Apr;65:105-110.

6. American Hospital Association. A patient's bill of rights. Chicago: American Hospital Association, 1973.

7. American Hospital Association. Health education: role and responsibility of health care institutions. Chicago: American Hospital Association, 1975.

8. Topper JM. Hospitals as centers for consumer health information. Bull Am Soc Inf Sci 1978 Apr;4:13-14.

9. West BP, Fink W. Community health education. In: Truelove JW, Linton CB, eds. Hospital-based education. New York: Arco, 1980: 95-113.

10. Gartenfeld E. The community health information network; a model for hospital and public library cooperation. Libr J 1978 Oct 1;103:1911-1914.

11. Van Gieson WR. The hospital library in transition. Hosp Prog 1978 Jun;59:66-69.

12. Mathes CB. Education as health care (letter). Libr J 1978 May 1; 103:909.

13. Davies NE. Bringing order to the literature of health education. N Eng J Med 1980 June 26;302:1476-1478.

14. Rickards DJ. Providing health care information to patients in small hospital. Bull Med Libr Assoc 1978 July;66:342-345.

15. Marshall JG, Hamilton JD. The clinical librarian and the patient; report of a project at McMaster University Medical Centre. Bull Med Libr Assoc 1978 Oct;66:420-425.

16. Eakin D, Jackson SJ, Hannigan GG. Consumer health information: libraries as partners. Bull Med Libr Assoc 1980, Apr;68: 220-229.

17. Foster EC. Patient/health information in the context of the consumer education movement. In: Larson MT, ed. Patient/health education: the librarian's role; proceedings of an invitational institute, February 5-9, 1979. Detroit: Wayne State University, 1979: 73-81.

18. Jeuell CA, Francisco CB, Port JS. Brief survey of public information services at privately-supported medical school libraries: comparison with publicly-supported medical school libraries. Bull Med Libr Assoc 1977 Apr;65:292-295.

19. College of Medicine and Dentistry of New Jersey, George F. Smith Library of the Health Sciences. Public services policy manual. Newark: College of Medicine and Dentistry of New Jersey, 1977.

20. Sorrentino S, Goodchild EY, Fierberg J. Cataloging procedures and catalog organization for patient education materials. Bull Med Libr Assoc 1979 Apr;67:257-260.

21. Goodchild EY, Furman JA, Addison BL, Umbarger HN. The CHIPS project: a health information network to serve the consumer. Bull Med Libr Assoc 1978 Oct;66:432-436.

22. Larson MT, Introduction. In: Larson MT, ed. Patient/health education: the librarian's role; proceedings of an invitational institute, February 5-9, 1979. Detroit: Wayne State University, 1979: xi-xvi.

23. Collen FB, Soghikian K. A health education library for patients: Kaiser-Permanente Health Education Research Center. Health Serv Rep 1974 May/June;89:236-243.

Archival Services in Hospital Libraries

Judith Overmier
Curator
Wangensteen Historical Library of
    Biology and Medicine
University of Minnesota
Minneapolis, Minnesota

and

Adele A. Lerner
Archivist
New York Hospital-Cornell
    Medical Center
New York, New York

CHAPTER 23

Archival Services in Hospital Libraries

Judith Overmier
Curator
Wangensteen Historical Library of Biology and Medicine
University of Minnesota
Minneapolis, Minnesota
and
Adele A. Lerner
Archivist
New York Hospital-Cornell Medical Center
New York, New York

Appendixes

Figures

Archives are "the noncurrent records of an organization or institution preserved because of their continuing value."* The records produced by a hospital may include correspondence, publications, reports, photographs, architects' blueprints, floor plans, subject files, and computer printouts. These records, which the hospital is often required to keep by law, are unique. They are primary source materials and provide documentation for current administrative action, legal and operational questions, public relations, and scholarly research.

Many hospitals do not have a formal system for organizing and preserving these documents. The decision to keep or discard them rests with the originating or the receiving department. This decision is frequently made on the basis of departmental requirements without considering the needs of the hospital as a whole.

A variety of people may be responsible for hospital records. Some hospitals have an archivist or a department responsible for records management. Others give part of this responsibility to medical records. In some cases, an administrative staff member may coordinate the retention of records. Different types of material may also be handled by different departments, with varying degrees of coordination and cooperation. Another alternative involves working with other hospitals to develop cooperative archives with shared services and staff.

Hospital libraries may sometimes become involved with archival services. The hospital administration may turn to the library for help with records management. Or the librarian may identify ways that an archival service based in the library might help to organize hospital records.

The rationale for library involvement with archival services is usually based on perceived similarities between libraries and archives. Librarians are experienced in using various methods to acquire and organize information in a variety of formats. Hospital libraries and archives require similar kinds of space, including reading areas, storage in stacks, and workrooms. They also require similar staff functions, particularly reference service. In many cases, the library is already collecting the publications of the hospital and its staff and thus may have the beginning of an archival collection. Burke discusses the similarities that might result in the assignment to the hospital librarian of the responsibility for collecting and caring for materials of an archival nature(1).

Libraries and archives differ in several important ways. Libraries purchase books and journals that other libraries may also own. Archives collect the unique materials produced by the hospital as a result of its daily operation.

These primary source materials include such documents as minutes, reports, and correspondence. Archival materials are usually boxed rather than bound in volumes. They are shelved in the order in which they are acquired and not according to a preconceived numeric system. It may be more difficult to provide reference services for archival materials because of their quantity and because they are usually not indexed in as much detail as library materials.

This chapter is intended for hospital librarians considering involvement with archival services. It presents an introduction to basic archival concepts and procedures.

ADMINISTRATION

Archival services involve a great deal of staff time. However, the librarian may feel that the benefits of such services justify the time and effort involved. The hospital administration must also be committeed to archival services. Ways of obtaining administrative support will be discussed later in the chapter.

Staffing

Library staff may receive training in archival techniques in courses or in continuing education programs. They may also visit other archives, attend meetings of professional associations, and read books and journals on the subject. A list of references appears in the Readings section at the end of the chapter.

Although library staff can become competent in archival procedures using these methods, hiring a trained archivist may be less expensive in the long run. When staffing is limited, the librarian might investigate various alternatives for supporting the beginnings of archival activities. Grant or gift funding from local organizations may be possible since hospital records reflect the development of health care in the community. Hospital funding for a pilot project to test the value of archival services might be arranged. Well-trained volunteers are sometimes available. The librarian may wish to develop a limited archival program and work toward adding an archivist to the staff.

As archival services develop, a professional archivist will probably be necessary either as a permanent staff member or on a consulting basis. However, the library staff can play an important role in limited archival services or in developing a larger program.

Space

Archival services require space for storing boxes, a stack area with shelving, and tables for processing. Processing involves accessioning, arranging, describing, cleaning, and preserving records. Thus long tables with a great deal of surface area are most desirable. Since hospital records grow at an alarming rate, providing enough

* Definitions used in this article are from "A Basic Glossary for Archivists, Manuscript Curators, and Records Managers," Evans FB, Harrison DF, Thompson EA, comps., Rofes WL, ed. *Amer Archivist* 1974 Jul;37:415-433., and used with the permission of the Society of American Archivists. Readers are referred to this publication for more complete definitions of terms and concepts discussed.

space for the closed stack area can be a problem. Inexpensive metal shelving like the kind used in warehouses is recommended for storing archival boxes. Both the stack area and the work area must be locked to ensure the security of the documents.

Legal Aspects

The legal ramifications of archival work are quite real. They include legal responsibility for records, problems of confidentiality, requirements for obtaining permission to use records, and the need to cite sources in published material. These considerations differ from problems that librarians typically encounter, and the hospital librarian must thoroughly understand them. Sources of information on the legal aspects of archive management are included in the Readings section at the end of the chapter.

Policies

Beginning an archival program involves deciding what records to collect, how they will be collected, and from whom. The process is similar to library acquisition except that a library buys materials but an archive collects them. Before an archival program is started, a formal policy statement approved by the hospital administration is needed. This statement should specify the purpose of the archives, the type of records to be acquired, and access and reference policies. This policy statement should be written in conjunction with the hospital administrative staff so that it accurately reflects its goals for the archives. Formulating policy in cooperation with the administration helps to ensure support for archival services. A sample policy statement appears in Appendix A.

Developing a formal archive policy requires a knowledge of the principles of archive management and a thorough understanding of the hospital's administrative structure. The librarian should carefully examine an organizational chart and the hospital directory. He or she should think about how departments have developed and how they are currently related.

After becoming thoroughly familiar with the hospital, the librarian is ready to develop the specifics of the collection policy. These decisions must be made in conjunction with the hospital administration and usually evolve during several discussions about expectations and objectives for the archives. Some questions to be considered appear below.

- Which departments will be emphasized because of the importance of their records?
- What records will be kept?
- How long will records be kept?
- Who will decide how long each record series will be retained?
- Will departments be required to deposit their records or will participation be optional?
- Will the archives include materials such as photo-

graphs, tapes, slides, hospital publications, newspaper clippings, and memorabilia?
- Will the archives include the personal papers of physicians and others affiliated with the hospital?
- Are there special areas like general medical history in which the archives will collect more widely?
- Is there interest in creating records through an oral history program?
- How will access and use be controlled?

It is recommended that the archives try to acquire the following types of hospital records.

- Founding documents or charter
- Bylaws and other legal documents
- Minutes, correspondence, reports, and memoranda of the hospital's governing board
- Official records of the administration and of other major departments, including correspondence files, subject files, manuals, and reports
- Accreditation reports and supporting documentation
- Minutes and reports of committees
- Annual budget, audit reports, and inventories
- Architectural drawings of the hospital, including any alterations
- Official hospital publications, such as annual reports, newsletters, bulletings, procedure manuals, directories, and brochures
- Audiovisual materials such as tapes of conferences held at the hospital
- Photographs of the housestaff and oral history interviews
- Memorabilia useful for exhibit purposes
- Biographial material on staff, including personnel records of retired or deceased staff

Librarians who wish to begin a limited archival program might start by collecting the records of the administrative offices. As the program develops, departmental records can be collected as well. Administrators may be interested in a collection that includes (1) founding and legal documents of the hospital; (2) official hospital policies; (3) annual reports; (4) budget, audit, space, and equipment reports; (5) accreditation documentation; and (6) official hospital publications.

The archives should not try to obtain the medical records of current patients, since these are usually handled by the medical records administrator. However, in large hospital archives, the librarian should work out a schedule with the medical records department for the eventual transfer of these records to the archives. Use of such records for scholarly research may be restricted for a long period of time because of the patient's right to confidentiality.

Small archives should probably not acquire patients' medical records, with the possible exception of landmark medical or surgical cases. The amount of space required for filing is very large compared with the relatively limited archival value of such records. Moreover, the legal problems of handling patient records are best avoided.

Once the collection development policy has full administrative support and approval, implementation can begin. The process will proceed much more smoothly if the administrative officers announce the policy and ask all departments to save their records. Departments should also be asked to cooperate with the library in working out the details for transfer of materials to the archives.

ACQUISITIONS

As Cavanagh points out, archival collecting is definitely the " . . . kind of acquisitions where persistence and personality take the place of money"(2). In addition to these qualities, a records management program can be very helpful in organizing archive acquisitions. "Records management [is] that area of general administrative management concerned with achieving economy and efficiency in the creation, use and maintenance, and disposition of records." Obviously a full-scale records management program extends beyond the domain of the archives themselves. However, even a small archival program can benefit from the efficient methods designed for a records management program.

Survey of Records

The librarian must first determine the amount and kinds of records being created by each department. The simplest way to obtain this information is to have each department complete a questionnaire. The questionnaire should cover the following information about each department's records: (1) type, (2) how records are being used, (3) location and amount of space occupied, (4) method of filing or organizing, (5) years covered, and (6) recommended retention period for each type of record.

Such a survey provides a quick overview of the records already in the hospital. The librarian can then examine the records in each department in more detail.

Records Scheduling

Next a records disposition schedule should be completed for each record type or series (see Figure 23-1). A record series is a set of materials, often of a common form, filed together because of a relationship resulting from their creation, receipt, or use.

The librarian should work with both the appropriate department head and the hospital's legal counsel to ensure that records are retained in accordance with legal requirements. The schedules should include a listing of all records that are created in a department, the length of time the department will retain each record in active use, and the final disposition of each record. If a record is placed in the archives, the schedule should specify the retention period. Some records are kept indefinitely, whereas others can be destroyed after a set period of time. For example, some fiscal records must be kept seven years, but have little value beyond that period.

It may be essential to preserve records of a sensitive nature. The archivist must point this out to the persons involved and offer to restrict access to these records for a designated period of time. These restrictions should be agreed upon and put in writing.

This process of evaluating records and deciding what should be done with them is called appraisal. It is one of the hardest parts of the professional archivist's job. When appraising records, the archivist must analyze not only possible uses but also volume, format, age, and availability of similar records. A knowledge of American medical history is often useful in judging the rarity of certain records.

The records disposition schedule thus provides the structure for the transfer of material to the archives. Each department is provided with a copy of its schedules and transmittal forms to facilitate the transfer of records. These forms are to be completed by the department and sent with the boxes of records. The librarian should acknowledge receipt of the records by returning a signed copy of the transmittal form to the department. These forms can serve as a reference guide to materials received by the archives and can also serve as a starting place for organizing records.

The Role of Persistence and Personality

The establishment of a collection policy and a records disposition schedule for each department would seem to assure easy acquisition of records and prevent the loss or destruction of important records. However, this is not always the case. The librarian must establish and maintain effective communication with those in charge of the creation of records in each department. The department secretary will often be a key contact.

It is often necessary to follow up the records survey and scheduling with reminders. Both memos and diplomatic personal contact are useful for this purpose. In addition to identifying a contact person in each department, informal contacts should be made whenever possible. During these informal encounters or at short training sessions, the librarian can educate the hospital staff about the advantages of keeping records in the archives. These advantages include preservation of the records, protection of restricted records from indiscriminate access, and ready access to reference services. Keeping records in the archives also saves space in departmental offices.

INTELLECTUAL AND PHYSICAL CONTROL

It is perhaps in the area of cataloging or bibliographic control that the purposes and practices of librarians and archivists differ the most. Archivists do not catalog. There are no specific schemes for classification, subject heading access, or descriptive cataloging. Intellectual and physical control of records is achieved by arrangement and description. The purpose of cataloging and classify-

Figure 23-1
Records Disposition Schedule

DATE: 1/14/1979	

RECORD SERIES TITLE and DESCRIPTION (CONTENTS, PURPOSE, USE) Medical Board, Transactions of Minutes of the monthly meetings of the Medical Board, with actions approved by said Board. The Medical Board has major authority for medically-related decisions, staffing, policies, etc.	VOLUME 44 bound vols., 5'4½"
	ARE FILES CUT-OFF PERIODICALLY? IF SO, WHEN & HOW? Yes, bound annually, Jan. thru Dec.

ARRANGEMENT: Chronologically, with pages numbered sequentially	INCLUSIVE DATES 1934-1978	IS RECORD SERIES MAINTAINED ELSEWHERE? IF SO, WHERE? Yes, latest 10 years are in Directors office
	IF INDEXES, DESCRIBE: Yes, each volume has a subject index at end.	

SUGGESTED RETENTION

IN ORIGINATING OFFICE 10 years	IN ARCHIVES/RECORDS CENTER Permanently	TOTAL RETENTION Permanent Retention
PERSON TO CONTACT Secretary to Medical Board	CURRENT LOCATION OF RECORD SERIES Office of the Medical Board	

COMMENTS, RESTRICTIONS, ETC.
The original, signed Transactions will, in the future, be typed on acid-free paper, and sent unbound to the Archives at the end of each year. The Archives will also receive a bound yearly volume for reference use.

*Note: Based on a form in use at The New York Hospital, Cornell Medical Center

ing library materials is to locate and describe each item. The purpose of arranging and describing archival materials is to locate and describe large units. These units are called record groups or record series and are made up of many related items.

Arrangement

Arrangement is "the process and results of organizing archives, records, and manuscripts in accordance with accepted archival principles." Arrangement is possible at several levels, including repository, record group or similar control unit, subgroup, series, file unit, and document. These levels represent the breakdown of each large group of related materials into smaller units until the level of an individual document is reached. Ideally,

the level of arrangement depends on the complexity and value of the records. In practice, it is often influenced by the amount of staff time available.

Most small hospital archives will not be able to proceed beyond the level of the file unit within the series. Thus records would be boxed by series. For example, the correspondence files of the medical director would be a series. The librarian would then list all the file units or folders in that series.

Provenance is the archival principle that states that the records of each department, person, or administrative entity should be kept together. Whenever possible, the order in which they were kept in the office of origin should be maintained. If there is no original order to follow, the librarian should impose a reasonable arrangement. When the principle of provenance is followed, the librarian can quickly determine where to look for certain information. For example, records regarding the care of infants would be created by the pediatrics department and thus would be found in that department's records.

The rule of maintenance of original order is designed to save time for the person organizing the archives. The librarian must resist the temptation to rearrange files or to remove papers to create a new file. This temptation may arise in connection with frequently asked reference questions. For example, the librarian may be repeatedly asked for information about the design of the new pediatrics wing. The temptation is to gather all the information on this subject from various files and to place it in a separate file. This is acceptable provided that the new file is made from photocopied documents. The original files should be left intact. A better solution, however, is to use description to provide access for reference purposes.

Description

Description is "the process of establishing intellectual control over holdings through the preparation of finding aids." Aids used to locate items include: guides, inventories, the card catalog, lists, and the accession register.

These finding aids provide access to the content of the archives and establish intellectual control over the neatly arranged records series. When the records are properly arranged—by provenance, in series with records in folders—the task of description through finding aids is minimal.

The level of descriptive finding aids needed by an archives should be determined by the value of the records, their size and complexity. Different types and levels of finding aids can be used for different records, depending on the librarian's assessment of the need. If certain records turn out to be used more frequently than expected, the librarian can always do a more detailed register.

Guides

At the repository level, the guide lists every record group or series in an archives. It gives a brief description of each item, including title, volume, dates, and availability of access. Appendix B is an example of one entry in a guide. Since a guide shows the total scope of holdings, it is of great value to the archives staff, scholars, hospital administrators, and potential donors.

Inventory

The inventory, or register, is the basic archival finding aid. A sample of such an inventory appears in Appendix C. The inventory should include a brief history of the department for which records are being inventoried. It lists each record series and provides title, dates, quantity, arrangement, and relationships to other series, as well as a description of the significant subject content. If the inventory is for the records of an individual, a biographical sketch rather than departmental history should be included. If a collection has great research value, a listing

of the titles of the file folders by box for the series should be made. This is called a container list, or folder list, and is the optimal level of description that a hospital librarian should attempt.

Card Catalog

The card catalog provides access to subject content from several in-house record series. For example, information by or about Dr. Jane Doe may be found in the records of the Medical Board, in the files of the Department of Surgery, in Administrative Correspondence files 1974-1976, and in the Office of Public Information Publications. A card on Doe, Jane, M.D., would direct the researcher to all four of these record series. Appendix D shows a typical subject card.

Cards can also be made for publications, cross-referencing of titles, or any other indexing function. A subject authority list can be created if the needs and subjects of a particular collection warrant it. The card catalog supplements but does not replace the inventory.

Lists

Lists are special finding aids that are developed to fill particular needs. Special lists can be compiled of items such as blueprints or people for whom the archives have biographical data, regardless of what record series the data belongs in or where it is located.

Accession Register

The least extensive finding aid, and the first to be created, is the accession register. When a collection of records is received, the following information should be written in an accession register:

- Date received
- Donor or source of records
- Quantity of records, given in general terms if the records are very disorganized
- Description, including titles of the records, the content, the physical condition, any restrictions on access, and other relevant data.

The information in the accession register can be as brief or as extensive as warranted. It provides fast information about the archival holdings. If possible, the librarian should assign a temporary location to these new records and indicate it in the accession register. A handwritten log of the holdings makes a useful register.

PRESERVATION OF MATERIALS

Many hospital administrative records are written on paper of poor quality, such as carbon second sheets, memo pad paper, or notebook paper. Librarians can slow the disintegration of these materials over time by providing proper physical care and optimum environmental controls.

Environmental Controls

The temperature in the closed stack storage area should be kept at 68° F. or below, year round. Relative humidity should be kept at 40-50 percent. Air filtration systems that reduce levels of sulfur dioxide, ozone, and particulate material are also desirable.

Storage Containers

The containers used for archival storage are usually 10½ inches by 12½ inches by 15½ inches. The boxes are made of acid-free, alkaline-buffered cardboard. Containers also come in different sizes and styles for archival materials of other shapes. Storage in a controlled environment in these boxes is the minimum level of preservation acceptable. File folders, insert sheets, and envelopes made of acid-free, alkaline-buffered materials are also available for use in separating materials within the boxes. These file folders and insert sheets prevent the migration of acidity from document to document and provide physical support to prevent sagging and buckling. The boxes also provide added protection during fire and water disasters.

Storage Preparation

When archival materials arrive in the library, they need to be processed and prepared for storage. This preparation involves several procedures.

Cleaning

Sometimes materials are delivered to the library dusty, even dirty. They may be cleaned by brushing gently with a soft brush. Very dusty materials can be vacuumed. Librarians should work very carefully with a brush attachment covered with cheesecloth to catch any loose pieces of paper. Although this method is time-consuming, librarians will find that they can organize materials without the irritation of loose dust and without adding dusty fingerprints to the papers.

These dusting methods suffice for removing loose surface dust, but if the materials are particularly dirty, and time permits, the librarian can erase light dirt with an Opaline dry-cleaning pad. Such work requires a gentle touch, erasing from the center of the document outward. If the paper is weakened at folds, extra caution must be taken. Librarians should also be careful when cleaning around signatures, typing, or printing. All of these can disappear during improper erasing. Finally, residue left from erasing should be brushed away. Some of these materials are harmful to paper. Vacuuming and cleaning of paper are described in detail in Banks(3) and Horton (4). Horton also provides illustrations of these procedures.

Only experts should attempt to clean paper by washing. Without professional experience, librarians using this method may wash away inks or damage the materials. Stain removal also should not be undertaken by the novice archivist. If the archival materials are so impor-

tant that they require sophisticated cleaning, they should be sent out to a professional conservator.

Removing Foreign Objects

While preparing to store materials in special containers, a librarian should gently remove metal paper clips, staples, pins, and rubber bands, if this can be done without damaging the document. Such materials can rust and stain the paper. Once the paper becomes brittle, it often disintegrates. Some archivists use plastic paper clips or Monel (rustproof) staples to replace metal ones. Adhesive tape or pressure sensitive tape should never be used on archival records. Unfortunately, materials can arrive with tape already on them. Since tape is difficult to remove, and the process requires experience, time, and the use of chemicals and fume hoods, librarians should not undertake the task.

Mending

Occasionally, a library receives torn, damaged, or ragged materials. These items should not be mended unless absolutely necessary. When necessary, some librarians use rice paper and a paste made of methyl cellulose paste powder. Care must be taken with water-base paste to prevent the inks, especially in signatures, from running. The tissue should be torn so that the ragged edges blend with the original document. Sometimes librarians are tempted to trim ragged edges to keep them from snagging or tearing further. This practice is a point of controversy even among professional archivists. Since the average librarian does not usually have the curatorial skills to make decisions about trimming, it should not be done.

Materials Requiring Special Care

Some archival materials require special care. This category includes oversize materials, fragile or disintegrating materials, scrapbooks, photographs, and newspaper clippings. Fortunately, conservators have addressed the special preservation needs of these materials.

Oversize Materials

Oversize documents should not be folded. Large papers, such as hospital floor plans or flow charts, should be stored flat. If materials are received folded, they should be flattened. This can be accomplished by opening the document and placing it under a light weight for a short time. During efforts to flatten paper, the temptation to reverse the fold should be resisted. This procedure only weakens the paper along the crease line. If the paper is brittle, it can be relaxed before opening by increasing its humidity level. This is often done by placing the paper in a closed container on a screen elevated over water, never touching the water. The document is left in this moist environment for several hours. Once the paper is relaxed and limp, it can be unfolded gently and placed between white, acid-free alkaline-buffered blotters.

Finally, a light weight is placed on it, and it is left in this condition for a period of several hours. Afterwards, refiling should be possible.

Fragile Materials

Fragile, historical documents should be encapsulated or enclosed in a protective envelope. Many conservators use polyester to encapsulate disintegrating or heavily used documents. Some conservators require the deacidification of the paper prior to encapsulation. However, this process is too involved to be practical in a hospital library. Since the materials needed for encapsulation are affordable, and the manual skills required for the process are minimal, the procedure is practical for most libraries. The method of polyester encapsulation is described in a pamphlet published by the Library of Congress (5).

Newspaper Clippings

Some librarians like to keep a file or a scrapbook of newspaper clippings about the hospital and its staff members. To avoid losing articles due to deterioration, librarians can photocopy the clippings on durable paper. The originals can then be discarded, and the permanent copies easily filed in acid-free folders in a standard filing cabinet. Newsprint, which is highly acidic, should never be filed with other documents. If the original clippings must be kept, they should be filed in a separate folder or encapsulated.

Photographs

Photographs and other iconographic records are usually removed from their record group and filed by subject for the archives. As they are removed, they should be identified on a "separation list" that remains in the record group to indicate the transfer of location. When filed by subject, each item is identified by subject, written lightly in pencil on the back of the print or on the slide sleeve. They are placed in acid-free folders, several pictures to each folder. Negatives are kept in a separate file and cross-referenced to the print. Placing negatives in acid-free envelopes, not in glassine envelopes, and filing them numerically in acid-free boxes, helps to preserve their quality.

On rare occasions, when the source of photographs is important, pictures are kept together as a record series with the appropriate subject file of photographs attached as a cross-reference. A cross-reference should also be used when a photograph contains several key hospital staff members whose pictures are requested frequently. For more details on the care and use of photographs, librarians can consult sources listed at the end of the chapter.

Professional Assistance

Librarians often seek professional assistance when planning for archival services, preserving items, or solving problems that arise from archival services. This assistance can come in the form of advice from nearby professional archivists in another large hospital or archives, from the Society of American Archivists, from local conservators, or from the Northeast Document Conservation Center. Information is also provided by suppliers who carry archival products, including the suppliers listed in Appendix E. Sophisticated protective and restorative projects also require professional assistance. The American Institute for Conservation certifies flat paper restorers who can be hired to carry out such projects.

REFERENCE SERVICES

Hospital use of the archives can serve many purposes. Administrators or legal officers may need to refer to details of previous decisions as background for current administrative action. The hospital public relations department will also use the archives heavily, especially for photographs of the hospital and staff, biographical information about staff members, and "first" dates of various hospital events.

Promoting Archival Services

Archival use and support can be increased by promoting these services. For example, materials from the archives, such as the following, might be exhibited:

- A series of photos showing changes in nursing uniforms in the hospital over the last 100 years
- A comparison of the first staff rules with the current ones
- A series of floor plans showing the physical changes in a popular department over a period of time
- Photos of the 1905 staff picnic
- Newspaper clippings and staff publications relating to an important medical advance.

In addition to exhibits, news notes or brief articles of a similar nature can be published in the hospital newsletter, town newspaper, or state medical journal. A small brochure describing the archives collection is also useful. Leaflets often travel far and may reach historians who travel to visit the collection. Scholars may also learn about the archives if the librarian lists any noninstitutional portions of the collection in the *National Union Catalog of Manuscript Collections* and in the *Directory of Archives and Manuscript Repositories*, a frequently updated directory and database maintained by the National Historical Publications and Records Commission.

Providing Reference Services

No matter how detailed the finding aids are in a hospital's archives, a researcher will need time to discuss information needs with a librarian and ascertain which record series will provide the most adequate information. While the card catalog can provide a subject guide for the researcher, it is impossible to put everything in the catalog or in a finding aid. In-depth knowledge of the archival collection acquired during years of experience enables the librarian to suggest the proper finding aids and records during the reference interview. At this time the librarian can also explain the rules and policies regarding access to original resource material. Often, the department that has supplied the records restricts access for a designated number of years, or requires that persons from outside the hospital have special permission to use the records. The librarian should strive for restricting as few records as possible since the goal should be equal access to information. It is understandable, however, that the administration may not want its recent records open. For this reason, the archives policy statement usually sets a reasonable period of time during which all records are closed, except to those departments that created the record or to individuals who have the department's permission to use them.

Writing Archival Policies

Rules and policies for the archives govern the use of the records. For reasons of security and preservation, most archives have the following policies:

• The researcher must show identification and sign a visitor's register.
• Large handbags and briefcases are not allowed in the reference room.
• A period of time is designated when records are closed to all departments except to the department where the record originated.
• Notes must be taken with pencil or typewriter. Pens are not allowed.
• Papers are to be handled with care, not folded or leaned upon.
• Papers are to be kept in the order in which they are found. If a document or folder seems misfiled, the user is to bring this to the attention of the librarian rather than refile.
• No eating or smoking is allowed.

• Photoduplication is allowed for the researcher's private study only. Photocopied records should not be passed on to any other person or institution. Also, photoduplication does not constitute permission to publish.
• Permission to publish must be requested in writing. The researcher is responsible for securing any copyright clearance, since the archives may not have the literary property rights. The copyright rules governing manuscripts are complex and should be studied by the librarian. These rules are available from the Copyright Office.

Providing Security and Access

Security and limited access to record files are necessary for maintaining the confidentiality of a collection. Usually the reference area is supervised and the stacks are closed to users. Materials are brought to the user a box at a time. This provides security for the unique, and often valuable, hospital records. Records of research requests from the hospital staff and from scholars are kept to help the librarian judge the value of the records. Frequently requested materials may be important enough to microfilm for research use. It is also useful to interview the researcher after he or she has used the archives to identify such things as weaknesses in finding aids or in service provided.

The question of confidentiality and privacy versus the scholar's right to know often challenges the accessibility of records in the archives. Because the archives have patient care records, personnel files, or other records containing confidential information about specific people, the archives may prefer to keep the records closed. An alternative approach requires users to sign an agreement stating that their research is of a general, demographic nature and that names of individuals will not be used. In such a case, a reference interview prior to actual use of records enables the librarian to know the researcher's qualifications and intentions. Generally, researchers are allowed access to case files after the death of the individual or 75 years after the file was created. When in doubt about record procedures, librarians should check with the hospital's legal counsel.

REFERENCES

1. Burke FG. Similarities and differences. In: Clark RL, Jr. ed. Archive-library relations. New York: RR Bowker, 1976:31-45.

2. Cavanagh GST. Rare books, archives, and the history of medicine. In: Annan GL, Felter JW, eds. Handbook of medical library practice. 3d ed. Chicago: Medical Library Association, 1970:254-283.

3. Banks PN. Paper cleaning. Restaurator 1969;1:52-66.

4. Horton C. Cleaning and preserving bindings and related materials 2d ed. Chicago: Library Technology Program, American Library Association, 1969.

5. Library of Congress. Preservation Office. Polyester film encapsulation. Washington, DC: Library of Congress, 1980.

READINGS

Banks PN. Environmental standards for the storage of books and manuscripts. Libr J 1974 Feb 1;99:339-343.

Bartkowski, P, Saffady W. Shelving and office furniture for archives buildings. Am Archivist 1974 Jan;37:55-66.

Baumann RM, ed. A manual of archival techniques. Harrisburg: Pennsylvania Historical and Museum Commission, 1979.

Bordin RB, Warner RM. Modern manuscript library. New York: Scarecrow Press, 1966.

Duckett KW. Modern manuscripts: a practical manual for their management, care and use. Nashville: American Association for State and Local History, 1975.

Hedlin E. Business archives: an introduction. Chicago: Society of American Archivists, 1978.

Kane LM. A guide to the care and administration of manuscripts. 2d ed. Nashville: American Association for State and Local History, 1966.

Lytle RH, ed. Management of archives and manuscript collections for librarians. Drexel Libr Q 1979 Jan;11:(entire issue).

Moss WW. Oral history program manual. New York: Praeger, 1974.

Society of American Archivists. Basic manual series. Chicago: Society of American Archivists, 1977.

    Brichford MJ. Archives & manuscripts: appraisal & accessioning, 1977.

    Fleckner JA. Archives & manuscripts: surveys, 1977.

    Gracy DB. Archives & manuscripts: arrangement & description. 1977.

    Holbert SE. Archives & manuscripts: reference & access, 1977.

    Walch T. Archives & manuscripts: security, 1977.

Society of American Archivists. College and University Archives Committee. Forms manual. Chicago: Society of American Archivists, 1973.

Society of American Archivists. College and University Archives Committee. Standards for college and university archives proposed. SAA Newsletter 1979 Jan:11-20.

Society of American Archivists. Committee on Finding Aids. Inventories and registers: a handbook of techniques and examples. Chicago: Society of American Archivists, 1976.

Society of American Archivists. Ethics Committee. A code of ethics for archivists; Commentary. SAA Newsletter 1979 Jul;:11-15.

Society of American Archivists. Report of the task force on institutional evaluation. SAA Newsletter 1980 Jan;:7-14.

Strassberg R, comp. Manual of archival and manuscript processing procedures. 2d ed. Ithaca: Cornell University Libraries, 1974.

Waters P. Procedures for salvage of water-damaged library materials. 2d ed. Washington, DC: Library of Congress, 1979.

Weinstein RA, Booth, L. Collection, use and care of historical photographs. Nashville: American Association for State and Local History, 1977.

APPENDIX A
Sample Policy Statement

NEW YORK HOSPITAL-CORNELL MEDICAL CENTER
Medical Archives
Policy Statement

Recognizing the need for a formal archival policy to insure the preservation and availability, for informational as well as historical purposes, of the official papers of

> The Society of the New York Hospital
> Cornell University Medical College
> Cornell University - New York Hospital School of Nursing
> Cornell University Graduate School of Medical Sciences

and of any institutions, foundations or corporate entities which have merged with or are part of the New York Hospital-Cornell Medical Center, the following policy for the collection and preservation of these vital records is hereby adopted.

The Medical Archives of the New York Hospital-Cornell Medical Center shall serve as a depository for all the institutions of the Center. The records which document the activities of the offices of the Center and its institutions are the property of these institutions.

Any records or papers generated or received by the administrative and academic offices of the Center in the conduct of their business are the property of the Center and constitute potential archival material. These records include all paper and correspondence regarding the functioning of the office, minutes of meetings, committee files, record books, reports and studies, official printed material, architectural and engineering plans. The private papers of faculty and staff are not included hereunder.

A Committee on Records Disposition shall be established to provide the authority for the destruction or retention of records according to their legal, administrative, fiscal, historical or other value. Said committee shall consist of

> 1) The Medical Archivist or a designated representative
> 2) A designated representative of the Society of the New York Hospital, of the Cornell University Medical College or of whatever Center institution is the primary creator or user of records being evaluated
> 3) Legal Counsel for said institution
> 4) An officer or designee of the department wherein the records under consideration originated and/or were housed.

All administrative officers as well as members of the faculty and staff who possess files and records relating to their official duties are requested to observe the following rules:

> 1) Institutional papers may not be destroyed or placed in "dead" storage without the approval of the Committee on Records Disposition. It is the responsibility of the officer in charge of each administrative office to notify the Medical Archivist regarding the need for evaluation of these institutional papers by the said Committee.
> 2) Records are to be considered for transfer to the Medical Archives when they are no longer in active use in their originating office. Materials designated by the Committee for preservation shall be transferred to the Medical Archives for processing and care.

The Medical Archives will actively seek the personal papers and other non-official records of those people connected with the Center and its institutions. These individuals have a place in our history, and the Medical Archives will solicit donations including:

> correspondence
> research notebooks
> office files (non-Center)
> lecture and course notes

financial records, grant applications, etc.
innovative or prototypical apparatus and documents associated with these artifacts
photographs and pictorial materials such as sketches
tape recordings
complete set of reprints/scientific papers
speeches
memorabilia/biographic material

All photographs, other visual material, and artifacts and apparatus significant to the Center and its institutions will be welcome in the Medical Archives as a part of the collection of iconography and of the "museum" collection.

The Medical Archives is the proper repository for all official records and manuscript material of the Center. As an adjunct to this, the printed material produced by the various departments of the Center and its institutions should also be centrally housed in the Medical Archives. These would include the formal publications of the various Center Departments such as:

annual reports
papers of the Department of _____ .
special studies and reports
history of the Department, etc.
announcements and catalogs
news releases

The purpose of the Medical Archives of the New York Hospital-Cornell Medical Center is to collect, organize, and preserve the records of the Center so as to make these records available for use. The Medical Archives is open for the service of all qualified researchers both within the Center and elsewhere. In view of this, the Medical Archivist shall consult with a representative of the originating office and with other interested parties to determine any restrictions that need be placed upon the use of confidential records. Additionally, access will not be permitted to records which are less than twenty-five years old.

Reproduced with permission of the Medical Archives of the New York Hospital-Cornell Medical Center.

APPENDIX B
Example of an Entry from a Guide

RECORD GROUP:
The Society of the Lying-In Hospital
of the City of New York

The materials in the Lying-In Hospital collection represent all extant records of an institution dedicated to the care of women. At its inception in 1799, the Lying-In Hospital was intended to aid poor women who couldn't get medical and nursing care during confinement for childbirth. Over the years, it was housed in several different buildings, including that of the New York Hospital (1801-1827), and had a period in which its only activity was fundraising and financial aid to women in confinement (1827-1892). In 1892, the Society took over the operation of the Midwifery Dispensary on Broome Street, and in 1894 moved into the Hamilton Fish mansion at Second Avenue and 17th Street. This building was demolished in 1899, and a new facility was erected on the same site. This new building, which opened in 1902, was the Lying-In's permanent home.

In 1928, the Lying-In Hospital and the New York Hospital affiliated, and Lying-In became the Obstetrics and Gynecology division of the New York Hospital-Cornell Medical Center when that medical complex opened in 1932. The focus of the Lying-In has, of course, changed over the years from care of the indigent only to general obstetrical and gynecological care and research. It presently occupies a wing of the Center and operates both as an extensive inpatient facility and as an outpatient unit.

The records of the Lying-In Hospital reflect the changes in the care of women in the past 150 years from both an administrative and a medical viewpoint, through the minutes of the Society of the Lying-In Hospital and the Medical Board, and the medical records of patients.

SELECTED RECORD SERIES:

Minutes of the Board of Governors, *1799-1947*
11 volumes   *18 inches*

Minutes of the Medical Board, *1896-1916*
13 volumes   *28 inches*

Annual Reports, *1890-1965*
unbound   *17-1/4 inches*

Midwifery Dispensary Histories, *1891-1892*
2 volumes   *5 inches*

Pregnancy Charts and Sheets, *1895-1932*
41 volumes   *16 feet*

General Histories, *1894-1931*
34 volumes   *10-1/2 feet*

Woman's Clinic, Register of Operations, *1932-1969, 1971-1972*
41 volumes   *3-1/2 feet*

Medical Board, Correspondence, *1895-1902*
2 volumes   *5-1/4 inches*

Reproduced with permission of the Medical Archives of the New York Hospital - Cornell Medical Center.

APPENDIX C
Example of Inventory at the Series Level

Ninth General Hospital. WWII. NYH.
Papers.
1942 - 1972.

3 boxes.   15 in.

Scope and Content

The Ninth General Hospital of World War II was comprised of the doctors and nurses from the New York Hospital who volunteered their services overseas during the war. This collection deals with the nurses' duties and activities, the bulk of it donated to the Medical Archives by Marie Troup, Chief Nurse of the Unit, Army Nurse Corps.

Materials dated 1942-47 are primarily military. Materials from the later years of this period include postwar correspondence from the nurses to Capt. Troup, newsletters, reunion materials, and reminiscences.

Nonmanuscript Material

Nonmanuscript material includes various scrapbooks and photographs depicting life at the Ninth General Hospital at sites in the United States, Australia and New Guinea between 1942 and 1945; monographs regarding Australia and New Guinea; six oversize display posters with photos mounted; and an ashtray donated by Margaret Pease Netsky.

Subjects

Nursing

Box Listing

Box 1:

Index cards: Set 1 - Memorandum of Designation or Change of Emergency Addressee Cards.   A-Z
             Set 2 - Vital Statistics file on Ninth General nurses noting addresses, promotions, allotments, etc.
                  A-Z
             Set 3 - File of Ninth General nurses by maiden names, cross-referencing to their married names,
                  addresses, and number of children.   A-Z

f.1 Fort Devons, Massachusetts. Station Hospital. Misc. Nov.-Dec. 1942.
  2 Embarkation Directives. Circulars, instructions, and passenger roster. 1942-45.
  3 Military correspondence. 1942-47.
  4 Rosters of Duty Assignments, leave, etc. 1943-45.
  5 Ward Routines, Administration and Procedures. Memos, circulars and notes. 1943-46.
  6 Staging Area Data. Memos and schedule. 1943-44.
  7 Expenses - "Kitty". Account book, misc. bills, etc. 1942-44.

APPENDIX D
Example of Subject Card from Card Catalog

Operating Rooms

see

1) Govs., Bd. of, NYH—Extracts from Minutes
   re. New Operating Theater, 1905-1907   71E

2) Operating Room Committee. Med. Bd. NYH.
   Minutes, agendas, correspondence etc.
   1960-.   41C

3) Operating Room Policies and Practices.
   NYH. Manual.   1970-.   53E

Reproduced with permission of the Medical Archives of the New York
Hospital - Cornell Medical Center.

APPENDIX E
Selected Suppliers of Archival Products

Conservation Resources International, Inc.
1111 North Royal Street
Alexandria, Virginia 22314

Hollinger Corporation
P.O. Box 6185
3810 South Four Mile Run Drive
Arlington, Virginia 22206

Light Impressions Corporation
Box 3012
Rochester, New York 14614

Pohlig Bros., Inc., Century Division
P.O. Box 8069
2419 East Franklin Street
Richmond, Virginia 23223

Process Materials Corporation
301 Veterans Boulevard
Rutherford, New Jersey 07070

TALAS
104 Fifth Avenue
New York, New York 10011

University Products, Inc.
P.O. Box 101
South Canal Street
Holyoke, Massachusetts 01040

Index

A

B

I

Q